**NUTRITION
AND
NATIONAL POLICY**

NUTRITION
AND
NATIONAL POLICY

**Beverly Winikoff,
editor**

The MIT Press
Cambridge, Massachusetts,
and
London, England

Second printing, 1979
Copyright © 1978 by
The Massachusetts Institute of Technology

This book was set in IBM Univers by Techdata Associates Inc., printed and bound by Halliday Lithograph Corporation in the United States of America

Library of Congress Cataloging in Publication Data
Main entry under title:

Nutrition and national policy.

  Bibliography: p.
  Includes index.
  1. Nutrition policy—Addresses, essays, lectures. 2. Nutrition—Addresses, essays, lectures. I. Winikoff, Beverly.
TX359.N87   362.5   78-19022
ISBN 0-262-23087-9

pd
6-7-84

CONTENTS

PREFACE

From lay publicists to scientific professionals, writers of the seventies have been increasingly concerned with the problem of feeding the world's growing population. The problem is presented as an overwhelming challenge to human ingenuity, and proponents of elaborate solutions invoke the glamor of high technology: the solution will rival the building of the pyramids or the Great Wall of China, or even the putting of an astronaut on the moon. Those who predict failure conjure up morbid but compelling scenarios of mass destruction: the black plague, the eruption of Krakatoa, the Deluge. Win or lose, there is drama in the outcome. A newsworthy, emotion-laden, and exciting topic to be sure.

Many of the works dealing with nutrition to date have taken a medical, agricultural, or technological perspective. Less has been written about the nutritional impact of political processes within countries. The present volume begins to outline the relationship between overall government activity and nutrition, attempting to enlarge the dimensions of what is already in the literature.

The book focuses on the relationships between different areas of government activity (health, agriculture, economic policy, etc.) and the nutritional status of populations, in an attempt to understand what happens when governments operate "in the real world." Instead of suggesting new, grandiose solutions to the problem of hunger, this collection looks at the old, seemingly sound, solutions and tries to discover why that which has seemed obvious and logical has usually proven ineffective. In the course of the conference upon which this book is based, it became clear that the questions traditionally asked about nutrition problems have not always been precise, appropriate, or adequately searching. Further work remains in the posing, and, it is to be hoped, the answering, of more relevant questions.

The major part of this book is composed of accounts of the histories of the attempts of eleven governments to grapple with nationwide problems of malnutrition. These studies were originally written for presentation at a conference on Nutrition and Government Policy, sponsored by the Rockefeller Foundation, and held in Bellagio, Italy, September 20-23, 1975. They were prepared from a common outline of questions designed to retrieve parallel information from all the authors (see Appendix). However, each study evolved differently within the given framework, reflecting personal as well as national differences in interpretation of the meaning of nutrition problems. Although the information and emphasis vary from case to case, all the papers do demonstrate, in historical context, key issues and stumbling blocks in national-level attempts to deal with nutrition problems.

The country papers were each written by prominent nationals who are, or have been, directly involved in the nutrition activities of their governments. The short commentaries (chs. 13-18), discussion sections, and the summary chapter were derived from the proceedings of the conference. Participants who contributed to these sections include professionals who have been deeply involved in both the medical and political aspects of nutrition planning.

Both the conference organizers and the other participants regret the absence of the nutrition stories of four countries in particular: Brazil, Cuba, India, and the People's Republic of China. It was felt by all the participants that discussion of the approaches and results in these four countries would have added immeasurably to the scope of the discussions. Unfortunately, although representatives were invited from each of the four countries, the individuals or governments concerned were unable to arrange attendance. Ultimately, the work of nutrition advocates, such as those in attendance at the Bellagio gathering, can be made more fruitful by broadening contacts and communications between different political and socioeconomic systems. We hope that in the future all will be able to benefit by wider participation in such discussions and by the freer exchange of ideas and experiences.

It should be emphasized that this book in no way pretends to cover its subject definitively. Rather, the volume should be viewed as a first attempt to describe various nutrition activities within their local political and historical contexts. It is a collection of a great deal of raw data, which can itself be studied by other students of the problem for new ideas and further analyses. But if this volume is in no way the final word, its authors hope that it is the beginning of a new perspective on the problems of hunger.

Special thanks are due to those who participated in the conference and its preparation for the willingness to give both time and thought to the enterprise. To say that this book could not have been compiled without them would be a gross understatement. All the authors participated willingly in the various stages of re-writing and editing, and this work is the product of many hours of advice and discussion cheerfully given with astounding openness.

The frank discussions central to a conference of this sort were made possible by the thoughtfulness and ready camaraderie of all the participants. This was all the more remarkable for the sensitive political nature of some of the topics discussed. Willingness to risk much in order to gain better insights and to perhaps find new, more fruitful paths was the underlying spirit which informed the entire endeavor.

In a large sense, then, this is the conferees' book, because they cared enough not only to write the papers but to share their very personal perceptions of problems encountered in the real world. That they did this at a public gathering of workers from all over the world, organized by a group of Americans, and not in private conversation with friends, is a manifestation of even greater trust and courage. It is a measure also of the acute importance that professionals attach to the development of realistic and workable solutions to one of mankind's great tragedies.

Allan C. Barnes, Vice-President of the Rockefeller Foundation, whose guidance and support have been invaluable from the inception of this project, deserves special mention and profound thanks. Without his help, this creation would never have been born intact.

Sol Chafkin and Derrick Jelliffe reviewed the manuscript and shared generously of their wisdom and good judgment. Their assistance was imaginative, reassuring, and greatly appreciated.

My colleagues at the Rockefeller Foundation were helpful in both large and small ways, contributing ideas, advice, and interest. I particularly appreciated the patience and humor of John Maier, Director of Health Sciences, and the enthusiasm and good cheer of John H. Knowles, President.

Helpful suggestions for organizing the Bellagio gathering were made by Alan Berg, John Field, Peter Hakim, Jim Levinson, Giorgio Solimano, and Joe Wray, many of whom also assisted with suggestions for editing the summary chapter. John Montgomery, Ewen Thomson, Fred Sai, and Soekirman also provided very useful commentary on the last chapter. Ann Swidler was a source of new ideas and fresh perspectives.

Endless resilience and good will, along with efficient and accurate secretarial work, were provided by Reinelda Moschner and Shirley Steinberg.

Most of all I was helped by my husband, Michael Alpert, whose warmth, encouragement, companionship, and sound advice are a constant joy.

1 INTRODUCTION   Beverly Winikoff

This book is the product of frustration. It was born of a perception of inadequacy. Millions of words have been written on the subject of nutrition while millions of people continue to die, some quickly, others more slowly, all as a result of undernutrition. What is wrong, then, that we humans cannot provide for a basic need of our own species? Is it an intellectual error? Do we misperceive the problem? Do we choose the wrong solutions? Do we ask the wrong questions? Is it a technological problem? Are we incapable of supplying the remedy? Is it a problem of judgment? Do we misinterpret, misconstrue, and misapply what we know? Is it a problem of motivation and political priorities? Or is it a moral problem? Do we, fundamentally, not care?

The paradox has recently seemed all the more poignant as Western technical advances and agricultural breakthroughs have increased productive capacity through such developments as high-yield grains. Yet, the results of the scientific advances do not fill the empty bellies. If anything, in general the problem of malnutrition has grown steadily more alarming in terms of the absolute numbers affected. On the other hand, the world has had before it the example of China, the most populous nation on earth—and one of the poorest—straining and reorganizing itself in previously untried ways, while apparently assuring an adequate diet for its many citizens. Why, then, do technologies which seem to make solutions near at hand fail so frequently to yield the promised benefits? How can a poor country nourish its citizens while so many richer countries see their people suffer the ravages of malnutrition?

Feeding populations is an old crisis, an early concern of all governments. It is also a question which presents new facets in every era. Now, in the late twentieth century, providing food for all is seen to affect, and in turn be affected by, crises of pollution, energy, and population growth. In times bounded by different political, social, and economic realities, Chinese dynasties rose and fell merely by virtue of their ability to provide for the distribution of the rice harvest. Later, but still long ago, Henry IV of France stated his intent to pursue a social policy with the aim that "there be no laborer in his kingdom so poor that he could not have boiled fowl for his Sunday meal."

In 1937 the League of Nations Committee on the Relations of Nutrition to Health, Agriculture, and Economic Policy concluded that "the ultimate responsibility for the nutrition and health policy of a nation must rest with that nation's Government."[1] Joseph Goldberger came to essentially the same conclusion when studying pellagra as part of a government commission in the American South.[2] So, both by tradition and the reports of commissions, the responsibility for nutrition is placed squarely on the shoulders of government.

Recently, governments have reacted consciously to this mandate—generally along one of two lines. These two approaches in their purest forms are based on two different perceptions of the roots of the nutrition problem. According to one school, malnutrition can best be understood as a result of grinding poverty. The remedy would lie, then, in increasing the overall productivity of society and improving income and food distribution patterns in order that the poorest might begin to participate, achieving reasonable levels of income generation and adequate diet. The second approach derives from the perception that many are malnourished simply because they do not use existing resources efficiently enough to provide themselves with proper diets and healthful environments. The implication is that eliminating malnutrition depends upon the elimination of nutritional ignorance, dietary superstition, and poor hygiene practices. Sometimes these approaches are seen as mutually exclusive; at other times they are melded by more "sophisticated" analysts into integrated solutions. Solutions based on each of these concepts often have been declared great successes in their own terms, yet they also often have done nothing to eliminate the basic problem of malnutrition. Let us take two examples.

The Chontalpa Plan[3] in Mexico was an important government project which aimed at improving the quality of life by raising agricultural production and increasing income in a rural tropical area. Indicators of quality of life were looked at before the inception of the program and thirteen years after it had started. At first glance, the statistics show impressive gains:

- population increased by 108%, but production of corn, the staple, increased by 116%
- cash crop increased between 118% and well over 1,000%, producing a large increas in per capita income
- per capita consumption of meat, eggs, and milk all increased significantly
- per capita consumption of calories and proteins increased
- adult illiteracy decreased from 60% to 28%
- in the beginning of the program, 40% of families owned radios; by the end of the program all had radios, and 38% had television sets as well!

And yet, the proportion of children moderately and severely malnourished (Gomez classification grades two and three*) had changed hardly at all over 13 years: 26% in these categories at the inception of the program; 22.5% thirteen years later. Perhaps most important, third degree malnutrition only changed from 4.4% to 4.1%. Because of population growth, this meant that, in absolute terms, there were twice as many hungry children in Chontalpa 13 years after the initiation of government effort as at the beginning.

The data give no indications of the dynamics behind these changing statistics. The implications in terms of altered family values, perceived improve-

---

*Gomez Classifications are a way of describing the nutritional status of children according to weight for age. The reference standard is the 50th percentile of weight for age. "Normal" is anything above 90% of this weight, 75-90% is designated first degree malnutrition, 60-75% is called second degree malnutrition, and a child whose weight for age is below 60% of the standard is said to suffer from third degree malnutrition.

ments in quality of life, or the potential for increased survival of children with poor health and nutritional status are not retrievable from the information given.

It is obvious, however, that dramatic changes in economic—and even some nutritional—indicators may mask an unchanging, or even worsening, malnutrition problem.

The second unfortunate example of a superficially successful program involves nutrition education as a strategy for overcoming malnutrition. Twenty Haitian mothers were taught how to choose and prepare the lowest-cost adequate diet available from their local marketplace. The cost was nine cents (US) per person per day. The mothers listened raptly to every word, and they repeated the lessons accurately. They were very good students and could prepare all the dishes properly. But they had only an average of eight cents per person per day to spend on food. Is this, then, a nutrition program? Would it have been rational policy if there had been ten cents per person per day to spend on food?

What does work? Or to turn the question around: Why have so many past efforts failed? Why are we so stymied? Why, finally, are so many of the world's citizens suffering from nutritional deprivation? It has seemed to many in thinking about these problems that there is insufficient understanding of the role of variables aside from food production in creating the nutrition environment for populations. Previous volumes on nutrition problems have dealt with scientific or technologic aspects or have attempted to define the scope and implications of widespread malnutrition. Now it seems necessary to explore the process of search for solution: to investigate the many variables that may bound and constrain the efforts to deal with malnutrition. Problems of cultural change, administration, economic policy, health policy, agricultural policy, and political philosophy, all seem to be fruitful areas for further exploration.

Among the questions needing investigation are:

- How do governments create policy which affects nutritional status?
- How are problems called to the attention of policymakers?
- What institutions can be brought to bear on a problem?
- What obstacles confront those who propose solutions?
- What is the relationship between the statements of governments and the results, intended and unintended, of government actions?
- How does a government's perceptions of a problem influence the solutions proposed to deal with that problem?
- How might the outcome of nutrition policy be measured?
- What is the most appropriate relationship between nutrition policy and the health sector?

Clearly, solutions cannot be attempted without the basic scientific underpinnings and the technological understanding appropriate to the problem. However, such knowledge has never been a *sufficient* condition for solution of any human problem. In part, this is because, for any given problem, choices must be made from among alternative technologies and solutions.

Application of the most recent advances or delegation of the problem to the best-established profession may be the instinctive reaction of policy-makers, and may, in fact, be the path of least resistance. However, such easy choices may result in suboptimal, perhaps not even appropriate, solutions which are not likely to produce the anticipated results.

Frequently, the technologies themselves are seen as solutions in toto, al-though it should be obvious that the environment in which a technology operates is critical to the outcome of its application. The automobile is no solution to the problem of mobility if there are no roads. It is also no solu-tion if there is no gasoline. In fact, it is no solution if there are no drivers. And certainly it is no solution if either no one knows how to obtain cars or can afford them. Yet we are still entertained by conversations such as the following, in which great hopes are expressed for the new high-protein vari-eties of grain:

Q Doesn't this approach still pose problems of distribution? Even if it is possible to improve the protein content of sorghum, for instance, the new seed variety must still be distributed to the farmer.

A Yes, but my point is that it doesn't raise some of the more difficult prob-lems of broadening income distribution, which is the other means of im-proving nutrition levels. It is *merely* a question of making the administrative arrangements to produce seeds of the new varieties and get them into the hands of farmers. This is easier on the whole than trying to change income distribution, which affects the whole social/power structure of a country. There are means by which the farmer now gets his seeds and a new seed vari-ety, instead of the old lower protein type, can be distributed through these channels.[4]

The assumption here is that, all things being equal, the one-for-one replace-ment of old seed by new will have a beneficial effect. But in human systems all things are *not* equal. Changing one part of a dynamic system influences the working of many, if not all, of the other components. It has become obvious, for instance, that changing seeds is not unrelated to changes in credit avail-ability, local political power, distribution of income, and resource use in farming techniques, to name only a few variables. What, then, is meant by the availability of technology? Is it "available" in any real sense without knowl-edge of the human aspects of the equation?

In planning this volume, some proposed that a compilation of all the solu-tions advanced in the field, either to increase food supply or to deal with malnutrition in its social and medical contexts, would be a worthwhile en-deavor for an international conference. The problem with such a compilation, however, is that no one really knows yet the true potential—for good and ill—of many of these alternatives. They have been worked out in theory or in the laboratory of the pilot project. Only in this sense are many of the "tech-nologies" available or able to be developed. Many of the human technologies, however, remain essentially unknown:

- how one can hasten the process by which nutrition problems are recognized and addressed
- how to convince political and social entities of the necessity to deal with nutrition as a high priority issue
- how to convince people to change old habits and adopt new ones
- how old habits *do* change rapidly in some circumstances
- how proven "good ideas" get used (Are they really "good ideas" if no one wants to adopt them?)

Obviously, an accurate compilation of current knowledge would be quite useful for planners and policymakers. Yet, until we learn how best to implement technical know-how, efforts will be based on half-truths and have only a fraction of their potential effectiveness.

Thus, in trying to understand more about how nutrition problems might be addressed, the conference planners did not choose to examine, in turn, each of the technologies used to address the problem: fortification, nutrient distribution, fertilization of soils, irrigation, improved seed varieties, agricultural credit, food coupon or ration plans, and so on. We also did not choose to divide the topic by medical definitions of the most common nutritional problems in the world: protein-calorie malnutrition, iron-deficiency anemia, hypovitaminosis A, goiter, B-vitamin deficiencies, and so forth. Attention to specific nutrient deficiencies received relatively little attention because of a consensus that many of these problems do lend themselves to known technological solutions not necessarily dependent on major social and political changes.

Since "good nutrition" is a functional outcome, the end-product of the functioning of many other systems, we chose to look at the problem from the point of view of some of those other systems: economics, culture, health, agriculture, administration, to name a few. It was understood by the participants that the entire topic of nutrition is intimately related to health and human well-being. In this sense, the book deals with fundamental problems of human health. This theme is not continually repeated, but it should be understood as the underpinning of all the discussions. Clearly, however, it is possible to achieve desired health effects by tackling problems either directly through a health system or indirectly and outside the conventional "health" superstructure. The major focus of the Bellagio conference was on the latter approach.

THE COUNTRY CASE STUDIES

The country case studies were designed to better define the specific environments in which all these systems function. Because each country has its own cultural, economic, and political context, as well as its own priorities and goals, there is great variety in both the problems themselves and the way these problems are perceived. There is variation, too, in the emphasis of each of the papers. Solimano and Hakim's work on Chile provides explicit hypotheses of how priorities in national political and health systems determine the nutritional status of different segments of the population. Lopez's study on Colombia, Soekirman's on Indonesia, and Maletnlema's on Tanzania, document the different ways in which three diverse governments attempt to integrate nutrition planning with overall national planning priorities. Ghana's story as told by Sai, Nigeria's by Omololu, the USA's by Schlossberg, and Zambia's by Vamoer, all demonstrate how nutrition problems, recognized over a substantial period of time, have been redefined by the changes in priorities and leadership within the political system. Perceptions of nutritional problems, in turn, appear to have affected the political process in different ways.

Antrobus's treatment of Jamaica's history falls somewhere in between, dealing partly with the overall process of government socioeconomic planning and partly with the changes over time in approaches to the Jamaican nutrition problem. It also reflects the influence on a small country of a well-established international nutrition-training institution, the Caribbean Food and Nutrition Institute.

Sandoval's paper on Panama and Solon's on the Philippines take a somewhat different approach. Sandoval explores the Panamanian government's new nutrition policy and program with specific reference to the food distribution scheme in one province. The rationale behind this scheme, its organization, and the government's hopes for its outcome are all related. Solon's paper also concentrates on the intricacies of one program; but, in this case, the overall nationwide program is described. The complex administrative structure and the roots of the program's power are related in detail.

The discussions following the presentation of papers revealed the extensive experience and well-considered ideas of participants from both developed and developing countries. Ideas and information were brought forward in such volume that they could not possibly be presented adequately in one book, and therefore only the most important and most thoroughly debated points have been included.

We have learned from the case studies and discussions that the current worries about malnutrition really are not so new, that many of the ideas about nutrition have been voiced repeatedly, and even that most of the methods of dealing with problems of malnutrition have been suggested before. We learned that, where politics and economics are concerned, money alone is not enough, leadership alone is not enough, and education alone is not enough.

THE COMMENTARIES

The short commentary papers (Part II) reveal both the multiplicity of factors necessary to deal with nutrition as well as varied methods of analysis of the problem. Often, experts from different fields start to tackle the same problem but, by analyzing it differently and using the jargons of different professions, they become unable to communicate. The summary of viewpoints to be found in the commentaries will help the reader to appreciate the contribution of each relevant profession to the understanding and solution of nutrition problems. In addition, in the discussions of government function, it becomes apparent that official actions themselves create complicated sets of incentive systems, some of which are harmful to nutrition goals. Understanding this dynamic makes it possible for nutrition planners to deal more effectively with other elements of the governmental structure.

THE SUMMARY

In a final day of deliberation, after discussion of the lessons to be learned from the country stories, the Bellagio conference participants moved to explore issues of general interest. Several concerns were expressed consistently, and these are summarized in the last chapter of this book. One set of topics relates to theoretical issues involved in deciding on approaches to nutrition problems, while another involves problems in the practice of nutrition interventions within countries.

Theoretical Issues

Political Commitment   Discussions frequently touched on the participants' deep, basic, and perhaps irreconcilable differences in world-view. When the nutrition issue is framed as a contest between pragmatism and ideology, which should come first in the solution of the problems? Ends and means, politics and philosophy, are always divisive subjects. Reconciliation of the points of view expressed was not attempted either in the discussions or in the summary. A subjective impression remains, however, that ideology plays a larger role in the Latin-American context—that it is more apparent and more important, more on the surface of consciousness there than in other regions.

The Role of Nutrition Advocates   The relationship between the nutrition advocate and the other government actors is also seen to rest partly on ideological considerations and partly on pragmatic political relationships. These interrelationships were explored by the participants in an attempt to understand how to increase the effectiveness of nutrition advocacy.

Targeting   The theoretical concerns of ideology are reflected also in discussions of specific program practices. Concern was expressed about targeting nutrition interventions to specific needy groups versus making programs part of overall nationwide action by the government without special reference to a group of "recipients." This discussion arose from the paradox that while malnutrition is clearly perceived as an overall social problem, it makes most sense from the point of view of efficient use of resources to target interventions as narrowly as possible. Targeting, of course, involves the redefinition of a program, usually making it more health- or medically oriented and thus may serve to remove it from the political and social realm. The entire problem then may become isolated from general social concerns, and, as Ivan Illich notes about other processes of "medicalization," it may become professionalized, mystified, bureaucratized, and essentially out of the reach of normal sociopolitical remedies.

Practical Issues in Nutrition Intervention

Role of Nutritional Scientists in Initiating Nutrition Drives The role of the medical and nutrition professions was also examined with much interest. Despite a recent tendency for scientists to throw up their hands and proclaim that the problem is basically political, it soon became apparent that the medical scientist's role is, in fact, crucial. Societies depend on those with professional expertise for a usable definition of the nutrition problem. Without the concerted support of medical professionals and biochemical nutritionists, the problem generally receives insufficient political backing. It is then not taken seriously enough for the political, social, and economic advocates to mount a sustained and effective attack.

This may be of some comfort to those medical experts who, although they have felt deeply concerned, have also felt "defined out" of the problem by its recent exposition as a social and economic predicament. In fact, this conference's perception of the process by which nutrition problems become public concerns places a special responsibility on the medical and nutrition communities to monitor, define, elaborate, and be society's gadfly generally as regards nutritional needs and nutritional problems. It seems that while the media can publicize and the politicians can make decisions, it takes the scientists—both researchers and clinicians—to formulate responsible definitions of the problem.

Nutrition Councils The role of national nutrition coordinating councils was also discussed. This topic has been the subject of debate over many years in several of the countries represented. All countries, once they are determined to tackle malnutrition, must be concerned with the problem of setting up institutions that are capable of functioning effectively and continuously. The Indonesian and Zambian case studies, for example, reflect enormous concerns over the proper method of organizing responsibility for nutrition within the governmental structure. Several alternative modes of organization have been tried in these countries, as well as in Ghana, the Philippines, and Colombia. Similar problems occurred in almost all of these cases—the individual form or flavor might differ, but the basic mechanisms were the same. The task of institution-building and bureaucratic reorganization is never simple and will continue, most probably, to prove troublesome in the future. Identification of the problems, however, helps to clarify some of the bottlenecks and, perhaps, to allow greater sophistication both in dealing with problems as they occur, and, even better, in creating situations to avoid some of them.

Professional Education   The education of professionals must also be of great concern in any ongoing program. In the African context, lack of personnel is a frequently mentioned problem. *Appropriate* training of professionals and lay personnel is a problem everywhere. Of course, appropriate training does not always result in a successful program; even very sophisticated thinking may not necessarily result in effective governmental action. Nonetheless, no program can function without adequate and appropriate manpower. Training must be adapted to local problems and needs, with particular attention to the interdisciplinary nature of nutrition intervention as well as the political context of possible solutions. Manpower constraints and the proper approach to manpower training must remain a large concern of any program developer or manager.

International Aid   For many years, nutrition programs (whether limited, as food distribution in times of famine, or long-term, such as school-feeding) have been dominated by international aid and assistance. More recently, nutrition planning and program development have also been dominated by an "international nutrition community" of sorts. The proper role of these international contributors was discussed quite feelingly by the participants. It was agreed that new programs and developing countries, in general, can benefit by contact with the international aid community—and not solely in terms of money, although this always helps. More important, perhaps, are the transfers of knowledge and experience, as well as the creation within the local political scene of a nucleus for the advocacy of nutrition programs.

On the other hand, at least three serious drawbacks were noted by all participants. First, there is the unfortunate but prevalent problem of introduction of inappropriate technology, as noted by Latham (ch. 14). Second, there are the adverse effects of centuries of "psychological dependence" on developed countries that the new ex-colonial countries are now making active efforts to escape. Third, and perhaps most administratively destructive, is the tendency for international organizations to reproduce interagency conflicts and other malfunctions of the international system within the recipient country. These reinforce existing ministry rivalries. This pattern was noted by many participants and suggestions were offered for overcoming the obstacles.

Those who sat round the conference table at Bellagio were working on a new and relatively unexplored field: nutrition planning. It was reassuring—in fact, encouraging—for all to discover similarities of goals, hopes, and many times, ideas for the future. Ironically, it was no less reassuring to find shared irritations, frustrations, and failures. The difficulties involved were found to be real, definable, and, it is to be hoped, soluble, rather than idiosyncratic perceptions or evidence of personal failure. The field is new and untested, and it is not clear yet whether this approach will succeed in filling the gaps which have become all too apparent in previous methods of tackling the problem.

Better definitions of the roles and purposes of "nutrition planning" remain to be worked out in practice. What is apparent from the case studies and discussions which follow, however, is that nutrition planning cannot be separated from the overall tasks of designing and implementing national goals. There may, in fact, be no professionals who can accurately be labeled "nutrition planners." Rather, there are nutrition advocates who have a dual task: (1) they must create awareness and sensitivity to nutrition problems within the ranks of government policymakers, and (2) they must help planners to understand the implications of their plans for the nutritional status of the population. In this case, nutritional and general government policy must proceed together, inextricably intertwined, to tackle the distressing problems of human deprivation.

CASE STUDIES

2 DEVELOPMENT, REFORM, AND MALNUTRITION IN CHILE

Giorgio R. Solimano
and
Peter Hakim

Giorgio R. Solimano of Chile was the Head of the Nutrition Division of the National Health Service in the Chilean Ministry of Health, from 1971 to 1973. Following the overthrow of the Allende government, Dr. Solimano was a Research Assistant at the Massachusetts Institute of Technology. At present, Dr. Solimano is Associate Professor of Public Health and Director of the Division of Community and International Nutrition, Institute of Human Nutrition, Columbia University. Dr. Solimano has been a frequent delegate to international conferences and symposia on nutrition planning and has also been active in the Pan American Health Organization. He was project director for a section of the United Nations World Food Program and represented Chile at the Third Western Hemisphere Congress on Nutrition. Publications by Dr. Solimano include articles on the biological as well as the policy aspects of nutrition and health.

Peter Hakim is currently a program officer of the Ford Foundation in its Office for Resources and the Environment. He also serves as a lecturer at Columbia University's Institute of Human Nutrition. Mr. Hakim previously occupied positions with the Ford Foundation in Brazil and in Chile; he has graduate degrees in both physics and public affairs. The present article was written while he was a visiting lecturer at MIT's International Nutrition Planning Program.

INTRODUCTION

The causality of malnutrition has conventionally been examined and explained in terms of individual and family characteristics of the malnourished, largely without reference to the social order in which they live. Nutrition analysts, for example, have given little attention to the effects of government economic and social policies or other broad socioeconomic influences on the incidence of malnutrition in a country.[1] Studies specifically concerned with the relationship between nutrition and national development have focused primarily on the implications of widespread malnutrition for economic growth and development (i.e., malnutrition as an obstacle to development), while neglecting the consequences of development and change for nutritional standards. Similarly, prescriptions for raising nutritional standards are invariably addressed to those suffering from or at risk of malnutrition, and rarely address changes in the rest of the society. It is apparently assumed that malnutrition can be alleviated in third world countries without altering economic growth patterns or transforming the social and political arrangements which underlie those patterns. The assumption is a questionable one, particularly as evidence increases that standard development strategies and growth-promoting mechanisms may also promote economic concentration and a worsening of the relative, if not absolute, position of the poor.

   This study explores, in the case of Chile, the influence that a country's development pattern has had on food consumption and nutrition among low income groups. The first section reviews the available information on Chile's food and nutrition situation during the period from 1930 to 1970 and concludes that nutritional standards probably did not improve significantly in that period, even as rates of infant mortality declined sharply. The second section examines the country's pattern of socioeconomic development in the same period, presenting the case that the continued prevalence of malnutrition was a consequence of the consistent discrimination against low income strata inherent in that pattern.

TRENDS IN NUTRITIONAL STATUS, FOOD CONSUMPTION, AND HEALTH

In the absence of any single source of continuing information on Chile's food and nutrition situation for the period under examination, it was necessary to compile data from a variety of disparate sources, including clinical investigations, food supply and consumption surveys, and infant mortality statistics, in an attempt to create a historical record. While we cannot attest to the reliability or accuracy of most of the specific references on which we have had to depend, the numerous studies and surveys that were conducted exhibit a remarkably high degree of consistency and, when taken together, provide considerable information on trends in food consumption and nutritional standards. On most questions, however, the available data are more suggestive than conclusive, and our interpretation cannot be regarded as definitive.

Clinical Surveys of Nutritional Status

Chilean researchers have more or less regularly carried out clinical surveys concerned with the nutritional status and growth of children since the early 1930s. As Cuminsky and Fleishman[2] noted in their review and summary of 21 such surveys done between 1940 and 1966, considerable variation exists in the quality and reliability of the different studies and the findings are not really comparable given differences in methodology, samples, and techniques of measurement. Moreover, with few exceptions, the available surveys did not specify adequately the population that their samples were supposed to represent.

Only one survey—done in 1960 by the Interdepartmental Committee on Nutrition for National Defense (ICNND)[3] —was performed on a nationwide sample.[4] Although large amounts of data were collected, the conclusions advanced by the authors of the ICNND survey were extremely tentative and cautious, and no estimates were provided on the extent of malnutrition in the country.

Overall clinical information was summarized as follows: full-term infants surviving for 48 hours are similar in size and weight to US infants, but they soon show retarded growth. By primary school age they have returned to US growth standards, but by nine or ten, the children's growth again slows and ceases at age 14 or 15. Our own reading of the original ICNND data yields a somewhat different interpretation, i.e., that Chilean growth rates are consistently below North American standards and the differences become increasingly accentuated between the ages of 10 and 14.

Specifically the ICNND survey found that the mean height of Chilean children at age 10 and 14 in each of the geographical areas sampled was beneath the 10th percentile of North American youngsters, while their average weight was between the 10th and 25th percentile. These findings suggest that nutritional deprivation had probably affected around 50% of the schoolchildren sampled.

One other clinical study was done on a representative sample of a defined population. Monckberg et al.[5] in 1966 examined a total of some 1,500 infants and preschool children in the province of Curico comprising about 13% of all children in those age groups.

As indicated in table 1, about 50% of urban and rural youngsters from ages one to seven in Curico fell beneath the third percentile of the Iowa Standard in height, while around 30% were beneath that percentile in weight, suggesting that upwards of 30% of the children were probably seriously malnourished. The numbers falling beneath the 10th percentile indicate that severe or moderate undernutrition probably affected 40% or more of the children surveyed.

Table 1
Height and weight distribution of children in Curico Province, Chile. Percent of Iowa standard

	Under 3rd Percentile				Under 10th Percentile			
Age	Height		Weight		Height		Weight	
(years)	Urban	Rural	Urban	Rural	Urban	Rural	Urban	Rural
0 - 1	32%	24%	27%	28%	55%	37%	37%	42%
1 - 2	50	43	30	37	67	61	47	48
2 - 3	48	54	26	30	61	77	45	44
3 - 4	55	57	21	27	64	71	39	47
4 - 5	57	58	27	33	73	72	43	47
5 - 6	48	57	29	33	55	79	42	55
6 - 7	47	58	28	37	58	73	47	62

The findings from Curico cannot, of course, be considered representative for Chile as a whole. The province includes less than 1.5% of the country's population, is one of Chile's least urbanized provinces, and according to most socioeconomic indicators, one of its poorest. The percentage of Curico's population classified as "poor" in a recent survey of poverty in Chile, however, was only slightly higher than that registered for the country as a whole, and among Chile's 25 provinces it ranked only twelfth in its incidence of poverty.[6] Moreover, using slightly lower reference standards of normality, Stegen and Barros, in a study in 1957 of 3,000 children in Valparaiso, one of Chile's more urban and richer provinces, reported incidences of malnutrition of a magnitude similar to those found in Curico, particularly for 4- to 12-year-old children.[7]

Almost all clinical studies in Chile, including those already cited, reached the following conclusions:

1 The average height and weight of Chilean children at birth conforms to US standards.

2 Rates of growth and development among infants and children from middle and upper class homes in Chile are equal to those observed for North American youngsters.

3 At approximately six months, there begin to appear significant differences in heights and weights among Chilean children from different socioeconomic levels, with lower and lower middle class children, as they get older, falling further and further behind those from upper and middle income households (tables 2, 3). The magnitude of the differences at each age is generally larger than those found among US children at different income levels.

Differential growth patterns were first observed by Mardones and Sepulveda in 1936[8] and similar results were reported by Riquelme in 1941.[9] And a survey in 1954 of 14,000 school children found that 10-year-old children

Table 2
Family income and child growth, Santiago, Chile, 1936

Family Income (in Multiples of Minimum Monthly Salary)	Weight (kg)		Height (cm)	
	9 years	14 years	9 years	14 years
Less than 1.0	23.5	35.0	122.5	140.0
1.0 - 1.5	24.5	35.6	125.0	142.0
1.5 - 2.0	25.2	42.5	124.8	146.0
2.0 - 2.5	25.8	41.6	124.3	147.8
2.5 - 3.0	25.0	44.4	123.1	149.0
3.0 - 3.5	25.3	44.5	124.8	149.3
3.5 - 4.0	25.6	45.3	125.6	153.3
4.0 - 5.0	25.7	47.5	125.2	151.5
greater than 5.0	26.6	47.0	127.8	150.0

Table 3
Average height and weight of schoolboys of high and low income levels, Chile, 1941

Age (years)	Height (cm)			Weight (kg)		
	High Income	Low Income	Difference	High Income	Low Income	Difference
10	135	125	10	31.5	25.2	6.3
14	157	144	13	48.5	37.0	11.5

attending public schools were some 10 cm shorter and 10 kg lighter than their counterparts enrolled in private schools charging tuition.[10]

There are no recent studies comparing growth rates of upper and lower class school children in Chile. Arraño et al.[11] observed in 1968, however, that children from a lower middle class school measured on the average 8 cm less than the Iowa standard at 10 years and 11 cm less at 14 years, and further, that the mean height corresponded to Iowa's 10th percentile. Several other studies done in 1968 and 1969 among public school students in different sectors of Santiago also observed that the average height of the children was at or below the 10th Iowa percentile, and average weight below the 25th percentile.[12]

Clinical survey findings for preschool children parallel those for school children. Montoya and Ipinza[13] in 1963 examined 712 children under age 7, about half from upper middle class backgrounds and the rest from working class families. Their results are reported in table 4.

Barja et al.,[14] in their survey of one to five year olds in 1964 and 1965, presented similar findings (tables 5, 6). The Barja study also revealed that, among low income children, the average height of 5-year-olds falls below the 3rd percentile of the Iowa scale, and the average weight below the 10th percentile. Among upper-income 5-year-old children, the average for both height

Table 4
Average height and weight of preschool children by age and socioeconomic class,
Santiago, Chile, 1963

Age (years)	Height (cm)			Weight (kg)	
	Upper Middle	Working	Difference	Upper Middle	Working
3½ - 4	99	94	5	16	13 - 14
4 - 4½	103	97	6	17	14 - 15
4½ - 5	105	99	6	18	15 - 16
5 - 5½	110	103	7	19	16 - 17
5½ - 6	113	107	6	20	18
6 - 6½	116	107	9	22	19

Table 5
Average weights (kg) of preschool children by age and socioeconomic class, Santiago,
Chile, 1964-65

Age (years)	Socioeconomic Class			Difference between Upper and Lower Class
	Upper (n=315)	Middle (n=3696)	Lower (n=1093)	
1.0	10.5	9.4	8.7	1.8
2.0	13.0	11.8	10.5	2.5
3.0	14.9	13.9	12.4	2.5
4.0	16.9	15.5	14.6	2.3
5.0	18.8	17.1	15.9	2.9

Table 6
Average heights (cm) of preschool children by age and socioeconomic class, Santiago,
Chile, 1964-65

Age (years)	Socioeconomic Class			Difference between Upper and Lower Class
	Upper (n=315)	Middle (n=3969)	Lower (n=1093)	
1.0	74.0	73.0	74.7	0.7
2.0	86.0	83.7	81.5	4.5
3.0	96.0	92.4	87.1	8.9
4.0	103.5	99.0	94.5	9.0
5.0	109.0	104.5	99.8	9.2

and weight was around the 50th Iowa percentile. Average height in the intermediate group was beneath the 10th percentile, and average weight around
the 25th percentile.

The available data do not reveal variations over time of nutritional standards in Chile. Indeed, they do not even provide the basis for estimating prevalence of malnutrition in the country for any single year. A few important inferences may nonetheless be drawn. First, malnutrition was long a characteristic of a portion of Chile's population, and persisted as a serious and widespread problem for the country as a whole through the 1960s. Secondly, a strong inverse relationship existed between nutritional vulnerability and socioeconomic status, i.e., the extent and seriousness of nutritional deprivations increased with declining income levels and other socioeconomic indicators.

The findings of Duarte[15] in 1951 and Avendaño[16] in 1969 underscore the latter inference. Comparing the family situations of normal and undernourished children from apparently similar class and cultural backgrounds, both authors reported sharp differences in a variety of socioeconomic measures. The comparisons revealed, for example, that families with malnourished children had lower incomes, less stable employment, higher rates of illiteracy, and less adequate housing conditions.

Food Availability and Consumption

Barja et al.,[17] using standard food balance techniques, provide the most complete statistics available on Chile's food supply for the period 1965-1969 (table 7). They estimated that approximately 2,400 kcal and 74 g of protein per day were available for human consumption.

Despite the care used in constructing these estimates, some margin of error may have resulted from inadequacies in the original data on food production obtained from the Ministry of Agriculture. The study overstates Chile's population by about 10%,[18] but this is balanced by a probable underestimation in the extent of wastage. Other estimates of caloric availability during approximately the same period range from a high of 2,860[19] per capita per day to a low of 2,310.[20] These data suggest that Chile was not, in the traditional

Table 7
Food availability in Chile, 1965-69

Food Group	Per Capita Per Year (kg)	Per Capita Per Day (g)	Per Capita kcal Per Day	Per Capita Protein Per Day
Cereals, pulses	138.1	378.4	1,230.2	37.8
Dairy Products, Eggs	115.2	315.6	191.3	11.5
Meat, Seafood	30.2	73.0	113.7	16.7
Potatoes	43.2	118.2	79.2	3.7
Fruits, Vegetables	121.3	332.2	139.7	4.0
Sugar, Fats, Oils	44.3	111.4	639.6	---
Miscellaneous	.5	1.4	4.6	.2
Total	492.8	1,330.2	2,398.3	73.9

sense, a food-short country in the late 1960s. Overall supply of both calories
and proteins approximated or exceeded estimated needs (of around 2,400
kcal and 65 g of protein per capita per day). Per capita availability was greater
than in all but three or four Latin American countries, and far above regional·
averages in Asia and Africa.[21]

These supply statistics, however, regardless of their accuracy, are not particularly useful indicators of the extent or nature of the country's nutrition
problems in the late 1960s since they provide no information concerning the
distribution of food or nutrients among different population groups. A consumer expenditure survey[22] conducted in Santiago in 1968 and 1969 on a
representative sample of some 1,800 households collected data on the variation of food expenditures with income level. The summary results, presented
in tables 8 and 9, conform to Engel's law—as income declines, an increasing
portion of total expenditures goes to food purchase, but absolute expenditures decrease.

On the basis of the food expenditures reported in the survey, Machicado[23]
calculated physical quantities purchased by consumers at each income level
and then translated these into caloric values.

Table 8
Food expenditure by family income level, Santiago, Chile, 1968-69

Family Income Level (Minimum Salary)	Expenditures on Food	
	Relative to Lowest Income Level	Percent of Total Expenditures
0 - 2	1.0	50
2 - 4	1.4	45
4 - 6	1.8	39
6 - 8	2.3	35
Greater than 8	3.1	26

Table 9
Per capita consumption by family income level, Santiago, Chile, 1968-69

Family Income Level (Minimum Salary)	Percent of all Families	Calorie Intake Intake (kcal)	Protein Intake (g)
0 - 2	54	1,600	39
2 - 4	26	2,100	52
4 - 6	8	2,150	57
6 - 8	3	2,200	65
Greater than 8	10	2,650	83
Weighted average		1,900	48

Given an approximate average per capita daily requirement of 2,400 kcal, it is reasonable to assume that families with per capita consumption levels below 2,000 kcal are nutritionally at serious risk, and, further, that one or more members are probably undernourished. Henceforth, these families will simply be designated "nutritionally vulnerable." Presuming some sort of normal distribution of consumption among households, Machicado's figures would place nearly all families earning less than two minimum salaries (representing some 54% of Santiago's families), along with some portion of families in the two to four minimum salary range, within the nutritionally vulnerable category. His study suggests that upwards of 60% of Santiago's families probably faced nutritional deprivation in 1968 and 1969.

Barja et al.,[24] working with a subsample of some 700 families from the same expenditure survey, made calculations similar to those of Machicado but arrived at significantly different results. They estimated that average per capita consumption among families earning less than two minimum salaries was on the order of 2,000 kcal daily (compared with Machicado's estimate of 1,600), and among families earning one minimum salary or less was approximately 1,800 kcal daily.

On the basis of the results from Barja, the estimates of food availability previously reported, and the negligible existence of second- and third-degree malnutrition in Chile, we are led to conclude that Machicado, in fact, seriously underestimated food consumption, particularly among low income groups. Potential sources of error in his calculations include an overstatement by about 10% in the average size of families earning less than two minimum salaries, and a failure to take into account meals consumed outside the home or wine consumption (which may average around 100 kcal per capita daily).[25] Correcting for these factors would raise Machicado's estimate by about 25% and bring them into line with the calculation of Barja and the estimates of food availability.

Conservatively interpreted, these studies suggest that roughly 30% of all families in Santiago consumed less than 2,000 kcal per day per capita in 1969. Since Santiago is one of Chile's more affluent and urbanized provinces,[26] food consumption levels there are probably somewhat higher than the national average. In per capita income, Santiago ranks fifth among Chile's twenty-five provinces[27] while only three other provinces had a lower percentage of families living in poverty in 1970.[28]

Comparing data from the late 1960s with earlier statistics on food availability and consumption is admittedly a risky and imprecise exercise; the recent data, as we have indicated, are not fully reliable, and we have even less confidence in the earlier information. We are unable to identify likely sources of error or to specify the magnitude and direction of inaccuracies. At best, our comparisons over time may yield evidence of some broad, general trends. Table 10 provides a compilation of estimates, based on food balance sheet techniques, of the average daily per capita availability of calories for human consumption in Chile for the period 1934-69.

Table 10
Daily per capita caloric availability, Chile, 1934-69

	Source	kcal
1934-38	FAO (1)	2,250
1948	FAO (1)	2,420
1947-51	Riquelme	2,127
1951-52	FAO (1)	2,450
1951-55	Arteaga and Santa Maria	2,613
1954-56	FAO (1)	2,550
1957-59	FAO (1)	2,380
1960	ICCND	2,600
1960-62	FAO (1)	2,430
1960-62	Donoso et al.	2,410
1960-64	Ministry of Agriculture (1)	2,797
1963-65	FAO (1)	2,660
1964-66	FAO (2)	2,516
1963-67	Soto and Arteaga	2,860
1968	Ministry of Agriculture (1)	2,540
1968	Autret et al.	2,310
1965-69	Barja	2,398

Sources: FAO (1): *The State of Food and Agriculture.* FAO, Rome, 1968, p. 179. FAO (2): Food Balance Sheets, 1964-1966 Average. FAO, Rome, 1971, p. 133. Riquelme: Alfredo Riquelme, Nutritional Problems of Chile and Their Implications with Public Health. Unpublished DPH dissertation, Harvard School of Public Health, 1955. Arteaga and Santa Maria: A. Arteaga and J.V. Santa Maria. Disponibilidad Promodio Estadistica de Alimentos en Chile, Quinquenio 1951-1955. *Acta de Sociedad Chilena de Diabetes y Enfermedades Metabolicas.* ICNND: Chile: Nutrition Survey, March-June 1960. Interdepartmental Committee on Nutrition for National Defense. Washington, DC: US Government Printing Office, 1971. Donoso et al.: G. Donoso, G. Solimano, 2nd M. A. Tagle. Politica Alimentaria y Nutricional a Nivel Nacional y a Nivel de Salud. Seccion Nutricion, Sub Departamento Fomento de la Salud (SNS), approved by Consejo Tecnico del Servicio Nacional de Salud, August 19, 1971. Ministry of Agriculture (1): Situacion de la Industria Alimentaria en Chile, 1960-1964, Seccion Fruiticultura y Tecnologia, Santiago, October 1965. Ministry of Agriculture (2): ODEPA-SAG, Santiago. Soto and Arteaga: S. Soto and A. Arteaga. *Estudio de Disponibilidad de Alimentos en Chile 1963-67.* Departamento de Nutricion, Facultad de Medicina, Universidad de Chile, Publicacion 16/70, 1970. Autret et al.: M. Autret et al., Protein Value of Different Types of Diet in the World: Their Approximate Supplementation. FAO *Nutrition Newsletter,* vol. 6 (1968). Barja: Ita Barja et al. *Disponibilidad de Alimentos en Chile, Quinquenio 1965-69.* Departamento de Nutricion, Facultad de Medicina, Universidad de Chile, Publicacion 25/71, 1971.

Although the data do not permit the drawing of any firm conclusions, it would appear that average caloric availability did not decline in Chile over the 35-year period. At the same time, however, it cannot be claimed that any important gains were made—especially since the prewar estimate was made while Chile was still suffering the effects of the world depression, which, according to a League of Nations study, was particularly severe in Chile.[29]

Only two studies—one done in 1935 under the auspices of the League of Nations[30] and the previously cited ICNND survey[31] —collected data on the frequency distribution of per capita caloric consumption among Chilean families. Their findings, presented in tables 11 and 12, suggest that the distribution of food consumption did not vary significantly over the 25-year period in question.

It is particularly striking that, in both studies, the percentage of families consuming less than 2,000 kcal per capita per day (and, therefore, nutritionally vulnerable) is essentially the same. These data would indicate that the prevalence of dietary inadequacies in Chile hardly diminished between 1935 and 1960. Our analysis of the findings of Barja[32] and Machicado[33] —although not strictly comparable to the earlier studies since they concern only Santiago and report consumption by income levels (rather than providing a frequency distribution) implied that in 1968 and 1969 a roughly similar percentage of families were nutritionally at risk.[34]

On the basis of these consumption surveys, which are not contradicted by the clinical findings or by the food-availability studies discussed previously, we would cautiously advance the proposition that food consumption among Chile's low-income groups probably did not increase by any significant extent between 1935 and 1970, and that nutritional deprivation consistently affected one-third or more of the country's families during that entire period.

Table 11
Calorie consumption, Chile, 1935

Daily Per Capita Consumption (kcal)	Percent of Families (n=593)
more than 3,000	27
2,400 - 3,000	23
2,000 - 2,400	11
1,500 - 2,000	27
less than 1,500	11

Table 12
Calorie consumption, Chile, 1960

Daily Per Capita Calorie Consumption (Percent of Recommended Allowance)	Percent of Families (n=278)
More than 134% (3,146)	10
115 - 133% (2,677 - 3,145)	14
85 - 114% (1,972 - 2,676)	39
65 - 84% (1,516 - 1,971)	24
Less than 65% (1,515)	13

Infant Mortality Studies

Infant mortality rates in Chile, as elsewhere in the third world, declined
sharply between 1927 and 1973. No improvements were registered in the first
12 years of that period, but, beginning around 1939 infant mortality showed
a steady downward trend, with the exception of the seven years from 1953 to
1960. Between 1938 and 1973, the number of infant deaths per 1,000 live
births dropped by more than 70% from 236 to 66 (table 13).

While malnutrition was a probable contributing cause in a majority of infant deaths throughout this period,[35] our previous analysis of food consumption and childhood growth statistics would suggest that reductions in the
mortality rate were not due to improvements in the country's food and nutrition situation. In the absence of contradictory data, we would argue that the
reductions can largely be explained by (1) the introduction of new methods
for the prevention, diagnosis, and cure of previously endemic diseases, and
(2) the extension and improvement of public health services in the country.
Stolnitz[36] has similarly interpreted evidence from other developing countries,
concluding that innovations in public health and sanitation, not increases in
overall income levels, were the direct and proximate cause of contemporary
mortality trends in the low-income world. According to Stolnitz, mortality
trends are "remarkably neutral with respect to economic events . . . [and]

Table 13
Infant mortality (per 1,000 live births), Chile, 1927-1973

Year	Rate	Year	Rate	Year	Rate
1927	226	1943	173	1959	118
1928	212	1944	162	1960	126
1929	224	1945	164	1961	114
1930	234	1946	143	1962	114
1931	232	1947	143	1963	106
1932	235	1948	146	1964	105
1933	258	1949	150	1965	100
1934	262	1950	136	1966	102
1935	251	1951	132	1967	98
1936	252	1952	118	1968	87
1937	241	1953	100	1969	79
1938	236	1954	116	1970	79
1939	201	1955	119	1971	71
1940	192	1956	109	1972	71
1941	179	1957	117	1973	66
1942	174	1958	123		

economic misery as such is no longer an effective barrier to the vast upsurge in survival opportunities in underdeveloped areas."

In the late 1930s important changes occurred in the concept and practice of medical attention in Chile. Increased emphasis was given the preventive aspects of medicine with greater attention to maternal and child health care. Authorities extended medical coverage under social security to spouses of insured workers and their dependent children under two years of age, launched an intensive campaign to eliminate tuberculosis (the single major contributor to adult mortality), and introduced antibiotics into common use. By 1952, the different government agencies responsible for health care were merged to form a unified National Health Service responsible for all of the country's preventive health activities and for the provision of curative services to families enrolled in social security and those classified as medically indigent.

The distribution of health services remained highly skewed throughout the period 1938-70, with particular prejudice toward lower income strata.[37] But by the late 1960s substantial gains had been made in extending attention throughout the country. More than a thousand clinics were operating in rural and urban areas, vaccinations were available to nearly all children, and almost 85% of births were attended by medically qualified individuals[38] (compared with less than 20% in 1938).[39] Several common infectious diseases (e.g., tuberculosis, polio, and diphtheria) were largely brought under control,[40] and general levels of sanitation and hygiene were considerably improved. Chile was a safer and cleaner place to live in 1970—even for marginal urban and rural dwellers—than it had been in 1939.

While infant mortality decreased among all social classes in Chile, strong positive correlations existed not only between survival chances and socioeconomic level, but also between the improvements registered in infant survival rates and socioeconomic level. This latter relationship suggests that the country's low income groups benefited least from advances in medical care and improvements in sanitary conditions. The findings of Behm et al.[41] regarding the interaction of social class, medical attention, and infant mortality are presented in table 14.

Table 14
Infant mortality by social class and medical attention, Chile, 1957

Children of:	Infant Mortality Rate Per 1,000 Live Births
Manual laborers	
without medical coverage	157
with medical coverage	102
Non-manual employees	
with medical coverage	57
National average	116

These differences in infant mortality rates between working-class and non-working-class families and also between the two categories of workers reflect the general stratification of Chilean society and the differential access to health services accorded to different socioeconomic groups. Those workers and their families who enjoyed medical coverage, besides receiving more and better medical attention, had higher incomes, more stable employment, and better living conditions than noninsured laborers.

There are no other studies, to our knowledge, directly relating mortality to socioeconomic status and medical attention in Chile. Available data at the provincial level, however, permit some further examination of the relationship among these variables. Marchant[42] in 1970 and Ugarte[43] in 1951 analyzed infant mortality trends by provinces. Using their findings and the income statistics prepared by Chile's National Planning Office,[44] we have constructed tables 15 and 16. The classification of the country's 25 provinces by income is our own: high income provinces had a gross product per capita which was above the national average in 1967; middle income provinces had per capita products ranging from 80 to 100% of the national average; and low income provinces from 40 to 79% of the average.

As can be observed, infant survival chances were consistently greater in higher income provinces, and the differences reported among high, middle, and low income provinces increased over time. Income was not the only fac-

Table 15
Infant mortality trends in high, middle, and low income provinces, Chile, 1940-47

| | Infant Mortality Rate Per 1,000 Live Births | | Percent Decrease |
	1940	1947	
High Income Provinces	179	144	20%
Middle Income Provinces	199	163	18%
Low Income Provinces	205	184	10%
National Average	197	167	15%

Table 16
Infant mortality trends in high, middle, and low income provinces, Chile, 1958/59 - 1968/1969

| | Infant Mortality Rate Per 1,000 Live Births | | Percent Decrease |
	1958/1959	1968/1969	
High Income Provinces	98	59	40%
Middle Income Provinces	130	96	26%
Low Income Provinces	136	105	23%
National Average	116	81	30%

tor influencing infant mortality rates, however: urbanization and medical attention are highly correlated with income at the provincial level as indicated in table 17.

PATTERNS OF DEVELOPMENT AND REFORM

Our analysis of the available data on food supply and consumption, clinical indicators of malnutrition, and infant mortality in Chile for the 40-year period 1930-70 has revealed marked and persistent inequalities in food consumption, growth rates, and survival chances among the country's different socioeconomic strata. Those inequalities, moreover, may have increased over time. It appears likely, although the evidence at our disposal is limited, that food consumption and nutritional standards among Chile's low income groups did not improve measurably and that the prevalence of malnutrition, affecting principally the poorest third or so of the country's families, did not diminish significantly over the period studied.

The country's food and nutrition situation cannot be attributed to a stagnant economy or to the absence of social reform. Chile experienced considerable economic growth and development as well as important social and political changes in the period under consideration. From 1930 to 1970, per capita income more than doubled, reaching more than US $500 per year by the latter date, and making Chile one of the more affluent third world countries. Per capita growth rates were uneven but averaged a reasonable 1.5% per year. Chile became a semi-industrialized country producing most of its own consumer items by 1970 and achieved a relatively high degree of modernization. Among developing countries, Chile had one of the most progressive records of social legislation—particularly in the areas of social security, health, and education.

If the continued high prevalence of malnutrition in Chile was not due to a lack of development or change, the explanation must then be sought in the type of development that took place, and in the underlying sociopolitical structures that conditioned its course and results. We will, therefore, turn our attention to the consequences of government policies in a few critical sectors in an effort to illustrate how such policies have consistently discriminated against low income groups and contributed to the maintenance of inequality and poverty in Chile. Without meaning to imply a lack of variation in the policies, priorities, and ideologies of different governments, we are suggesting the existence of an identifiable pattern of political and economic decision which characterized Chilean development efforts in the period 1930-70.

The Industrial Sector

The year 1930 marked the beginning of a rapid expansion in Chilean industrial production. The world depression had produced a sharp contraction of

Table 17
Income, urbanization, medical attention, and infant mortality by provinces, Chile[45]

	Gross Product per Capita (relative to national average for Chile) (1967)	% of Population Classified as Urban (1970)	% of births without Medical Attention (1970)	Infant Mortality Per 1,000 Live Births (1968/69)	% Decrease in Infant Mortality Rates (1958/59-60)
High Income Provinces					
Magallanes	2.08	86.3%	2.1%	47.3	41.2%
Antofagasta	1.54	96.5	5.2	88.0	34.1
Atacama	1.54	83.3	18.2	88.3	22.7
Tarapaca	1.25	91.0	7.1	65.3	24.8
Santiago	1.24	93.3	6.6	55.7	38.2
O'Higgins	1.22	54.1	20.9	80.2	37.8
Valparaiso	1.04	91.4	5.8	55.7	45.4
Middle Income Provinces					
Concepcion	0.89	85.0	20.7	99.6	29.2
Acencagua	0.89	60.5	27.2	72.7	28.9
Osorn	0.83	53.7	31.3	110.3	20.1
Aysen	0.81	64.4	28.2	103.6	(3.6)
Low Income Provinces					
Talca	0.74	52.6	34.4	94.2	36.3
Llanquihue	0.69	51.2	34.8	116.9	1.0

Bio-Bio	0.68	47.9	36.2	112.1	27.4
Coquimbo	0.64	59.5	32.3	84.7	31.9
Valdivia	0.63	52.3	32.6	121.5	10.0
Maule	0.61	44.8	39.9	95.5	25.9
Curico	0.57	45.7	29.0	97.8	37.2
Colchagua	0.57	38.0	31.1	72.2	38.2
Linares	0.54	41.7	30.4	101.4	22.9
Nuble	0.51	46.6	42.5	114.2	16.6
Malleco	0.47	51.9	35.8	125.2	13.1
Arauco	0.47	50.5	47.1	139.2	3.7
Cautin	0.43	48.9	38.2	100.9	24.2
Chiloe	0.42	31.6	49.1	107.9	30.6
Chile	1.00	75.0	30.2	81.0	31.3

the international market for Chile's exports, and with it a dramatic reduction of nearly 70% in the country's capacity to import.[46] The resulting government measures to maintain internal demand, prohibit most imports except for capital goods, and control exchange operations created conditions for a rapid growth in the internal production of manufactured goods to substitute for lost imports. In 1938 a more deliberate policy of industrialization was initiated by the Popular Front government. Private entrepenuers were encouraged by continued protection, tax exemptions, and special credit facilities, and the government organized a State Development Corporation (CORFO) to guide and promote industrial growth. Through CORFO, efforts were made to create a modern infrastructure for industry, state enterprises were established in such basic areas as steel, electricity, petroleum, and rubber, and investment funds were made available to stimulate private ventures.

Successive governments continued to give emphasis to industrial development, which advanced steadily through 1954—with particularly rapid growth registered during World War II and the Korean War. As possibilities for replacing imports with domestic production became increasingly scarce, however, industrial activity along with the economy as a whole entered into a ten-year period of stagnation, with negative per capita growth rates in five of those ten years. Finally, during the Frei government (1965-70), a small resurgence of industrial expansion took place. Throughout the period 1930-70 industrial production grew at a rate which was approximately three or four times faster than the rest of the economy.[47]

The process of industrialization, however, failed to lead to a dynamic economy or to provide the basis for a more egalitarian society. Sunkel, in 1965, concluded that:

The emphasis placed on industrial development has left untouched the traditional system of land-ownership while new forms of high concentration of capital have been created in industry (and other sectors) . . . As a result income distribution has remained markedly unequal and savings have therefore also tended to be highly concentrated . . . Because of this high degree of concentration of economic power and the growing association of the higher echelons of the bureaucracy with the industrial and financial groups, the state has increasingly come under the control of private interests.[48]

Chilean industry, although by far the fastest growing economic sector, was limited in its expansion by a small internal market and an inability to compete overseas. It was able to absorb only a portion of the country's rapidly increasing urban workforce. Workers employed in larger and more productive enterprises were organized into labor unions and enjoyed adequate living conditions, reasonable salaries, and considerable social benefits. These unions, which enrolled less than 15% of the economically active population, achieved an important measure of political influence, primarily through the left-wing political parties of which they formed the core support.

Conditions were more difficult for the rest of the workforce, much of which was engaged in the so-called service sector occupations. These workers frequently lacked steady employment, earned low wages when working, were excluded from many social services, and remained largely without political representation. On the whole, these nonindustrial laborers appear not to have benefited significantly from economic growth, and indications are that their real incomes may have declined as development progressed in Chile. It is among these groups which emerged as an outgrowth of industrialization and the accompanying urbanization in Chile, that nutritional vulnerability was highest.

Data from 1940 to 1957 indicate a general decline in the earnings of manual workers relative to white-collar employees.[49] A subsequent study for the period 1950-60 showed gains for manual laborers compared to white collar workers, and further that the 30% lowest paid manual workers improved relative to all manual workers.[50] This study, however, was based on social security statistics and did not take into account those workers (representing some 30% of all workers) outside of the social security system, among whom individuals from the lowest income strata predominate. One direct indicator of the economic situation of Chile's poorest families is the legal minimum wage—which declined in purchasing power by more than one-third between 1952 and 1970,[51] while the percentage of income recipients earning one minimum salary or less remained approximately the same during that period.[52,53]

Agriculture and the Rural Sector

In Chile's rural areas, where the incidence of malnutrition is consistently higher than in urban communities, the structure of class power remained largely unchanged until the mid-1960s when the Frei government initiated the country's first serious efforts at reforming land tenure patterns. Rural areas were characterized by extreme concentration of land ownership and sharp inequalities in the distribution of wealth and income. In 1960 large landowners, comprising approximately 2% of the rural population, controlled more than 65% of the country's arable land. Less than 10% of rural residents owned nearly 90% of agricultural land, earned upwards of 50% of the income generated by agriculture, and received more than 90% of available credit. Subsistence farmers, representing some 25% of the rural population, held only about 1% of the land under cultivation. These farmers seldom cultivated more than five hectares, were virtually excluded from government and private credit, and were generally forced to sell some of their labor to maintain themselves and their families.[54]

Large- and middle-size holders, through their control of resources and their national political connections, dominated the political and economic life of the countryside and were able to prevent any effective challenges to their authority until the mid-1960s. Voting rights were virtually denied peasants until the 1950s, union organization was prohibited by law until 1965, and a minimum wage for agricultural workers, established only in 1952, was set at one-third the urban wage (and widely disregarded in practice). Most important, landowners were able to forestall any changes in land tenure arrangements until 1965.

At the bottom of the socioeconomic scale were the tenant farmers (*inquilinos*) and the landless wage laborers (*afuerinos*). The inquilinos lived and worked on large agricultural holdings and were economically dependent on their landlords. As a group, however, they were somewhat more privileged than the afuerinos who, contracting their labor by the day, were frequently unemployed and excluded from most types of social services and benefits. It was among the afuerinos that poverty and social disruption were most intense.

In 1930 the population of tenant farmers exceeded that of afuerinos by about two to one, but by 1955 the latter outnumbered the former by approximately 34 to 30% of the active rural population. [55] The expansion of this subclass of free laborers has been explained by a combination of factors—the development of commercialized agriculture, the general weakening of ties between owners and workers, the sharp increase of absentee ownership, and the growing population pressures on available land.

The country's first workable agrarian reform law was passed in 1967 and the Chilean government began the expropriation and distribution of private agricultural property. Passage of the law was made possible by changes in the rural areas themselves, shifts in the national balance of power (reflected, in part, by the election of Frei) and the increasing acceptance of the structuralist view of the Chilean economy (i.e., that low productivity in agriculture was a prime obstacle to economic growth and stability, and was basically caused by the outmoded structure of land tenure).

The Frei reform managed to settle some 28,000 peasant families on newly expropriated land. [56] This number, however, was far short of the government's own goal of 100,000 families, and represented less than 8% of all rural households. The principal beneficiaries of the reform were tenant farmers who were given the estates on which they had previously worked. Conditions of the more impoverished afuerinos, who were not attached to any specific agricultural holdings, were by and large not improved.

Throughout the period 1930-70, government policies designed to promote industrialization and satisfy urban demands discriminated against the agricultural sector. Foreign food imports were subsidized, domestic farm prices controlled, and few investments made in rural areas. Large landowners were able to defend themselves by shifting resources and profits into industry and commerce, maintaining their workers at low wages, and avoiding taxes. Many of the traditional landowning families sold their land to newly wealthy urban buyers, whose interest was often land for prestige or as a hedge against inflation. Typically the new owners were not interested in introducing technical or other changes for increased production, or even fully cultivating their land.[57] These land purchases tended to strengthen further the community of interests between upper income groups in rural and urban areas, and contributed to the growth of absentee ownership, which, in turn, probably led to deteriorating conditions for agrarian labor.

Marmalakis and Reynolds[58] reported that unskilled agricultural workers "suffered close to a 20% decline in real wages between 1940 and 1952," while "salaried employees and proprietors . . . experienced an increase of more than 40% in the same period." Only after 1964 did real wage rates in agriculture improve measurably, but, in 1967, nearly 90% of rural workers (compared to 55% of urban workers) still earned one minimum salary or less.

Whether because of the land tenure system and rural social structure or general government discrimination against the agricultural sector (or more likely some combination of both), the performance of Chilean agriculture was unsatisfactory for the entire period 1930-1970. Production barely kept pace with population growth and fell far behind rising demand for food as national income expanded. Agricultural imports rose sharply and placed an increasingly heavy burden on the country's scarce supply of foreign exchange. In short, government policies and priorities resulted in an agrarian structure which failed to satisfy the needs of an urban- and industrial-oriented development process, and, at the same time, kept an overwhelming majority of the rural population in poverty.

Social Services

Since the 1920s there has been a continuous expansion of government-provided social services in Chile—reflecting in large measure the growing political influence of the Chilean middle class and organized sectors of the working class. Expenditures on health, education, social security, and other social services increased from some 28% of total government expenditures in 1940 to 37% by 1954,[59] and to around 50% by 1970. But the country's social legislation, which was one of Latin America's most progressive, rather than reducing inequalities and assisting low income groups, tended to reinforce existing socioeconomic inequalities. The main beneficiaries of social programs were white-collar employees, other middle income earners, and organized workers. Chile's lowest income groups, which were largely without political representation, had only limited access to most public services and welfare benefits. At the same time, these groups may have borne a disproportionate share of the financing of the programs through the country's regressive tax system.

The single most important component of Chile's social welfare structure was the social security system. Considering all sources of contributions and income, the amount of funds flowing through the system exceeded 90% of the entire national budget in some years.[60] Through pensions, medical facilities, unemployment and disability insurance, and family allowances, the social security system was intended to help insure minimum standards of living for Chilean families and protect them against unexpected misfortune. The first social security legislation was enacted in 1924, and since then the system experienced steady growth in both the range and level of benefits provided and the number of its participants.

As late as 1970, however, social security provided coverage to only 70% of the economically active population.[61] Upper income families who had little need for the kinds of services provided accounted for some portion of the 30% not covered, but the majority of those excluded were from lower income strata—rural workers, recent migrants to cities, persons generally without stable employment, or individuals working in marginal jobs where social security payments, as well as minimum wage requirements, could be avoided. These individuals and their families received no dependent allowances, unemployment benefits, old age pensions, or the like. Moreover, those families lacking social security took far less advantage than did participants in the system of other social services such as medical care and free milk distribution to which they were legally entitled.

For participants in the social security system, benefits varied sharply, depending in most cases on income and job status. A basic distinction was established between white-collar employees (*empleados*) and blue-collar workers (*obreros*), with the former enjoying a wider range of benefits in almost all categories. Retirement pensions, for example, were granted to empleados on the basis of years of service, while obreros could only receive their pensions at a designated age regardless of their length of service. Differences, typically favoring those of higher occupational status, also existed in the methods used in calculating the size of pensions, in awarding disability pensions, computing readjustments in pension rates with rises in the cost of living, and in determining family allowances and qualifications for eligibility as a dependent.[62]

Medical service was included among the benefits provided to workers under social security. Initially such services were restricted to the workers themselves, but subsequently were extended to dependents. Families lacking coverage and unable to afford private care were attended by another set of institutions until 1952, when the National Health Service was established. The new health service assumed responsibility for the provision of direct care to families under social security (except for white-collar employees who elected to remain apart and eventually evolved their own medical insurance scheme) and those classified as medical indigents. While legal discrimination between beneficiaries and nonbeneficiaries of social security (although not between empleados and obreros) was eliminated from Chile's health care system, the former, in fact, consistently received higher levels of attention.

Despite some real gains in the quality and extent of health care available to low income groups in Chile between 1930 and 1970, sharp inequalities persisted in the medical attention provided to different socioeconomic groups. De Kadt, in a recent study of health services in Chile, concluded that "the inhabitants of rural areas, those with very low income, and people without social security benefits make less use of health services and have a greater unsatisfied demand, i.e., they are more frequently unable to use the services of the health system for reasons of distance, for lack of time or money, or for failure to be attended"[63] (table 18). Public expenditures on health—which in principle were supposed to reduce inequalities in access to medical care—were approximately evenly distributed among different socioeconomic strata[64] (table 19), even though lower income groups had greater need for government-provided care because of their inability to purchase private care and their greater susceptibility to disease (as a result of adverse living conditions, more dangerous occupations, and poorer diets).

Table 18
Utilization of medical services, Chile, 1968

Medical Insurance Coverage	Medical Visits Per Capita Per Year
None	1.5
Social Security	2.1
Other forms of coverage (largely white collar employees)	2.6
Family Income Per Capita	
0.0 - 0.19 (minimum salaries)	1.5
0.2 - 0.39	2.1
0.4 - 0.59	2.3
0.6 - 0.99	2.5
Greater than 1.0	3.0
Residence	
Santiago	3.0
Other urban areas	1.9
Other rural areas	1.5

Table 19
Public and private health expenditures, Chile, 1969

Family Income Stratum	% of the Population	Public Expenditure on Health (Relative to Lowest Income Group)	Total Expenditure on Health (Relative to Lowest Income Group)
0 - 1 (minimum salary)	30	1.00	1.00
1 - 2	32	1.03	1.29
2 - 3	18	0.94	1.68
3 - 5	12	0.92	2.24
5	9	0.88	3.16

Education was also thought to be a factor promoting equality and social mobility in Chilean society. Considerable progress had been made in expanding educational opportunities by 1970 when approximately 90% of all 7- to 14-year-olds were enrolled in school and illiteracy had been reduced to around 15%.[65] Substantial growth was also registered in secondary, technical, and university training. Dropout and repetition rates, however, remained high, so that only approximately 40% of Chilean children reached secondary school and less than 10% graduated. The rate of failure was highest among rural and poor urban groups: only 2 or 3% of university students were from working class families, which comprised about 70% of the country's population. In 1968 some 55% of public expenditures on education were allocated to secondary and university education, which enrolled only 13% of all students.[66] Sunkel[67] argued that "the educational system, far from fulfilling a function of democratization and equalization, has become organized in such a way that it segregates classes and discriminates heavily against the lower and in favor of the upper middle and higher income groups."

One can only conclude that government-provided social services tended to reinforce and perpetuate, rather than alleviate, inequalities among different socioeconomic groups in Chile. Middle class, white-collar sectors were the major beneficiaries of the country's panoply of social legislation, followed by organized sectors of the working class; far fewer benefits were extended to Chile's lowest income groups, who often were partially or fully excluded from social assistance programs. Moreover, given the regressive nature of Chile's tax structures, lower income groups probably bore an important share of the costs of the country's social legislation. Indeed, as numerous observers have commented, the system of welfare and social services in Chile, ostensibly designed to assist the poor, turned out, in fact, to be a device for redistributing resources from lower to middle class groups—or for the exploitation of the lower class by the middle class.[68]

Overall, Chile's pattern of development during the period from 1930 to 1970 was characterized by a high concentration of economic resources under private control, a sharp degree of stratification among different social classes, and the virtual exclusion of a significant portion of the population from the benefits of economic growth. Government policies in the period, even those designed to improve the situation of the disadvantaged, by and large acted to reinforce and sustain these processes of concentration, stratification, and exclusion. The evidence suggests that persistence of low levels of food consumption and a high incidence of malnutrition among the poorest third or so of the population was a direct consequence of this development pattern. Significant improvements in the nutrition standards in Chile would probably have required fundamental changes in the development policies and strategies. These changes, however, probably could not have been achieved under the existing balance of political forces.

EPILOGUE: THE ALLENDE AND POST-ALLENDE YEARS

Salvador Allende, the Marxist candidate of the Popular Unity Coalition, was elected to the Chilean presidency by a narrow plurality of votes in 1970. His program called for a restructuring of established economic, social, and political relationships in Chile with the stated goal of moving toward some form of socialism: in short, a breaking of the country's established development pattern. The Allende government sought to end the high concentration of private ownership and control in Chile by expanding public control over basic sectors of the economy, and to achieve a relatively rapid redistribution of income in favor of the working class.

During its short term in power, the government nationalized an important share of the country's foreign and domestically owned industry, brought most mining and banking operations under state ownership, fostered the concept of worker-managed enterprises, and extended land reform to the point where nearly all legally expropriable land had been expropriated. At the same time, a general redistribution of income was achieved as the government decreed wages and salary adjustments in excess of inflation rates, reduced unemployment to historically low levels, controlled the prices of numbers of basic items, and expanded health care and other social services available to low income groups.

No extensive evaluation has been done concerning the impact of these measures on different socioeconomic sectors, let alone of their consequences for nutritional standards. The redistribution of income, however, did result in a sharp upswing in demand, particularly for food. Tagle et al.,[69] using the same methodology employed by Barja et al.,[70] estimated an increase in caloric availability of approximately 8% for the period 1971-72 over the period 1965-69. Barraclough and Affonso[71] estimated even higher increases in food consumption: 14% in 1971 and an additional 12% in 1972 relative to the period 1966-70. These increments were made possible by a sharp rise in food imports, since agricultural production within Chile probably decreased during the Allende government.

There is no specific data from the Allende years on the distribution of food consumption by income level. By using available income and price statistics and calculating expenditure elasticities for a wide variety of food items, Machicado[72] estimated that consumption had increased by approximately 10% from 1969 to 1971 among Chile's lowest income group (earning two minimum salaries or less), compared with an average increase for all income strata of about 7%.

This expansion of the food supply was, however, insufficient to satisfy the growth in demand, and food shortages, hoarding, and black marketing assumed increasingly serious proportions. Food import and distribution policies, moreover, contributed substantially to a worsening balance of payments and a deteriorating overall economic situation.

The military junta that toppled Allende in September 1973 has established
a highly repressive, authoritarian regime. Economic policy, based on ortho-
dox free-market principles, has transferred most state-operated enterprises to
the private sector and reduced government controls on prices and imports.
Social changes and reform have been assigned low priority and government
expenditures and services have decreased sharply. These policies have resulted
in a severe decline in purchasing power among lower and middle income
groups, a high concentration of economic resources, a contraction of industrial production, and extremely high levels of unemployment in both urban and
rural areas (estimated at between 20 and 30% of the workforce in mid-
1976).[73]

Nutritional standards have suffered. Medical doctors and others[74] working
in public clinics have observed marked increases in the number of malnourished infants—including those affected by second- and third-degree malnutrition. Although there were no studies[75] to confirm these observations of
medical personnel, the available evidence does suggest that food consumption—particularly of low income families—has declined precipitously. Food
imports in 1975, for example, were nearly 50% lower than they had been in
1972, while domestic agricultural production was virtually the same.[76]

Chossudovsky[77] estimated in November 1973 (two months after the fall of
Allende) that the purchasing power of families earning less than two minimum salaries had dropped by nearly 50% from 1968/69 levels. Meller and
Ruiz Tagle[78] repeating the Chossudovsky study in December 1974 calculated
a decline of some 37% for the same income group. Since low income families
spent upwards of 50% of their income on food, it is probable that this decline
in real income forced a deterioration in diet quality and quantity. One example taken from Meller is illustrative. In 1968/69 bread purchases—which provided some 38% of all calories—amounted to 1.8 kg per day and accounted
for 7.3% of the monthly expenditures of families earning less than two minimum salaries; to purchase the same quantity of bread in December 1974
would have required 22% of these families' budgets.

DISCUSSION (CHILE)

Solimano

In sum, the Chilean experience has been examined in this paper as an initial exercise in the study of how food and nutrition situations relate to the patterns of economic, political, and social development of a country. We were able to start around 1930 and move from there to the present. Chile has had a long experience in developing nutrition activities throughout this entire period of 40 to 45 years. This period saw the initiatives for creation of several national food councils, the first one in 1942, the second one during the Frei period in '64 to '70, the third one, during the Allende period, '70-'73, and the fourth one recently, under the military junta. Looking back, though, we realize that when the government supported this formal and institutional approach, not much really happened to change nutritional status.

Chile provides a good case because Chile has had, since 1925, increasingly progressive social legislation. Basically we see that nutrition problems are no more than the consequence or output of the patterns of development of a society. This, I think, needs to be discussed, analyzed, and developed further. By looking at the problem in this way, we will see what is needed in order really to solve the problem.

The basic hypothesis in this paper is that Chile followed a certain pattern of development, which continued through time, sometimes steadily, sometimes not, but this development didn't mean that the food and nutrition situation of all groups in our society improved. On the contrary, what we demonstrate here is that, consistently, during that whole period, the type of development that the country followed *systemically excluded the groups that were undernourished and were vulnerable to the risk of malnutrition.*

I think we have started to make this case although we are not completely satisfied yet. We *can* show, in terms of nutritional status and food consumption, that at least a third of the population of Chile was discriminated against and, as a result, had nutritional problems.

Total infant mortality in Chile, from 1937 to 1970, and, later on, to '73, decreased significantly in the time period. Yet, the food and nutrition situation for some people did not improve significantly. I'm not saying it didn't improve, but it didn't improve *significantly.* Yet, there are changes in terms of health. What happened?

How much do food and nutrition influence the improvement of health in the country? Although health of the country improved as a whole, we can demonstrate that this improvement was mostly for the middle and upper classes. There was not the same amount or same percentage improvement for the lower class, or for the rural, as compared to urban population. When we deal with the health system, again, the pattern of development was very uneven, although there was some growth in the amount and in the quality of the health services provided for poor people.

Montgomery
Do you have longitudinal data showing calorie and protein consumption by income level over a period of time?

Solimano
We have two studies [see pp. 15-17] : one in 1935 by the League of Nations and one in 1960 by the ICNND. You can see that over a 25-year time span, very little changed: 38% of the population in 1935 and 37% of the population in 1960 were consuming less than 2,000 calories.

Levinson
I wonder if these two sets of statistics are using comparable population groups. One looks like it might be taking children into equal account with the adult population in calculating per capita calories. Is that possible?

Solimano
No. As we mentioned in the paper, the first figures are low because they leave out some consumption. A figure between 1,800 and 2,000 is more accurate.

We advance the proposition that food consumption among Chile's low income group probably didn't increase in any significant degree between 1935 and 1970 and that nutritional deprivation consistently affected one-third or more of the country's population during that entire period. This is something which would be interesting to examine in other countries. It is shown strikingly in the trends in daily per capita caloric availability in Chile from 1934 to 1969. There are some differences, but not many in that thirty-year period, in terms of theoretical per capita availability of calories.

The table showing infant mortality by social class and medical coverage in Chile in 1957 reveals that manual laborers without medical coverage have a rate of 157 deaths per thousand live births and nonmanual employees with medical coverage have only 57. That represents real discrimination by social class.

Wray
Before you leave infant mortality, is there any data at all which sheds light on the cause of death in those three groups? What were the differences?

Solimano
It's very, very clear that, in the group with higher infant mortality, infection is a primary cause. In Chile, gastrointestinal and respiratory infections are very important. All this has as a base line: malnutrition. We're fairly sure of these factors because we participated in the inter-American research on mortality in childhood. In the more economically favored groups, the problem was much more akin to that in the developed countries: neonatal mortality is proportionately more important than late infant mortality. Quite a different pattern.

Mellor

In your estimates of food availability under Allende, you are simply taking the total supply of food and relating it to the total population?

Solimano

Yes.

Mellor

Do you know whether the PL 480 aid is significant in that figure? It was presumably cut off during the Allende period, with very serious subsequent results. Would imports of food explain most of the difference? Do you know?

Solimano

PL 480 was almost all cut. Assistance only continued for the school feeding program, but all other types of aid were rapidly discontinued. The increase in food availability during the Allende period was due mainly to the importation of food. In 1971, food production was more or less on the same level as earlier, but it decreased in '72 and '73 because there was an extensive agrarian reform taking place. As a result, the country was putting a lot of money into food imports.

Schlossberg

In that case, the price must have been considerably higher.

Solimano

Yes, the prices went up, but not as severely as later on. Machicado's estimate that consumption had increased by approximately 10% from 1969 to 1971 among Chile's lowest income group was not a study; he was simply trying to translate the data from '69 to what was going on in '71.

Wray

Two things were operating in Chile: they were importing more food, but also they had substantially adjusted the salaries of that lowest third.

Solimano

Yes. What is clear, although we cannot demonstrate it with data, is that a better redistribution of that food was occurring in the country.

Mellor

And that, at a time when domestic food availability was reduced and the United States was working very hard to reduce Chile's foreign exchange availability, pressing for cancellation of World Bank missions, etc.

Solimano

In '72 and early '73, if you had gone to Chile, you would have seen an apparent food shortage, with a food "black market." But, actually, there is a different explanation in terms of what happens between competing groups when political change occurs: since more poor people were buying more food in the marketplace, there was less available for the middle and upper classes. In the end, because of political considerations, the Allende government was unable to establish food rationing, even though there was enough food available in the country. This became one of the basic points in the struggle against the Allende regime: a very well-organized campaign to demonstrate that people were eating less!

We have some figures about malnutrition in that epoch mainly from the preschool children served by the National Health Service. These children are from the lowest socioeconomic group. In table 1, the right column shows the percentage of preschool children who were found to be malnourished. How this changed after the anti-Allende coup is very hard to know. Unfortunately, for the people living through it, this period will probably provide another big contrast, an extreme case of what occurs when you shift the type of economy and your goals and your priorities.

Table 1
Studies of children under six: prevalence of malnutrition[a]

Year	Total Studied	With Malnutrition: All Grades	Percent
1970	241,547	42,432	17.6[b]
1971	262,086	41,782	15.9[b]
1973[c]	578,597	83,721	14.5[d]

[a]Population seen in SNS (National Health Service).
[b]Nutritional status, according to Mardones chart in use at that date.
[c]From nutritional status survey, completed October 30, 1973.
[d]Nutritional status, according to SNS norms, used from 1973 on.

A centrist weekly magazine published an article entitled "How Much Are We Spending to Eat?" in Chile in August, 1975. In it, there are graphs showing that, while the minimum salary now is about 250,000 escudos, people earning between 300,000 and 400,000 escudos are expending 87% of their budget on food. Fifty percent of the population earn less than two minimum salaries, or 500,000 escudos per month. People earning less than one minimum salary make up around 30% of the population. So the group earning less than 300-400,000 escudos per month accounts for at least 30 to 40% of the employed population. This survey does not even consider the unemployed and unsalaried.

Mellor
Does this include rural people?

Solimano
From what I read, I believe it is mostly urban. The figures are from areas all around the country, but mostly urban and employed people. According to the last survey, around 19% of the population is currently unemployed.

Levinson

That's really an incredible figure: 87% of the budget on food is higher than John's figures for India.

Wray

Giorgio, do we have any knowledge of the proportion of families in each of these income groups? You mentioned maybe 30 or 40% in this bottom group, but how about the others?

Solimano

Yes, I have that based on '68-'69 figures. Below two minimum salaries, in 1968/69, included 54% of the entire population. If you look just at the workers, around 80% were below two minimum salaries.

Perhaps the Chilean case—in some sense, unfortunately—provides an interesting example from which conclusions can be drawn and studies devised, trying to relate the food and nutrition situation to social, economic, and political changes occurring in a developing country. This, I think, will be useful to one of our main aims: to examine the areas of research that need to be developed in this field.

Montgomery

Do any specific interventions, such as land reform, have measurable outputs in terms of nutritional change for identifiable target groups? For example, there are no data about the land reform in the paper because, apparently, the land reform was overtaken by general agricultural policy. So I couldn't tell from this if the beneficiaries of land reform necessarily improved their nutritional status.

Solimano

Land reform was initiated around '67 during the Frei government. At that time there was a big change, not in terms of land ownership, but mostly in the expectations of the rural people, in regard to wages and their inclusion in the modernization and change in society. It is clear that the rural workers started to earn more at that time although the goals of the agrarian reform were not achieved by either the Frei or Allende governments. Finally, in terms of food production, there was not a significant increase in total production.

Latham

This examination of the Chilean case is very interesting and very important, and the approach is very exciting. Infant mortality rates, I think, are a very good health indicator, and for Chile, maybe, are a good indicator of malnutrition, but for many other countries, infant mortality rates are maybe not the best indicators of malnutrition. Do you have any figures for toddler mortality rates? For the preschool age children? I think most people know that, in Chile, the main form of protein-calorie malnutrition is marasmus, occurring in much younger age groups than in many other developing countries.

Also, in your earlier figures, you showed what I thought was the rather surprising figure that the income groups below two minimum salaries were only spending 50% of their income on food. In most other developing countries, it would be 60% or 70% or even 80%. So there seems more flexibility in those income groups in Chile than in some other developing countries.

Solimano

Let me start with your specific question about health indicators. General mortality has gone down: the last figure for 1973 is 8 per thousand in terms of crude death rate. The figures for one-to-four-year-olds are as follows: in '64, it was 69.9 per 10,000 children of that age group and, in 1972, it was 28.0 per 10,000. So Chile, according to the Punta del Este Charter, was doing well in terms of the one-to-four-year-old mortality, but not in terms of infant mortality, which, in '73, was 65.3 per thousand live births. With the high level of urbanization in Chile, these figures are quite reliable. Only 25% of the population is rural, but rural in a very narrow country, where the most distant rural place is 60 kilometers from the main city. There's no rural area, except in the farthest South, that is not accessible to the roads and to services.

Vamoer

You mentioned four nutrition councils from the four periods. What are the reasons for the failures of these councils? Why did they have to be created four times?

Solimano

The main failure is that these were nutrition councils established through the health ministry. They were really unable, in Chile, to influence the pattern of socioeconomic development, especially economic policies and social development. Such councils have always been given a sort of advisory status that prevented them from making any important decisions. That's my own interpretation.

I have the four organizing documents and the best one is the one from 1942 because that, at least, tried to look carefully at the nature of the problem. Most of the councils were established through the social sector or the health sector, trying to use the traditional types of interventions. The only difference is that, instead of being done by health or education ministries, now the activity is being carried out by a council. So supplementary feeding, enrichment, and nutrition education are run by the council, but the president of the council has nothing to do with the Ministry of Finance or the Ministry of Economics, where most of the policies are devised.

I would like to add a final point about my own experience being in office in the government. It turns out that things are quite different from what the textbooks or the conferences or the scholars say. Even if you intend to do your best, what we call the "real world" is very, very important in modifying your actions. Even without being a politician, you have to understand very clearly the political significance of any plan or policy to the government or to groups within the government.

The period when I was in the government in Chile corresponded to what I call the "fashion" of developing food and nutrition policies all around the world. In Latin America, there has been strong involvement of international agencies trying, with the mandate of the governments, of course, to develop food and nutrition policies. In Chile, where revolutionary change was occurring, one could attempt to work out very clear, well-planned and -defined objectives for food and nutrition policies and take into consideration those basic changes that were occurring in the country.

In the world of international nutrition planning, there are a lot of experts, but, to put it bluntly, the question remains, how much empirical evidence is available to support this exercise of nutrition planning? In writing this paper, we realized that, first, there is not enough empirical evidence to link food and nutrition factors with national development in different settings. And, second, something more needs to be done, in terms of the conceptual framework, taking into consideration all the factors that different people claim are important. What we are arguing here is that some of the people that have written in this area very clearly define the factors involved, but, later, in order to decide what needs to be done, analysis must come down to the micro level. There is as yet no serious confrontation in terms of the social, institutional, economic, and political factors of critical importance.

3 NUTRITION AND GOVERNMENT POLICY IN COLOMBIA

Clara Eugenia López

Clara Eugenia López is Special Assistant for Economic Affairs to the President of the Republic of Colombia. In this capacity, she attends cabinet meetings, and serves as a member of the National Council for Nutrition Policy, of the National Council for Economic and Social Policy, and of the Monetary Board. The author is also Professor of Economic Policy in the Business Administration Faculty of Rosario University in Bogotá. Ms. López was born and raised in Bogotá, and educated at the Madeira School and Radcliffe. Her knowledge of the inner workings of the Government of Colombia is enhanced by her close contact with the present president and other high officials of the Republic.

INTRODUCTION

This paper describes the evolution of concern for the problem of malnutrition in Colombia. Starting in the mid-1940s and continuing through the 1960s, serious studies were carried out by nutritionists which revealed the magnitude of the problem as well as its interdependence with income distribution, education, health, and agricultural production.

It is presently estimated that for 30% of the Colombian population, income is a barrier to proper nutrition. Furthermore, there is evidence that about 60% of the children in Colombia suffer from some degree of malnutrition, with consequent irreversible effects on physical and intellectual development.

The present government has identified the problem of malnutrition as the one that requires the most urgent attention among the priorities for development policy. The government is therefore in the process of designing an integral food and nutrition plan which will be the axis of the country's development policy for the next four years. This plan will affect the entire economy, as it calls for the execution of concrete projects in just about every sector of economic and social activity: education, health, agriculture, industry, commerce, transportation, public construction, and so forth.

This paper outlines the problem of malnutrition in Colombia, and the solutions that have been attempted in the past. The final pages describe the process by which the present government decided to design and implement a national food and nutrition plan, the problems encountered in designing it, and its major components.

THE NUTRITIONALLY VULNERABLE

Malnutrition is a component, as well as a consequence, of the poor socioeconomic status of the lower income groups in society. It arises from the interplay of insufficient incomes, poor education, and deficient health and sanitary conditions, among other factors.

The Problem

Studies of malnutrition in Colombia have identified, in order of importance, the following principal types of problems: (1) protein-calorie malnutrition in infants and children; (2) chronic subnutrition in adults; (3) widespread vitamin A and some vitamin B deficiencies; (4) anemia caused by iron deficiency and (5) dental caries.[1]

Magnitude of the Problem

The latest available food balance sheet, based on 1972 data, shows a significant deficit of the major foodstuffs and nutrients on a per capita basis.

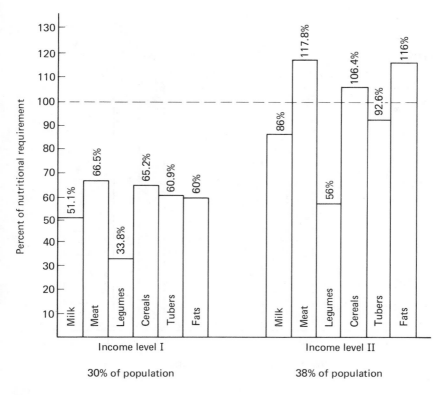

Figure 1
Food consumption for two income groups. Source: DANE (Household Survey, 1970),
ICBF (Provisional Recommendations of Food Consumption, 1975)

Figures of actual consumption as a percentage of recommended levels for the
same year reveal:[2]

A   In terms of foodstuffs:

Milk	90%	Green and yellow vegetables	62%
Meats, fish, eggs	76%	Fruit	83%
Legumes	41%	Fats	63%

B   In terms of nutrients:

Calories	104%	Vitamin A	73%
Protein	83%	Thiamin	95%
Calcium	91%	Riboflavin	77%
Iron	100%	Niacin	78%
		Vitamin C	213%

Viewed in the context of the existing income distribution of the country,

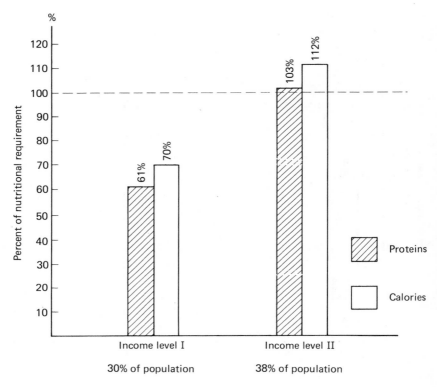

Figure 2
Protein and calorie consumption for two income groups. Source: As figure 1

the food and nutrient situation is even more critical for the members of the lower income groups of society who have their income level, and not overall food availability, as the principal barrier to adequate nutrition.

By comparing consumption data by income from the National Household Survey (1970) with the Family Welfare Institute's (*Instituto Colombiano de Bienestar Familiar*, ICBF) minimum consumption recommendations (1975), figures 1 and 2 were obtained.[3]

As can be seen, families in income level I (0-Col$18,000 annually in 1970 or US$940), consumed only 61% of the minimum recommended level of protein and 70% of that of calories. This income group represents 30% of the country's population. Families in income groups earning above Col$18,000 annually, as a whole, do not show consumption deficiencies in terms of calories and protein, although some underconsumption of specific foods is observed.

Malnutrition in children, however, does not respect the above family classification. Results from the nine nutrition surveys carried out by the Nutrition Institute in the 1960s showed that 66% of children under 5 years of age suf-

fered from some degree of malnutrition as follows: first degree malnutrition
45.6%, second degree 19.3%, third degree 1.7%.[4] Of the undernourished
children, 51.6% were under one year old and 73.6% were under four. Absolute numbers show that some 90,000 children under five die each year, more
than one-third of these from malnutrition-related causes.

Of the total number of deaths that occur in the country each year, 43.1%
are of children under five years old, an age group which represents only 18%
of the population. Although children under one year old make up only 3.9%
of the population, 27.6% of registered deaths occur in this age group.[5]

Malnutrition exerts a negative effect on a person's intellectual and physical
potential, and, therefore, on general welfare and productivity. Adult subnutrition in Colombia represents the second most important nutrition problem,
and it is manifested in work absenteeism, lack of initiative and ambition, and
in other measures of labor productivity. The health ministry has estimated
that about 96 million work days are lost each year due to illness, which, at
the present minimum salary, represents the sum of Col$3,840 million
(US$128 million), without calculating costs of medical care, reduced worker
efficiency, residual crippling, and years lost through premature death.

RELATIONSHIP OF THE HEALTH SYSTEM TO THE NUTRITIONALLY
VULNERABLE

The associated problems of malnutrition and infectious diseases, and their
mutually reinforcing mechanisms, constitute the principal causes of mortality
and morbidity in younger age groups.

The principal cause of death in children under 14 years of age is the group
of gastrointestinal and diarrheal illnesses (see table 1). Since most of these
diseases are transmitted by water, inadequate provision of aqueduct and sewage services has serious effects on the health status of the population, especially in rural areas. At present, only 29% of the rural population has access
to potable water as compared to 73% of the urban population.

Immunization services for children are provided against measles, whooping
cough, tuberculosis, poliomyelitis, tetanus, diphtheria, yellow fever and smallpox. In 1974, coverage extended from a low of 31.2% of children under 5
years old immunized against poliomyelitis to 88.0% against smallpox. The
immunization service against measles only started in 1973, although this
illness represents one of the ten most important causes of death in children.
However, by 1974, 22.1% of children under 5 were already covered, up from
5.7% in 1973, the first year of the program (table 2).

The effect of immunization services can be measured by the occurrence of
the illnesses these services seek to prevent. In spite of the progress in coverage
between 1972 and 1974, the incidence of these illnesses, with the exception
of measles and smallpox (and there have been no reported cases of the latter
since 1971) has not greatly diminished and in some cases has even increased.

Table 1
Principal causes of mortality in children from 1 to 14 years of age, Colombia, 1972 (as percent of deaths in each age group)

	Age (Years)			
	1-2	2-4	5-9	10-14
Gastroenteritis and other diarrheal diseases	27.50	19.62	13.40	5.15
Vitamin and other nutritional deficiencies	12.05	10.67	7.60	2.92
Pneumonias	11.51	9.68	6.32	4.53
Bronchitis, emphysema, and asthma	8.65	7.29	3.76	1.68
Measles	3.92	4.92	3.36	1.64
Parasitic diseases	3.14	3.65	2.99	1.60
Whooping cough	2.76	2.52	1.29	0.62
Anemias	1.74	3.34	5.27	4.02
Meningitis	1.81	1.81	2.48	1.60
Percent of national total	7.60	7.11	3.55	1.70

Table 2
Immunizations, Colombia, 1972-74

Year	DPT (2 Doses) % Covered (0-5 Years)	Polio (2 Doses) % Covered (0-5 Years)	Measles % Covered (0-5 Years)	BCG % Covered (0-15 Years)	Smallpox % Covered (Entire Population)
1972	56.2	17.9	—	68.9	80.0
1973	55.7	26.31	5.7	72.2	84.0
1974	56.8	31.15	22.1	76.0	88.0

Table 3
Incidence of diseases that can be prevented through immunization, Colombia, 1971-74 (rates per 100,000 inhabitants)

Illness	1971	1972	1973	1974
Measles	148.4	125.8	127.7	122.5
Whooping cough	73.4	84.7	79.5	82.7
Tuberculosis	54.7	56.7	53.5	60.15
Poliomyelitis	2.3	2.1	1.4	2.2
Tetanus	2.9	2.5	2.6	2.1
Diphtheria	3.1	3.2	2.2	1.4
Yellow fever	0.01	0.01	0.05	0.14
Smallpox	0.0	0.0	0.0	0.0

Source: Ministry of Health, Republic of Colombia

It is important to note, however, that most of these illnesses are not among the ten principal causes of mortality in children under 15 years old (table 3).

In Colombia, the private sector provides medical attention to 15% of the population and social security institutions provide care for another 10%. The remaining 75% of the population is, in theory, covered by the government health services. In fact, however, these services at present reach only 39% of the total population.[6]

The country has 12,000 doctors, or one for every 2,083 persons. Their geographical distribution is so uneven that 74.2% of them provide their services in departmental (state) capitals that contain only 35% of the total population. Likewise, 80% of the dentists and 86% of the trained nurses are located in these cities. Although a large effort has been directed in the last few years to the training of paramedical and auxiliary personnel, these workers cover only 1/3 of the rural population.

The health ministry's budgets for the last five years and the proposed budget for 1976 are listed in tables 4 and 5. As can be seen, expenditures in 1976 will be 80% higher than in 1975, with considerable increases particularly in curative medicine and infrastructure.

FOOD AND AGRICULTURAL SYSTEM

The agricultural sector is of primary importance to the country's economy. Although its contribution to the gross national product has decreased somewhat, from 28.4% in 1969 to 25.9% in 1973,[7] it is still the highest of any sector in the economy. Furthermore, agricultural products, such as coffee, cotton, sugar, meat and bananas, account for more than 60% of the country's total exports. Coffee is by far the largest single export crop, accounting for almost 2/3 of all agricultural exports.

With the exception of wheat and fats, Colombia is practically self-sufficient in food commodities. Small quantities of corn, barley and cacao are imported yearly, but do not require a substantial expenditure of foreign exchange earnings.

Table 4
National budget and Ministry of Health budget, Colombia, 1971-76 (Col$ millions)

	National Budget	Ministry of Health Budget	Percent
1971	17,700	1,522	8.6
1972	21,422	1,524	7.1
1973	26,212	2,051	7.8
1974	30,303	2,681	8.8
1975	34,854	2,819	8.1
1976	51,332	5,087	9.8

Sources: 1971-75, Ley de Presupuesto; 1976, Proyecto de Ley de Presupuesto

Table 5
Ministry of Health budget by category, Colombia, 1972-76 (Col$ millions)

	1971	1972	%	1973	1974	%	1975	1976	%
Preventive Medicine	169	185	12.2	175	302	11.3	311	484	9.5
Curative Medicine	354	340	22.3	611	804	30.0	1,094	2,376	46.7
Investment in Hospitals	155	80	5.3	212	282	10.5	280	364	7.2
Infrastructure[a]	763	833	54.7	972	1,201	44.8	1,031	1,670	32.8
Current Expenditure	82	84	5.5	81	92	3.4	103	193	3.8
Total	1,522	1,524	100.0	2,051	2,681	100.0	2,819	5,087	100.0

[a] Infrastructure includes investment expenditures for the Family Welfare Institute, construction of aqueducts and sewage treatment plants, and the training of personnel.
Sources: As in table 3

Food imports represented 11.3% of total imports in 1973, the year food imports reached their highest percentages of the total. In that same year, agricultural imports were only 17.4% of total agricultural exports.

Furthermore, price policies have recently been rationalized, abolishing a government subsidy for the price of imported wheat. This measure should stimulate internal production and diminish the need to import.

Colombia has great agricultural potential, so that an adequate food supply need never be a limiting factor in proper nutrition for the entire population. On the other hand, the agricultural sector has grown at a relatively slow pace, averaging an annual growth rate of 3.2% between 1950 and 1974. More recently, however, agricultural production has grown at a faster pace: 5.5% in 1972, 4.5% in 1973, and 5.0% in 1974.[8]

The two subsectors of agriculture, modern and traditional, have had very unequal development since 1950. The modern subsector, in which crops are grown on a commercial farming basis, primarily for industrial use and for export, has experienced a rapid growth rate, between 7% and 8% annually since 1950.[9] This high growth rate has resulted primarily from the ample credit available to this subsector, the development and adoption of high-yield technologies and the application of modern management skills.

On the other hand, the traditional subsector, which produces 55% of the foodstuffs consumed by the population, is characterized by low productivity, poor soil, small land holdings, scarce credit, and scarcer application of modern technologies. As a consequence, the traditional sector has tended towards stagnation, with consequent negative effects on food production. Since 1973, despite a 5.0% annual growth of agricultural production, the increase of commodities destined primarily for domestic consumption barely exceeded the estimated 3.2% rate of population growth, and food price rises were one of the major components of inflation.

Since 1950 the traditional sector has grown at an average rate of 2.7% annually, and since 1972 high and rising food prices have underlined the inadequacy of food production.[9] In this context, it is worthwhile to point out that in 1974, 94% of the growth in production of the 16 most important agricultural products was concentrated in only three commercial crops: rice, cotton, and sugar. Important staple foods, such as corn, beans, cacao, panela (block brown sugar) and meat, registered only slight increases. Thus, along with the stagnation of traditional agriculture has come stagnation in food production, rural incomes, and rural employment.

Colombia has had a policy of agricultural support prices since 1944. The primary objectives of this policy have been: (1) to stimulate production by assuring farmers a minimum income and (2) to stabilize food prices through the accumulation of buffer stocks at the support prices. Although the state agricultural marketing agency (INA between 1944 and 1968; IDEMA since 1968) buys part of the production of crops such as rice, wheat, corn, beans, soybeans, sorghum, and sesame, its limited financial and storage capacity has resulted in effective intervention only in the case of rice. A recent study shows that government intervention in this instance increased production by 10% annually since 1960, and managed to stabilize incomes received by rice farmers.[10] It is important to point out, however, that rice in Colombia is a commercial crop, belonging primarily to the modern subsector of agriculture.

State intervention also occurred, but with negative results, in the case of wheat. Because it was initially imported cheaply under the US PL 480 program, the internal price became increasingly unappealing for local farmers. As world wheat prices jumped in 1972 and PL 480 dispatches were discontinued, the government adopted a policy of subsidizing internal consumption by keeping internal prices below those of the world markets. Internal production therefore diminished further; consumption increased as a result of the subsidy, which grew considerably as world prices kept rising and the internal price was kept constant. As previously mentioned, this subsidy was recently eliminated and wheat production as well as consumption appears to have responded to the rationalization of this product's price.

True price controls, on the other hand, exist only for sugar, milk, and coffee. In the case of sugar, the Price Board fixes a ceiling for the price at which sugar can be sold to the public. Although this ceiling proved effective between 1960 and 1972, the rise in international prices placed heavy pressure on the frozen internal price. Consumers, however, only pay prices 13% above the ceiling, while international prices have risen to more than double the internal price.[11]

In the case of milk, IDEMA buys 20% of production, at a price frozen at one-half the market price, for sale in low income areas of the main cities. The rest of the milk is marketed through private commercial channels and no limit is placed on its sale price.

The coffee price policy is aimed at assuring adequate incomes to coffee growers by mitigating the effects of the great fluctuations in international prices.

Data on rural employment is sparse, but about half of the country's labor is employed in the agricultural sector. Over 70% of these live on sub-family-sized farms or are workers without land.[12] About 25% of the agricultural working people are unemployed or work in marginally productive jobs.[13]

INCOME DISTRIBUTION

Income distribution in rural Colombia is uneven and skewed. The upper 10% of the rural working population earn 51% of the agricultural sector's income, whereas the lowest 10% earn only 1.4% of that income. A comparable situation is found in urban areas, although urban income is more evenly distributed (table 6). Furthermore, any analysis of income distribution should also take into account the fact that services such as health and education are more readily available in the cities than in the countryside.

Table 6
Average income by deciles of the labor force, Colombia, 1974

Decile	Rural Sector Agri and Non-Agri (% of Total Income)	Urban Sector (% of Total Income)
1	1.40	0.9
2	3.10	3.3
3	3.60	4.3
4	3.90	5.0
5	4.50	5.5
6	5.50	7.0
7	6.00	8.0
8	8.00	11.0
9	13.00	14.5
10	51.00	40.5

Source: See ref. 14

In the most comprehensive study to date on income distribution in Colombia, recently published by Albert Berry and Miguel Urrutia, the authors reached the conclusion that the uneven distribution of income in the agricultural sector is due to the uneven distribution of land.[14] The ownership of rural property is highly concentrated; despite the fact that comprehensive agrarian reform legislation was enacted in 1961 and a number of land reform projects have been undertaken since that date, these have not been ambitious enough to improve the existing patterns of land tenure (table 7).

It is useful to look at comparative data in order to understand the problem of income distribution in Colombia. In Great Britain, for example, the lowest 25% on the income scale earn 8% of the total income, whereas in Colombia this same group earns only 4%. On the upper side of the scale, the top 7% of the labor force earn 22% of the income in Britain, compared to 40% in Colombia.[15]

The 30% of the population labeled "Income Level I" in figures 1 and 2 earn only 4.5% of the total income. It is only above this level that incomes allow for nutritional intake at the minimum consumption requirements recommended by the Family Welfare Institute.

Colombia's present government is headed by a president who was elected on the basis of a social platform founded on the belief that economic development practices of the past, with primary emphasis on growth and only secondary importance given to income distribution, constituted a mistaken approach. The president, in his electoral campaign, advocated growth accompanied by income distribution in the present and not at some undefined future date.

Table 7
Number of Land-Holdings and Total Area, Colombia, 1960, 1970 (distribution by size)

Size of Land-Holdings (Hectares)	Number of Land-Holdings				Area and % of Total			
	1960		1970		1960		1970	
	No.	%	No.	%	Thousands of Hectares	%	Thousands of Hectares	%
Less than 1	298,071	24.7	251,262	22.1	132	0.5	119.5	0.4
1 - 3	306,352	25.5	278,555	24.4	546	2.0	484.2	1.5
3 - 5	150,182	12.4	36,490	12.0	561	2.0	505.8	1.6
5 - 10	169,145	14.0	55,547	13.7	1,165	4.3	1,067.2	3.4
10 - 50	201,020	16.6	217,236	19.0	4,211	15.4	4,685.7	15.0
50 - 100	39,990	3.3	48,788	4.3	2,680	9.8	3,267.1	10.4
100 - 500	36,010	3.0	43,415	3.8	6,990	25.6	8,420.8	26.9
500 - 1,000	4,141	0.3	4,887	0.4	2,771	10.0	3,229.7	10.2
Over 1,000	2,761	0.2	3,322	0.3	8,322	30.4	9,598.7	30.6
Total	209,672	100.0	1,139,502	100.0	27,338	100.0	31,378.7	100.0

Source: DANE (Departamento Administrativo Naciónal de Estadística), Agricultural Sector Census

Thus, in one of the first presentations of the principles of the administration's development plan, the president announced: "The national purpose should be that of bettering the standard of living of the poorer 50% of the population, and, in order to reach this end it is necessary to stimulate the maximum economic growth rate possible, in the context of a process of development which will guarantee that this growth will more than proportionately benefit that 50% of the population which has been least favored by the country's development until now."[16]

The presentation was made following the enactment of a tax reform which a World Bank study deemed "a landmark in the recent history of such undertakings, both among developing and developed nations."[17] Aside from the distributive effects of making the tax system more progressive through the abolition of tax exemptions, the introduction of capital gains taxes, and a presumptive tax on wealth, the reform has also substantially improved government revenues, absolutely and in relative terms, thus helping to solve the problem of chronic deficits in government finances. The government is, therefore, in a better position to fulfill many of the country's expectations and needs through increased public expenditures. These additional expenditures, in turn, will not be inflationary because of the increased revenues produced by the new tax reform.[18] Following the criteria mentioned above of giving priority to projects which benefit the poorer 50% of the population, the national development plan is being designed to redistribute income through public expenditure—with emphasis on health, education, and nutrition.

EXPERIENCE WITH NUTRITION (1943-74)

Although preoccupation with the problems of malnutrition is not new in Colombia, the latest plan for the first time envisages the involvement of all sectors of the economy: agriculture, health, education, industry, and public works, at a national level, on a massive scale.

Existing Nutrition Programs*

Iodization of Salt Although made mandatory by Law 44 of 1947, provisions for its enforcement were only introduced in 1963. Since that date, endemic goiter, previously quite widely distributed, has disappeared, ceasing to be one of the primary health and nutritional problems of the country.[19]

Nutrition Institute Originally created as a Division of the Health Ministry in 1947, the Nutrition Institute became an independent entity in 1963 with its own funds, derived from a percentage of the revenue from sales of iodized salt. In 1968, it was incorporated as a division of the newly created Institute of Family Welfare (*Instituto Colombiano de Bienestar Familiar,* or ICBF). By

*Only the principal programs are described here.

conducting many studies of the problems of malnutrition, the Institute created public consciousness of this problem throughout the '60s.

The growth of attention to malnutrition can be measured by the budget of
funds for the Nutrition Institute. In 1963, its receipts from salt sales amounted to Col$1 million (US$111,111). In 1968, its budget had risen to only
Col$16 million. In 1970, the budget of the Nutrition Division of the Family
Welfare Institute (former Nutrition Institute) rose to Col$200 million,
Col$155 million of which represented WFP food aid and UNICEF equipment,
and Col$45 million national government transfers. By 1974, the budget rose
to Col$1,500 million (US$50 million), Col$800 million (US$27 million)
representing food aid.[20]

PINA   The contribution of international organizations to nutrition programs
in Colombia has been substantial, both in terms of resources and of encouragement. Because food aid was given in kind, it predetermined to a great extent
the actual scope of the programs initiated, limiting them primarily to supplementary feeding. Substantial local resources were not forthcoming, originally,
for nutrition programs.

This process can be seen in the Integrated Program of Applied Nutrition
(known as PINA). The programs of applied nutrition, initiated in some 70
nations during the '60s, were designed with a multisectoral approach by food
and nutrition experts from various countries and from the United Nations
specialized agencies (FAO, WHO, and UNICEF). In Colombia, the first PINA
project was initiated in 1960 in Caldas and slowly spread to cover 14 departments by 1970. It now includes all 22 departments (table 8).[21]

The objectives were (1) to define the nutritional problems of the population; (2) to encourage agricultural production and the improvement of family
life through the promotion and development of agricultural extension activities and home economics; (3) to promote and develop nutrition education
activities through health, agricultural, educational, and communal action;
(4) to improve the health status of the population through the prevention and
treatment of malnutrition; and (5) to integrate all activities in the field of
nutrition, throughout the country, by coordinating existing programs run by
different official and private entities.

The first of these objectives was fully achieved by the execution of surveys
and studies. These studies still represent the basic sources on nutrition in the
country.

Success in areas such as the improvement of family life is hard to measure.
Nonetheless, reviewing the personnel sheets of PINA, we find, in 1974, that
of a total of 51,788 persons participating in the program, 35,280 were volunteer mothers, the real link between the program and the community. Such
collaboration cannot but have a positive effect on family life within the communities involved.

Agricultural credit and extension has had limited application due primarily to limited financing. Nonetheless, by December of 1973, there had been 1,400 beneficiaries in five departments who received credits totalling Col$8,404,262. During 1974, seven more departments appear on the credit list, with 1,303 beneficiaries of credits amounting to Col$23,045,215.[21]

The major achievements of the PINA programs are in the fields of nutrition education and distribution of food supplements to mothers and children under seven years old. According to the PINA statistics, 37% of those attending primary school receive a food supplement in school. The program covers 44% of all official primary schools. The food supplement provides 35% of the child's daily requirements and consists of milk, fish, corn and wheat meal, oil, and vegetable mixtures.

Preschool children receive their food supplements through the health posts. In 1974, 38% of the total number of preschool children who went to a health post for the first time benefited from the program (table 8). The food supplement for these children represents 45% of their daily requirements and consists of milk, legumes, vegetable mixtures, and oil. Since its distribution is accompanied by health and nutrition education, as well as by a food supplement for mothers, the effect on the child's diet may be of even greater impact. The mothers' supplement covers 30% of daily requirements.

Supplements are distributed to school children throughout the school year (190 days). Preschoolers receive food supplement for 180 days, but if nutritional status remains inadequate, the supplement is continued until a satisfactory condition is achieved. Mothers receive food during the last three months of pregnancy and for six months following delivery.[20]

The food supplements are mainly composed of food aid from WFP, CARITAS, and CARE. For the period 1970-74, this aid amounted to about Col$800 million (US$27 million) yearly.[20]

Between 1975 and 1978 the food aid received will decrease gradually, ceasing altogether by December 1978. Colombia is taking the necessary steps to substitute domestic production for all foreign food aid. This process is part of the National Food and Nutrition Plan, examined below.

National Food and Nutrition Plan[22]   The innumerable studies and observations made about the gravity of the problem of malnutrition in Colombia over the past two decades have demonstrated to nutritionists and policymakers alike the close interdependence between nutrition, health, and the country's social and economic development processes. It is clear that malnutrition and associated illnesses have severe impact, not only on the health sector, but also on the whole economy, especially on the agricultural and educational sectors.

Thus, attempts at confronting the problem of malnutrition have always been multisectoral in their approach. The programs have had components from the agricultural, health, and educational sectors in conjunction with the food supplement distribution activities. Until the present, however, no plans

Table 8
Preschool population (under 7 years of age) served by PINA, 1974

Department	Number of Preschoolers Served for the First Time by Health Services	Number of Preschoolers Served by the Program	Coverage (%)	Number of Health Agencies Aided by the Program
Antioquia	479,750	115,199	24	219
Atlántico	95,083	4,000	4	45
Bogotá D. E.	115,654	86,814	75	75
Bolívar	91,693	45,942	50	85
Boyacá	46,356	11,348	24	226
Caldas	56,427	15,913	28	100
Cauca	24,982	7,945	31	93
Cesar	22,660	16,950	74	57
Córdoba	27,442	20,760	75	58
Cundinamarca	36,760	36,760	100	150
Chocó	4,217	3,590	85	51
Huila	37,400	32,900	87	414
Guajira	19,995	7,354	36	30
Magdalena	22,518	1,396	6	21
Meta	8,558	8,558	100	69
Nariño	37,589	16,000	42	81
Norte de Santander	24,049	14,489	60	78
Quindío	39,505	4,880	12	44
Risaralda	35,600	17,091	48	60
Santander	62,000	36,700	59	195

Sucre	27,661	1,116	4	46
Tolima	39,000	22,230	57	103
Valle	135,840	63,444	46	176
Caquetá	2,150	1,905	88	2
San Andrés	3,765	1,950	51	6
Total	1,496,654	575,241	38	2,484

have approached the problem with the integrated nationwide effort of the present National Food and Nutrition Plan.

The growing interest in nutrition is seen through the progressive resources allotted to programs in this field: from a budget of Col$1 million (US$111,111) in 1960 to one of Col$1,500 million (US$50 million) in 1974, the budget will now leap to Col$17,178 million (US$572 million) for the four-year period 1975-78. This statistic alone is indicative of the current importance given in Colombia to an integrated solution of the problem of malnutrition.

The economic development process that took off in Colombia in the '50s and continued until the present was industrial. The agricultural sector was not given adequate attention, as its slow growth and the increasing exodus from the countryside to the cities amply testify. From the beginning of his political career, President Alfonso López-Michelsen advocated a fairer treatment of rural Colombia, especially of the traditional sector which had been kept on the fringe of the country's development process.

When elected in April 1974, Dr. López called together a team of Colombian experts composed primarily of economists and engineers to study specific national questions: among others, the problems of malnutrition, of incorporating the traditional farm sector into the country's development process, and of raising *minifundista* (small farmer) incomes.

Heavy emphasis was placed on the inequity of malnutrition for the children who will suffer its irreversible effects. This is a special burden to low income families, and is particularly prevalent in the rural sector where the problem of poverty is more pervasive.

By putting these two major problems—nutrition and rural income—together, the idea of the National Food and Nutrition Plan was conceived. To raise minifundista incomes, substantial resources were to be directed to the traditional sector in the form of credit, technical assistance, and services (health, education, etc.) all aimed to raise labor productivity. In order to avoid a scenario of increased productivity, leading to higher production, falling prices, and thence lowered income, a market had to be found for the additional foodstuffs that would be produced. This market would be provided by a nationwide effort to improve nutrition, where the state could be one of the future buyers. The program aims to assure a market for the additional produce generated by the transfer of resources to the traditional agricultural sector.

Previous experience with nutrition, as well as the personnel of high quality trained by the Nutrition and Family Welfare Institute over the preceding years, provided the elements necessary to translate this conception into a reality in a short period of time. Only one year after the new administration was in office, an all-encompassing plan (figure 3) had been designed.

The political will and high level decisions necessary to channel efforts and funds to an integrated attack on malnutrition were the principle elements

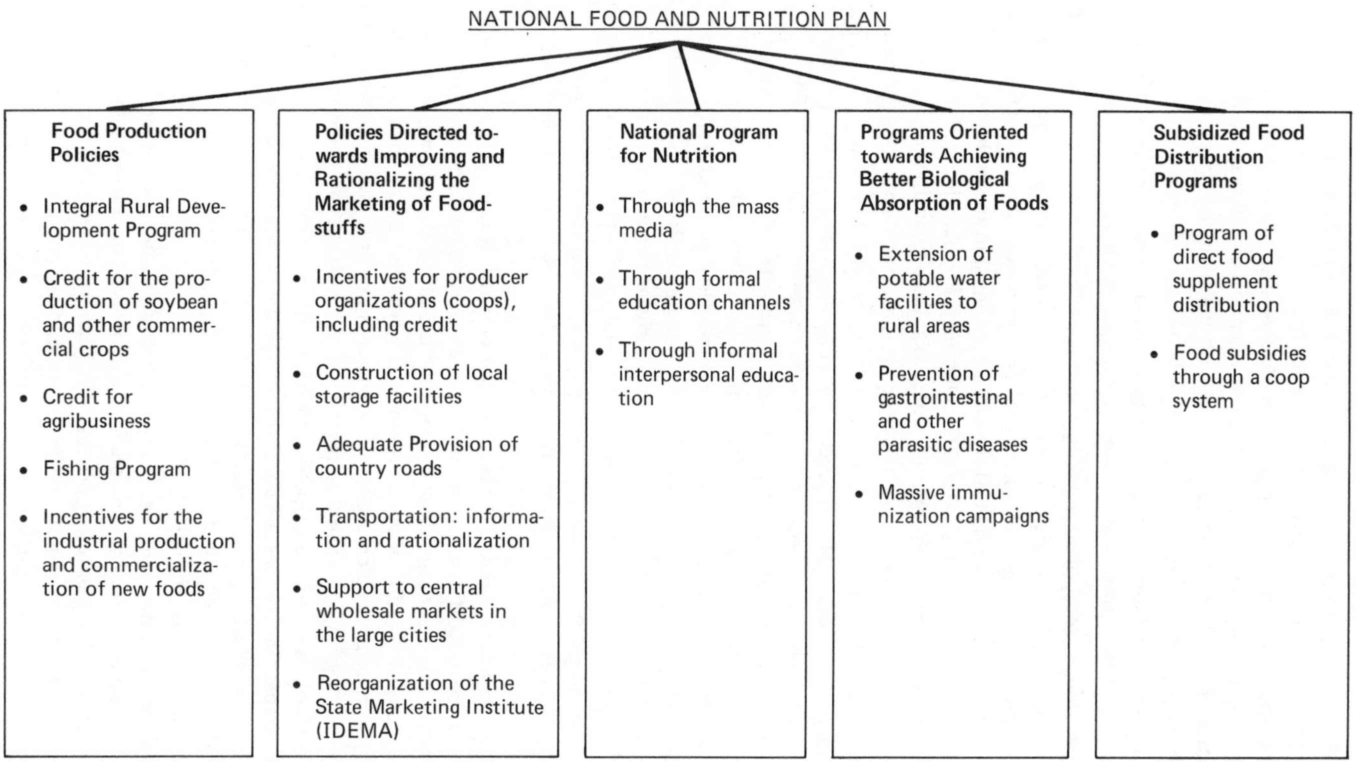

NATIONAL FOOD AND NUTRITION PLAN

Food Production Policies

- Integral Rural Development Program

- Credit for the production of soybean and other commercial crops

- Credit for agribusiness

- Fishing Program

- Incentives for the industrial production and commercialization of new foods

Policies Directed towards Improving and Rationalizing the Marketing of Foodstuffs

- Incentives for producer organizations (coops), including credit

- Construction of local storage facilities

- Adequate Provision of country roads

- Transportation: information and rationalization

- Support to central wholesale markets in the large cities

- Reorganization of the State Marketing Institute (IDEMA)

National Program for Nutrition

- Through the mass media

- Through formal education channels

- Through informal interpersonal education

Programs Oriented towards Achieving Better Biological Absorption of Foods

- Extension of potable water facilities to rural areas

- Prevention of gastrointestinal and other parasitic diseases

- Massive immunization campaigns

Subsidized Food Distribution Programs

- Program of direct food supplement distribution

- Food subsidies through a coop system

Figure 3
National Food and Nutrition Plan.

lacking in the past; the consciousness of malnutrition and the necessity to deal with it in a comprehensive way had never been consolidated into action. The Food and Nutrition Plan represents a massive effort to eradicate malnutrition through concrete actions carried out in an integrated way by the various entities of the Colombian government with the financial collaboration of international agencies (World Bank, IDB. AID, etc.).

Primary effort will be directed to the agricultural sector in order to increase the output of food (particularly beans, green peas, soybeans, rice, corn, wheat, potatoes, yucca, plantain, fish, poultry, and pork as well as other small farm animals.) This strategy will be oriented specifically towards increasing the productivity of farmers with little land, the minifundistas of the traditional sector who produce over half of the food consumed in the country. Through a series of Integrated Rural Development Projects, located in the minifundio and poorest areas of rural Colombia, large quantities of resources are to be invested where the state has been conspicuously absent in the past. Projects include the building of basic infrastructure such as country roads, local storage facilities, rural aqueducts, and rural electric networks, and the extension of the basic government services of health and education. These facilities will be accompanied by both massive transfers of credit and technology to the small farmer sector and land reform, which will undoubtedly increase the production of food, both through increased productivity per acre and increased area cultivated. Alongside the Integrated Rural Development Projects which benefit the poorest areas, a massive extension of credit is planned at the national level for the entire agricultural sector, including the commercial subsector. Through these projects, a partial solution is reached for both urban and rural areas, as more foodstuffs reach the cities and small farmer incomes grow.

The second main area of emphasis for the Food and Nutrition Plan is nutrition education. Traditional Colombian diets are surprisingly good in nutritional terms, but due to artificial pricing mechanisms and consumer-oriented propaganda on the radio, many of these diets have been abandoned. A return to tradition may prove a considerable nutritional bonus in the short run without requiring increased expenditures on food. A nutrition campaign through the mass media is therefore being designed which will compete with nutritionally counterproductive messages and encourage the return to traditional consumption and breast-feeding practices. Concurrently, programs of interpersonal and institutional education are being started, through the health personnel and at all levels of formal education.

A third field of action will be that of marketing. As in most developing countries, great quantities of food are lost, with a resulting rise in prices, due to imperfections of the marketing process. Through the construction of local storage facilities and the improvement of transportation, as well as through the encouragement of central wholesale markets in the cities, increases in the food supply and decreases in marketing costs will be sought.

Both the industrial and commercial sectors have an important role to play in the production and commercialization of highly nutritive, low cost new foods. The Institute of Technological Investigation has developed and adapted technologies for the production of texturized vegetable protein, vegetable mixtures, fortified pastas, soybean milk, and so on. The government will provide financial and technological assistance to the private sector in order to stimulate the production of these new foods and their distribution through existing commercial channels. Part of the mass media campaign will be directed to the introduction of the new foods in family diets. Legislation will be proposed to Congress which will control advertising, protecting both the consumer and the new food producers from false claims of a product's nutritional value. State purchase and subsidy of a proportion of the production of these products will provide a guaranteed market for the industrialists. This is perhaps the most important element in securing the private sector's collaboration with the plan.

The raw materials required for the production of the new foods will all be produced in sufficient quantities in Colombia (soybean, corn, wheat and rice meals, skim milk) as a result of the agricultural sector strategies. The use of these products in the production of new foods will absorb a proportion of the increased food production by the traditional agricultural subsector, thus helping to prevent price declines. These new products will substitute, to a great extent, for the food aid presently provided by international agencies.

Another important component of the Food and Nutrition Plan is the extension of health services and the provision of clean water. Not only are intestinal diseases an important cause of mortality, but they limit the efficiency of nutrient absorption. Since the principal source of these diseases is contaminated water, a great effort is planned to bring potable water to small rural villages and to the countryside.

Furthermore, the Ministry of Health is planning a massive extension of services. Health posts are to be brought to remote rural areas and some 6,000 paramedical and rural promoter personnel are to be trained. This latter group is made up mostly of women trained in basic health, sanitation, and nutrition practices who work in the communities or at health stations. They relay sick people and expectant mothers to the health posts where auxiliary personnel diagnose and give treatment. Serious cases can then be sent either to hospitals or to health centers which have permanent doctors and more sophisticated equipment, depending on the gravity of the patient's condition.

Finally, the Food and Nutrition Plan contains a supplementary food distribution program as a component of health services. Food supplements are for children under two years old and expectant and lactating mothers in the 10 to 20% poorest segment of the population. This is considered a temporary subsidy, amply justified until family incomes of this group rise to an adequate level. Food distribution will be carried out through the channels developed in the past with the support of the World Food Program, the Catholic Relief

Service, and the other international food donor agencies mentioned above.

A second part of the food supplement program consists of the distribution of new foods through the commercial channels, to be purchased by mothers with a subsidy in the form of a coupon. The coupons will be distributed by the health personnel to mothers who have children under two years of age, or who are pregnant, and whose income does not permit an adequate level of nourishment. The coupon will represent a proportion of the purchase value of any of the new foods placed on the market.

The store owner will in turn use the coupon he has received as partial payment to restock his supply of new foods. The industrialist will be able to exchange the coupons he receives from intermediaries for money at any of the state-owned financial institutions. Aside from guaranteeing a market for the new foods, the coupon system will be an effective tool in transferring resources to the poorest members of society. Even if it is "misused" by resale, it will still represent a net resource transfer, a large proportion of which will be spent on food.

Table 9 contains the expected costs of the different programs of the National Food and Nutrition Plan. Many of the projects will be presented to international agencies (World Bank, IDB, etc.) for financing. Although substantial external resources will be secured, national resources will represent at least 50%, and in many cases more, of each individual project or program. Initial contacts by the government with the international financial institutions have elicited a very favorable response to the National Food and Nutrition Plan.

National Food and Nutrition Council[24]   The coordination of all these programs is complex since they involve a great number of ministries and institutions of the state as well as the private sector. The National Food and Nutrition Council was set up with the primary function of coordinating, through the National Planning Department, the action of all entities involved in the execution of the programs of the National Food and Nutrition Plan. The members of the Council include all the ministries and main government institutions involved with the plan's execution. In this way, problems of authority arising at lower levels can be solved at a ministerial level. The council is an advisory body in charge of recommending to the government the measures necessary for effective execution of the plan. It is, in a sense, the body in charge of enforcing the decisions taken. Each agency is the executive agency in its field with the National Planning Department coordinating all activities at the national level.

PROBLEMS ENCOUNTERED AT THE PLANNING STAGE

Although the Food and Nutrition Plan is still in its planning stage, many problems have arisen.

Table 9
Summary of estimated total costs of the national food and nutrition plan

	Col$ Millions	US$ Millions
I Production of New Foods and Agribusiness	1,568.0	52.3
II Subsidized Food Distribution	1,538.0	51.3
A Direct food distribution[a]	538.0	17.9
B Coupon system	1,000.0	33.3
III Continental Fishing	109.3	3.6
IV Agricultural Credit	2,400.0	80.0
V Nutrition Education	520.0	17.3
A Interpersonal	215.2	7.2
B Institutional	71.4	2.4
C Mass media	26.2	0.9
D Production of educational aids	207.2	6.9
VI Health	2,942.7	98.1
A Aqueducts and sewage	1,300.0	43.3
B National health system	1,502.7	50.0
C Health centers and posts	140.0	4.7
VII Integrated Rural Development Program	8,100.0	27.0
Total	17,178.0	572.6

[a] Additional to ICBF Nutrition Division budget.
Source: DNP

Diagnosis of the Problem

The nutritional status of the population and the medical factors with which it meshes are known through indirect health indicators, such as mortality and morbidity rates, causes of death, etc., but there exists little data about the exact effect on nutrition of other socioeconomic factors such as production, distribution, consumption, sociocultural patterns by regions, or of some specific health problems that prevent optimum biological use of the foods consumed.

A major problem arose with the form and quality of existing statistics. Production, distribution, and consumption data, for instance, were available, but not in a disaggregated form nor analyzed in terms of specific aspects of nutrition. Sociocultural studies were completely absent as were studies related to problems of food absorption. The most recent data about protein-calorie malnutrition date from 1966. In order to close these gaps, a National Morbidity Survey will be carried out to provide up-to-date information on nutrition and health problems.

At the same time that the National Food and Nutrition Plan was adopted (March 1975), many studies were undertaken. However, it was decided to proceed with the Nutrition Plan simultaneously instead of losing valuable time awaiting the results. When data becomes available, alterations will be made in the specific programs affected.

Personnel

At present, technicians such as doctors and nutritionists are at work within the medical field. Rapid training of additional personnel in nutrition-related fields, therefore, has had to be started without delay. In the meantime, shortages of personnel were unavoidable. These have been partially overcome through external technical assistance. Although valuable, some problems have been encountered with this technical assistance, due to some experts' erroneous conceptions of local conditions.

First Actions and Elaboration of the Plan

At first, little interest in nutrition activity was shown by sectors other than health. The first interdisciplinary groups organized by the National Planning Department in late 1974 encountered problems because of the voluntary nature of each institution's participation. This led to intermittent rather than continuous activity, depending on the interest the plan elicited in each institution.

Once the plan was adopted by the Council for Socio-Economic Policies in March 1975, the principle problems that arose were the following:

a   Absence of a timetable and clear definition of the human, physical, and financial resources available for the elaboration of the programs and projects of the plan.

b   Shortage of time and of interdisciplinary personnel expert in the problem of nutrition made it necessary to improvise schemes which often resulted in a disorderly planning process. For example, the presence of the same individual was sometimes required in two different places at the same time.

c   Absence of administrative agility, which delayed the incorporation of personnel both at the professional and auxiliary levels.

d   Rotation of personnel and the assignment of multiple functions to one person led to inefficiency and dispersion of efforts.

e   Absence of an overall coordinating body with decisionmaking power and the authority to enforce the cooperation of all entities involved created difficulties, since the plan requires close coordination among sectors. This problem was solved to a great extent with the creation of the National Food and Nutrition Council in June 1975.

f   Institutional and professional jealousies among the participating entities and disciplines were aroused by the new multisectoral and integral approach,

thus making coordination difficult at the beginning. The favorable and enthusiastic response that the plan has had, both inside and outside the country,
has helped to overcome this difficulty and has created an element of cohesive-
ness among the different participants.

g The multiplicity of projects and areas covered, as well as the necessity of
granting independence and individual treatment to different projects, has
made it difficult to fulfill the requirements of presenting projects for partial
financing by international institutions.

h The rapidity with which the planning process is being implemented has
made it impossible to carry out certain investigations where gaps in knowledge exist. The necessary studies require long periods of time and high spe-
cialization, but they have been or will be undertaken promptly in order to
include the results in the final formulations of the projects.

Finally, the plan is itself part of the income distribution strategy of the
government. As such, it addresses the problem of income as a barrier to adequate nutrition for 30% of the population. It is not, however, the only program which is designed to solve this problem: land reform, as well as education and health services, will be extended. The Food and Nutrition Plan is
perhaps one of the primary motors of income distribution through public
expenditures, but it will not bear total responsibility for this accomplishment
in the vast field of growth, development, and income redistribution.

DISCUSSION (COLOMBIA)

Schlossberg

How did the president come to his own personal belief that there had to be a major agricultural development and nutrition program, as opposed to the previous kind of development policy that had been followed? What was the process that resulted in that commitment? Second, how was that translated into a political success? Third, what is the assurance that there will be financial commitment over the necessary time period? And fourth, does the administrative capacity in fact exist to provide the technical assistance required to make it a success?

López

The first part is very hard to answer because it relates to one person's political career over many years. Originally, the president's political support came from his discussion of precisely these views, and, in the recent election he obtained three million of the four million votes cast, with a platform based on the idea that economic growth had to go hand in hand and was compatible with income redistribution. It is a long story of political process, which I think goes outside the bounds of this conference.

Schlossberg

I don't think that it does go beyond our bounds. In a country where the government has not yet turned its development policy around, how that can take place would be among the very most important things to discuss in terms of developing a national policy. If development policy is oriented towards one part of the society, industry, for example, how that can be changed is a very important question.

Solimano

That is one of the basic questions we have to try to understand.

Montgomery

The question might be: Do the very poor people, the ones who are most disadvantaged in the society create a sufficiently powerful political force so that the president's career and the future of his regime depend upon some success in this? I think that is what we are talking about.

López

That is true in the sense of political support interpreted as a mandate for social change. If the campaign had taken place without the social overtones, the "silent majority" would have remained silent, and there would have been widespread abstention as has often been the case in the past. It is perhaps a sad reflection that so much depends on so few people: one man can mobilize a country around an idea, but the idea has to be born in him and is not necessarily born of the disadvantaged classes. It is still a very paternalistic society in that sense.

Barnes*

Can you identify those who did not vote for him? Are they the upper classes? industry? the military?

López

Industry, primarily. In this context, it has been very surprising that the reaction has not been more negative to the new tax reform, which represents a real change of the power structure. Only about 10 or 15% of the population declares income tax, and with the new tax reform, only 10% of those 10% do most of the taxpaying.

Solimano

Ken's original question related to how you create consciousness and where. One level is that of the presidency. Another important issue is the consciousness of the base: how much do people understand what is going on and why? Food is very easy to understand, but nutrition policy is not easily comprehended by the people most in need. In Chile, in the last election in 1970, all three candidates, from the left to the extreme right, were offering something in terms of nutrition because it had appeal to the people. But that is not enough. You have to analyze exactly what is going on and how much the program really does for whom.

López

In Colombia, nutrition is a new topic in terms of its political presence. Campaigns had previously centered around economic growth, controlling inflation, stopping the rise in food prices, but not nutrition per se. Now, nutrition has become an instrument to explain the government policy because it is very difficult for a great number of people to understand the tax legislation and fiscal reforms. For example a lot of road-building has stopped, which has created conflict. The government intends to switch its emphasis from highways to small roads, but the worker doesn't understand why the big highway project that had provided employment is suddenly stopped. So there's a bit of a demogogic counterplay, but it does have social content in the sense that it is backed by a budget with heavy expenditures in services such as health and education, and it is backed by government policy.

Barnes

And backed by the legislature?

López

Yes, because the Liberal party has a vast majority in Congress, and the development plan is presented to the Congress, where suggestions for changes are made. However, these are not substantial because the initiative in public expenditure comes from the Executive.

   The present government is only in office for three more years, and we expect that the loans from the World Bank and other international lending

*Dr. Allan C. Barnes.

agencies will be signed in one year. That then constitutes a contract, and for
the duration of the loans you have tied the budget of any government to the
nutrition projects. Furthermore, once a program shows its benefits, I venture
to say it would be hard to find a government in Colombia which would abandon them.

Schlossberg

I see; in other words, the government has made a commitment that the next
government cannot undo.

López

Yes. At least insofar as the foreign finance goes. So, there is some continuity
to be expected.

Levinson

It seems clear that we have, in this area, the grist for some of the most important hypotheses that will be emerging from this meeting. We must try to
determine, historically, the process of policy formation and also try to understand how, as in the Colombia situation, when there is interest and commitment by a small group of individuals, the roots can be sunk. In Chile, I think,
there was a somewhat different situation. There was a longer period of historical evolution, as opposed to a more recent emergence of the issue in Colombia. It appears from Chile's story that the roots were so deeply embedded in
the political system, in the bureaucratic and administrative systems, from the
early years, that when this most recent government came into power, despite
everything that government stood for and despite the exodus of everyone
from the previous government, the milk program continued. I find it absolutely remarkable that the milk program continues on almost the same level.
In some sense, it isn't only a matter of who sits in the key positions.

López

I would suggest that, once you arouse the consciousness of people by ex-
pounding certain ideas, you can never go back. In a way, continuity is bound
to be there, even if you don't want it to be.

Schlossberg

Part of the problem when you announce a major national nutrition program
is that it requires considerable funding and large-scale administrative capacity.
Yet, there must also be some sort of immediate delivery on the promises.

López

And electorates are becoming much more sophisticated than they were before.

Schlossberg

My point is, between the cup and the lip there is often a slip. The final result
of your plan has to be a farmer on a piece of land with a loan and with a

technical assistant to help him use his new seed, his fertilizer, and everything else.

López

Yes, so you have to mobilize yourself.

Montgomery

No, no. You have to mobilize *him*.

Schlossberg

But can you do that within the period of time that you have? These things rely finally on human factors.

López

Well, you can't do it in one year; you can't do it in two years. But you can start in one year. You can start with credit. You can start with building country roads. You can start rural electrification. The government is conscious of the fact that these are long-term projects, the full benefits of which probably will not show themselves before 1978, the year the government's mandate terminates.

Sandoval

I would say it depends on the social price you want to pay. It's not free. You want it quickly: you can use the Cuban style.

Schlossberg

Or else, the government has to be very sophisticated and take the limited progress achieved in the short run and somehow convince people that the limited progress represents a real step in the right direction and is not simply a token.

Barnes

Clara. what is the real clout of the Nutrition Council? Are they merely advisory, or have they some power? If they have, where did that power come from?

López

Actually, the real power is in the National Planning Department. The council's main purpose is surveillance and coordination. The only way to have the members of the different state entities collaborate without claiming that they have more important things to do, for instance, is to have each minister participate directly in the council where these types of problems are analyzed and the decisions communicated directly from the top level to the different government officials and entities. The council has members from at least five ministries as well as several decentralized state agencies.

Latham

You show, in figure 2, that 30% of your population is only getting 70% of its calorie needs. Where are you going to find those 30% of calories? This represents a huge amount of food. Since you have no plan to take that food from the wealthiest 30% of the population, you are obviously going to need a lot more food in Colombia.

Incidentally, calculations of nutrition based on a percentage of the required consumption of a specific foodstuff are probably not very helpful. In the last three days, I got 0% of my "milk requirement," but I have certainly had adequate nutrition. I think it's probably better to talk in terms of nutrients rather than foods.

Mellor
To expand on Michael's question, do you believe, in Colombia, that you can have significant improvement in nutrition of the lower income people without, in the short run, a massive allocation of foreign exchange to the import of food, as happened in Chile?

López
In Colombia, we are pretty much self-sufficient in food, except for wheat.

Mellor
Yes, with the bulk of the poor starving, you're self-sufficient.

López
The statistics show that 30% of the population do not consume an adequate amount of nutrients, that is, that malnutrition is widespread, but not that the bulk of the population is starving. The idea is not to solve the problem of malnutrition through imports of food but through increases in internal production. In fact, all foreign donor food aid is going to end by 1978. Note that there is a huge injection of straight agricultural credit, which we estimate will stimulate food production. You can talk about technology and other things, but the really important input is credit. If people just have enough credit, they might double the area that they are cultivating, from the small farmer to the very large landowners.

Levinson
This term "self-sufficiency," on the whole, does us more harm than good. It is a terribly, terribly misleading term. FAO uses the same terminology in calculating its food gaps for countries. All it really means is *effective demand*. If the price of wheat is $100 a pound, and only two people can afford to pay that $100, and each one were willing to buy a pound, then the effective demand for wheat would be two pounds for Colombia. If you produced two pounds, you would be self-sufficient. That is the extreme case, but that really is what that word "self-sufficiency" means as it's used. Yet there is an enormous difference between effective demand and nutritional needs. When we take into account the distributional factors, "self-sufficiency" means a lot of hungry people.

López
In Colombia, 60% of our exports originate in the agricultural sector. Of course, that includes coffee, which is our main foreign exchange item. However, I don't see the necessity of importing increasing amounts of food. It just doesn't seem natural to me as an incentive to agricultural production, which is, in the end, what you are going to depend on, especially given the often quoted predictions of food scarcity on a worldwide scale. Colombia, next year, will need to start importing petroleum, and that bill is going to rise, so that we will not be able to afford massive food imports. It will be better to depend on internal production.

Mellor
But that means you are not going to do anything for the poor for five or ten years.

López
Just by raising the small farmer's productivity, you raise his income, and his family's food consumption. A great proportion of the undernourished population belongs precisely to the group of people the Integrated Rural Development Projects are directed to.

Levinson
How can you run that food coupon program you mentioned without imports?

López
That's going to be done with the new mixtures and protein blends. Basically, we will produce a weaning food. Inputs for the new foods will come from increases in internal production resulting from the agricultural sector strategies that are planned. The new foods will go primarily to consumption by the young.

Schlossberg
Please explain who will get the coupons.

López
Coupons will go to the mothers that the health personnel decide seem to need it the most. In rural areas this means just about every mother that the health personnel approach.

Schlossberg
It's a supplemental-feeding food coupon program then and not a general food coupon program?

López
It's a subsidy for one product through commercial channels. In the long run, this is cheaper than direct distribution, which never reaches the remote coun-

tryside, and it does not have the psychological effects of a charitable give-away.

Wray
But will it be based on the nutritional status of the children?

López
Yes, in theory. But the decision will be based on an eyeball judgement and not a measure of weight.

Wray
Why not?

López
Because we are talking about the remotest rural areas in Colombia. We are talking about the judgment of a rural "promotora," a woman who may not even have primary school education, but who will be trained in very basic nutrition education, sanitation, and so on. Promotoras will be taught certain indications of poor nutrition, but we do not think they will be making a traditional professional choice based on calculations.

Solimano
Almost universally, every new government tries to discover and initiate new things: "We are the first to do this." I've learned recently, by looking backward in Chile, that things do not in fact happen de novo. They happen because something has happened before. Such analysis, based on past experience, is necessary to develop your plan. Even more important, at this stage of planning, is to devise how you're going to measure and evaluate. This is useful even for the next government.

López
That is being done. I just failed to make a point of it.

Montgomery
In your paper, you mentioned at least two different specific policies which were indirectly addressed toward food supply, though not necessarily nutrition. You also have a number of very specific programs that are identifiably distinct in your new multisectorial policy. The question is: What instruments do you have available for examining the consequences of the previous policies for low income groups and for following the consequences of these new interventions so that you can find out which ones are most effective and build on experience?

López
The old distribution programs get their funding from a percentage of the salt sales, and they will be continued. Evaluation is done as in most other countries: checking children's height and weight monthly. Over the years the ration which is distributed has been improved, and this will continue. We are

not expecting to be able to evaluate the food policies because the personnel
in charge of choosing who gets coupons will not be professional and will not
be in a good position to evaluate the results. They will, however, collect information on the health status of the population which will be relayed to the
Ministry of Health for evaluation.

Montgomery
I would worry about that. I do not think that macro data about changing
rates and other medical measures are adequate evaluation outputs for specific
interventions. You must get closer to the program in order to find out what
you're doing. It seems to me that this question is important enough, so that
when you start a major undertaking, you should allocate a portion of your
funds, as I understand is now being done in Indonesia, to the problem of
following through.

It is not only useful to know what you're doing and useful to the next
government, but it also keeps your people on the job while they are actually
"out there." They know that they are being valued by their output, and that
changes their whole attitude toward their work.

López
Yes. For instance, in small farmer credit and technical assistance, if an agency
doesn't follow through on its technical assistance, it will lose money because
it will have to pay to the farmer a minimum of what the farmer was producing before, plus a certain percentage of what it had promised the farmer in
increased production. So, whether the farmer produces or doesn't produce,
the agency itself will be financially responsible.

Mellor
Better move the programs to the bigger farmers, then, because the small ones
won't make their targets.

López
That is not true, in fact. We've done a pilot project with about 300 small
farmers, and it worked very well. They have increased their production by
substantial percentages.

Wray
In the description of the program, a lot of emphasis was placed on nutrition
education, backed up by $17 million in the budget. Why such heavy invest-
ment in this one area?

López
Because nutrition education is a program that didn't exist before. If you
notice, this nutrition plan is mainly an extension, although in an integrated
fashion, of things that have been going on before, such as rural development,
health, subsidized food distribution. So those budget items are additional

investment, whereas nutrition education through the mass media and at all levels of institutional education is totally new.

Wray
Someone once asked me why I insisted on data. Well, here is an area where I wonder what evidence the policy planning people have about the effectiveness of nutrition education to justify that kind of expenditure.

As for the provision of health services and clean water, I have heard that before in Colombia, over many years. Health plans have been generated with each new election and the same things have been said: extension of health services, development of health centers in rural areas. What's different now?

López
The definition of rural has been changing over the years. Previously small cities were 300,000 people. Now we're talking about delivery of service to cities under 10,000 people, and to truly rural areas.

Wray
Now, what has really changed that makes you think this is going to be possible?

López
The response to political pressure. In spite of all the pronouncements in the past, rural areas got some health posts here and there, but they didn't really have health services. We hope, finally, to take them out there. Maybe we will fail like all other governments, but a new system has been designed to extend coverage, which makes it a more realistic possibility.

The new system is based on paramedical personnel. You don't need to have a doctor in a rural post, as had been attempted in the past when, obviously, no doctor wanted to go there. The idea now is to take people from the area, train them with minimum knowledge, and then have them return to their own town or rural area where they're more likely to stay than a doctor who is sent out as an obligation. Higher levels of care, with permanent doctors in the health posts and local hospitals, will be available so that patients can be relayed and treated with the sophistication necessary for serious conditions. But the new system maintains the theory that paramedic personnel can be trained to cure the most widespread cause of mortality and morbidity, the group of gastrointestinal diseases.

Montgomery
Remember, too, that you have not always failed, even in Colombia, if you consider the salt iodization program which, in fact, eliminated disease for an identifiable target group.

4 NUTRITION IN GHANA   Fred T. Sai

Fred T. Sai was born in Accra, Ghana, and attended secondary school and college there. He studied medicine in University College Hospital, London, where he received his MB BS in 1953. He is also an FRCP (Edin.) and holds a Harvard MPH degree. Dr. Sai has been Deputy Director and Director of Medical Services in his country. From 1963 to 1966 he was FAO's Regional Nutrition Advisor in Africa. From 1966 to 1972 he was Professor of Preventive and Social Medicine in the Ghana Medical School, where he started the Comprehensive Rural Health Research and Training Program known as the Danfa Project. He has consulted for various UN and bilateral agencies, and is at present Assistant Secretary General, Forward Planning and International Liaison, International Planned Parenthood Federation. His publications range over human nutrition, preventive medicine, family planning, medical education, and health services administration. Dr. Sai's high-level and long-term involvement with the Ghanaian government makes him uniquely able to speak out about government relationships with a perspective that few other Ghanaians and no foreigner could possibly duplicate.

INTRODUCTION

Ghana is a relatively small tropical coastal African country, with an area of 92 thousand square miles, lying north of the equator. The country, previously under British colonial rule, has been independent since early 1957. It is surrounded on the east, west, and north by French-speaking nations. At present it has a nonrepresentative military government which cannot be described as a dictatorship.

DEMOGRAPHY

The total population grew from 6.7 million in 1960, to an estimated 8.5 million at the time of the 1970 census. In 1973, the population was estimated at 9.35 million. The population growth rate has been, therefore, 2.7 to 2.9% per annum in recent years. Twenty percent of the population is still under 5 years of age and 48% is under 15. Including the 4% over the age of 64, there is thus a very high dependency ratio. The percentage of women in the reproductive ages—15 to 44—is about 20%, crude birth rate is between 44 and 48 per thousand, and the crude death rate is about 17 or 18 per thousand. Ghana thus ranks among countries with a very high birth rate and a relatively high death rate.

Urbanization is proceeding very rapidly. The major cities of Sekondi, Takoradi, and Accra are growing at rates of between 7 and 12% per annum. According to the 1970 census, about 30% of all Ghanaians live in towns and cities of 5,000 or more persons. This level of urbanization is higher than that of most African countries and is maintained by the migration of young, mostly male, adults from the rural areas.

This migration has several implications for food production and nutrition. A disproportionate number of children, women, and older men are left to do the agricultural work, with a resulting loss of efficiency. More important, those migrating frequently remain unemployed or else employed as casual labor with no job security. They receive minimal wages. Their lack of education and skills and their initial inability to understand town life and expenditure patterns adversely influence their nutrition as well as that of their families.

In towns, cash is the main basis of good nutrition. "New townsmen" and their families have little cash and at the same time have fixed expenditures which they did not have in their rural environment. When budget cuts become necessary, it is the food budget that suffers. So, while food may be plentiful and varied in town markets, those with low earnings in peri-urban or decaying parts of big towns, have quite serious nutrition problems. Fiawoo found that school children in peri-urban areas grew less well than those from the settled parts of the towns or the rural areas.[1] It has been noticed in Accra that children from peri-urban families are represented disproportionately among cases of PCM.[2]

To improve the nutrition of rural families, diversification of local food production and emphasis on underutilized foods, such as pulses, legumes, eggs, and fresh vegetables and fruits, plus basic education in physiological needs and methods of food preservation is fundamental. In the case of urban/peri-urban nutrition, providing good job opportunities, education in budgeting for city living, health and welfare services for wives, and cooperatives where foods can be obtained at reasonable prices, may all take precedence over any nutrition education in regard to the needs of individual members of families.

ECONOMY

Unfortunately, Ghana, until recently, has been mainly dependent on a single agricultural crop. The major base of the economy is cocoa. The export of this crop generates almost two-thirds of the country's foreign exchange. Other sources of foreign exchange earning are minerals, including gold, bauxite, manganese and industrial diamonds, and, to a small extent, timber.

The distribution of the gross national product throughout the population shows the same disturbing features as in many other developing and industrial countries. About 20% of the population absorbs 40-50% of the total gross national product; the lowest earning group, 40% of the population, consumes less than 20% of the gross national product.

Sixty to 70% of Ghana's population earns a living from agriculture, mostly peasant agriculture. On the coast, fishing is a major occupation. Casual labor, both in agriculture and in building and industrial concerns, is a common occupation for people with little education who migrate to developing towns. Among such people, unemployment is a great problem. Underemployment can be observed in both the agricultural and the industrial/commercial sectors. Table 1 shows the growth of Ghana's gross national product from 1960 to 1969.

EDUCATION

Primary education has been free and compulsory since 1960. However, the availability of school places is so tight and the rate of growth of the population is so rapid, that in 1971 only 64% of all eligible children 6 to 10 years old were actually attending school. Of those completing their secondary education, at most 4 or 5% get a university place. Both primary and university education are completely or nearly free. However, the secondary-school sector is still operated largely on a fee-paying basis and thus constitutes a block in the country's realization of its goal of universal education.

Table 1
Gross national product of Ghana

	1960	1961	1962	1963	1964	1965	1966	1967	1968	1969
Gross national product (¢ millions)										
At current market prices	946	1,008	1,084	1,190	1,345	1,589	1,779	1,757	2,028	2,285
At 1960 prices	946	976	1,028	1,056	1,085	1,093	1,099	1,116	1,120	1,158
Per capita gross national product (¢)										
At current prices	141	146	153	164	180	207	224	216	242	266
At 1960 prices	141	142	145	145	145	142	138	137	137	135

¢ = new cedi. At 1 December 1972, £ 1 sterling = 3.02 ¢; US $1 = ¢1.28.
Source: *Economic Survey*, 1969. Central Bureau of Statistics, Accra

THE NUTRITIONALLY VULNERABLE GROUPS

Studies have been carried out to identify nutritionally vulnerable groups as well as the total nutritional status of the country. One of the most recent comprehensive studies is the National Food and Nutrition Survey undertaken by Davey and the staff of the National Food and Nutrition Council in 1960-62.[3] Prior to that, there had been qualitative surveys undertaken by individuals and isolated studies on smaller populations. Information on the nutritional status of the people can also be gleaned from hospital data and death registrations. From the surveys and statistics, it is clear that the major nutrition problems in Ghana can be divided into two groups: (1) Under-nutrition, and (2) Various types of specific deficiency malnutrition.

From estimates of the National Food Balance Sheet, it can be inferred that there is almost enough food in the country to feed the population satisfactorily; there seems to be enough for 90-105% of the calorie requirements of the population, based on recommended allowances, and about 90% of the protein requirements.

MALNUTRITION

Malnutrition due to gross lack of food—either year-round or cyclic—is found most often in the Northern and Upper regions. Davey found that in these regions adult males lost between 5 and 6 pounds in weight during the hungry seasons, and put this weight back on again after the harvest. On the whole, people of these regions have a smaller weight/height ratio than those in other parts of the country. In the forest belt, the adults also show some seasonal weight fluctuations, but the amounts involved, 2 to 3 pounds, are not particularly significant. Coastal dwellers seem to fare best. In all areas, however, there is a tendency for undernutrition to occur in large numbers of children, especially those under 5 years of age. Where weight alone is used as an index, about 30 to 40% of Ghanaian children under 5 years of age deviate from the accepted norm by significant amounts. Women, especially those who are pregnant or lactating, are also found to have signs suggestive of inadequate total nutrition. Many women were found to go through pregnancy without putting on weight commensurate with the physiological needs, although lactating women, aside from grand multiparas, in the majority of forest-belt/coastal areas seemed to maintain their weight well.

Children from about 6 months until they are ready to hold their own in the household eating system are the most nutritionally vulnerable group in Ghana, as in the majority of developing countries. Two to 9% of these at any given time have signs of overt protein-calorie malnutrition (PCM). These children are found mainly in the forest belt and in the coastal savannah. To a large extent, this problem is due more to poverty, lack of knowledge, and poor household food practices, than to nonavailability of the right foods. In

addition, children in the Northern and Upper regions show a general deficiency in growth patterns. In her first descriptions of PCM, or kwashiorkor, from
Accra, Cecily Williams[4] pointed out that this condition which occurred in
weanlings seemed especially related to the maize gruel that was fed to children. This has been borne out by all later findings. PCM has a mortality of
almost 50% when untreated and 10-20% with vigorous treatment. Thus, malnutrition is both a direct and indirect cause of the high young-child mortality
in Ghana.

SPECIFIC NUTRIENT DEFICIENCY DISEASES

Goiter has been found to be highly prevalent in the Northern and Upper
regions, affecting between 5 and 33% of the population with the highest
occurrence in adolescent and young adult women. So far, not much government attention has been devoted to this. Among the vitamin deficiencies, the
most overt are riboflavin deficiency, mainly in pregnant women and children,
and folic acid deficiency in the form of macrocytic anemia. This anemia may
be aggravated by malaria, which is more common and more severe in the
pregnant and the very young. Vitamin A deficiency, with high rates of night
blindness and xerophthalmia, is observed in Upper and Northern Ghana. The
direct relation of the high incidence of blindness to vitamin A deficiency
alone has been questioned because in these same areas there is a high prevalence of other eye conditions, such as trachoma and onchocerciasis. Low
dietary calcium levels have been observed and this may be related to poor
pelvic development which may become an obstetrical problem later in life.

THE RELATIONSHIP OF THE HEALTH SYSTEM TO THE
NUTRITIONALLY VULNERABLE GROUP

Health Coverage

The government intends to offer total health care for the entire population.
However, the present situation is very far from the ideal, except in isolated
instances. Isolated coverage success has been achieved by the Medical Field
Units, where multipurpose disease diagnosis and treatment units use very
simply trained personnel with very specific tasks. These personnel usually had
only 8-10 years of formal education and a year of on-the-job training, but
they did a thorough job and were able to hold the major diseases under control. Recently, their mobility has been checked and the units have been made
to respond to the needs of static centers and the hospitals.

In actual fact, probably only 20% of the population has health coverage on
anything like a continuous scale, as pointed out by Sai.[5] The treatment
meted out to women and children, nutritionally the most vulnerable group, is
even more episodic than that provided to the other members of the popula-

tion. The fact that those in greatest need tend to have least health care is brought out graphically when one looks at the distribution of health facilities, hospital attendance rates, death rates, and the population by geographic regions (figure 1).

Infant mortality rates are very high, varying from about 70 per thousand in the big centers (Accra, Kumasi, etc.) to about 150-200 per thousand in the more rural areas. The preschool child, only 20% of the population, contributes 50% of the total deaths, as recorded by Saakwa Mante in 1967, from postmortem and hospital death reports.

The maternal and child health services are the most backward. There is very little development of these services outside of the main towns. The major thrust, at present, is to attract the women and children to come to static clinics, although it is well known that these people cannot travel the long distances frequently. Efforts are being made to test alternative strategies; among these the most comprehensive is the Danfa project.

Antenatal attendance appears to be reasonable in many areas, although delivery usually takes place outside the formal health care system. Postnatal attendance is very poor. Family planning services were officially introduced through the National Family Planning Program of the Planned Parenthood Association of Ghana. Although there are ambitious plans to extend coverage, the percentage of the population which has so far received family planning, in relation to those in need, must be considered relatively small. Figures in an International Planned Parenthood Federation study[6] show that only 30.6% of women at risk are covered. This is probably an overestimate, based on inadequate data.

Health Budget

The government budgetary support for direct health services is 2-3₵ per capita. The recurrent health budget has risen from ₵ 15 million to almost ₵ 93 million from 1967 to 1975. Of this, 80% goes to curative services. The maintenance of already existing institutions and wrongly trained personnel, badly motivated, supported, and deployed, as well as political decisions unrelated to needs, all help to maintain the status quo.

Ghana has been training its own doctors since 1964 and other health workers even before then. However, the curricula and syllabi, as well as the approaches to education and training of all health workers, were based on the British pattern. In a country in which children under 15 comprise 48% of the population, and where diseases of infancy and childhood and problems related to childbirth are the most serious and important, internal medicine and surgery were, until very recently, still receiving the greatest attention in teaching and student clerkship.

Despite all the promises to hold down the expenditures on hospital beds, successive governments have gone ahead with prestige hospital construction.

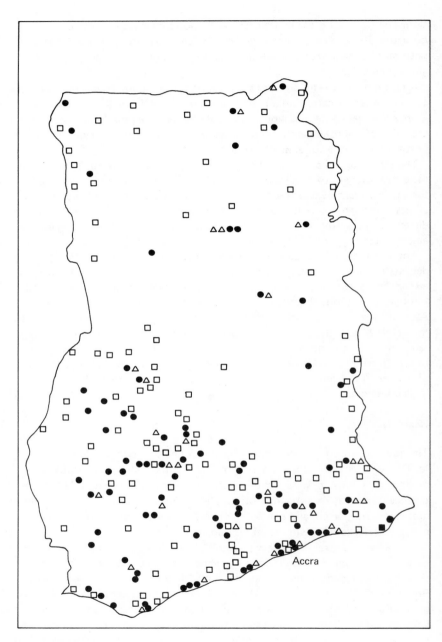

Figure 1
Health services in Ghana. ●, hospitals; □, health centers; △, MCH clinics.

Health centers have been altered into cottage-type hospitals to satisfy purely political motives. Even where health posts have been considered for the expansion of primary medical care, the siting of these has been based on the possible political returns rather than on the needs of the population. In all of these decisions, the senior doctors, as leaders of the medical profession, have not played a very worthy role. Their own training, background, and aspirations often mislead them into thinking that "excellence" in their own small practice of a specialty in the city is making a great contribution to national health needs.[5]

When corrected for inflation the budget given in table 2 shows a relatively modest rise up to 1975. This is due to deliberate policy after January 1972 to deemphasize the creation of expensive facilities. It would appear that from 1975 there is a reversal of the policy to emphasize promotive and protective health care; large sums of money are again being given over to the development of hospital facilities that provide little or no input into nutrition activities.

The Ministry of Health includes a division responsible for human nutrition with a total strength on paper of 188:

Senior Medical Officer (Nutrition)	1
Chief Nutrition Officer	1
Principal Nutrition Officer	1
Senior Nutrition Officers	2
Nutrition Officers	6
Assistant Nutrition Officers	3
Senior Technical Officers	40
Technical Officers	134

Table 2
Health budget of Ghana (¢ thousands)

Year	Recurrent	Capital	Total health budget	% of national budget	% of capital health budget
1967/68	15,000	2,159	17,159	4.78	12.58
1968/69	17,258	3,459	20.727	5.61	16.74
1969/70	20,400	4,207	24,607	5.25	17.1
1970/71	21,956	9,530	31,486	6.06	30.27
1971/72	27,163	9,236	36,399	6.26	25.37
1972/73	33,356	7,177	40,533	6.44	17.71
1973/74	45,000	9,500	54,500	7.14	17.43
1974/75	68,943	12,723	81,666	8.06	15.58
1975/76	93,032	19,063	112,095	11.08	16.61

Source: Dr. Ofosu-Amaah;[7] Ministry of Economic Affairs

Health Facilities and Personnel and Their Geographic Distribution

The total numbers of health facilities, doctors, and other health personnel, together with their distribution, are shown in tables 3 and 4. Ofosu-Amaah[7] showed that 40% of all doctors practising in Ghana in 1973 were in the Accra area.

From all evidence, there is a maldistribution and maldeployment of facilities as well as of staff, and there is discrimination against those geographic areas where health needs are greatest. The type of staff employed and the method of their deployment are such that infants and young children, followed by women, get the least continuous care. Those least in need, such as office clerks and senior-level personnel in the civil services and armed forces, get the most health care.

FOOD AND AGRICULTURE

Food production in Ghana is widely distributed throughout the country. Table 5 shows the amounts of the major crops produced.
Total arable land is about 75,000 square miles, but it is important to consider food production in relation to the major geographic and climatic regions. The country divides naturally into three geographic regions: a coastal belt, a forest

Table 3
General-hospital beds

Region	Population Total (thousands)	%	Hospital beds Total	% of national total	Bed ratios Population per bed	Comparison with national average (%)
Greater Accra	650	3.1	2,230	23.2	290.1	+183
Eastern	1,337	17.0	1,402	14.5	967.9	−15
Volta	871	10.9	1,201	12.5	725.2	+14
Central	1,650	20.7	656	6.8	−	−
Western	−	−	994	10.3	1,000	−17
Ashanti	1,331	16.7	1,502	15.6	886.2	−7
Brong-Ahafo	682	8.5	449	4.7	1,518.9	−45
Northern	−	−	443	4.6	−	−
Upper	1,444	18.1	751	7.8	1,209.3	−31
Total	7,985	100.0	9,628	100.0	829.4	100

Population figures are 1968 estimates.
Source: Ghana Medical Facilities. Data presented at 2nd Ghana International Trade Fair, February 1971

Table 4
Regional distribution of doctors and nurses in government service, December 1970

Region	Population (1970)	No. of doctors	Doctor/ population ratio	Nurses and midwives
Greater Accra	848,825	134	1/6,000	895
Eastern	1,262,882	28	1/43,000	315
Velta	947,012	17	1/55,000	233
Central	892,593	16	1/55,000	272
Western	768,312	59	1/13,000	341
Ashanti	1,477,397	78	1/19,000	244
Brong-Ahafo	762,673	12	1/63,000	88
Northern	728,572	17	1/43,000	221
Upper	857,295	8	1/100,000	159
Total	—	369	—	2,768

Source: Report of Health Sector Committee, October 1971

Table 5
Production of various crops in Ghana, 1968-72 (thousands of long tons)

Crop	1968	1969	1970	1971	1972
Maize	301	303	435	378	396
Rice	64	60	64	68	69
Groundnuts	37	37	36	49	54
Cassava	1,423	1,485	1,618	1,782	2,047
Sugar cane	500	250	250	250	500
Plantain	750	805	920	1065	1168
Oil palm	225	270	283	298	313

Source: Economics and Marketing Division, Ministry of Agriculture

belt, and a (northern) savannah belt. The first two have two rainy seasons each year, whereas the savannah has only one. In the coastal belt the basic staple is maize, with cassava and some plantain as supporting staples. Other foods include tomatoes, okra, and green leafy vegetables and pulses. In the forest belt, tubers and starchy fruit such as cassava, plantain, and yams and coco yams constitute the major staples, and maize is only very rarely grown. In the savannah, millets, sorghums and, to some extent, yams constitute the major staples. Supplementary food production is poor, even though a variety of wild green leafy vegetables are included in the diet. Fruits such as oranges, limes, mangoes, and pawpaw grow well in the coastal and forest parts of the country.

The extent of cultivation and use of vegetables and fruit, in conjunction with the type of staple, determine the nutritional status of the population. In the Northern Region, for example, because of prolonged dry periods and a relative lack of vegetables and fruit, vitamin A deficiency tends to be prominent. One-season cropping is also, to a certain extent, responsible for the seasonal calorie shortages that occur in the North. In the Central Region, the abundant use of foods poor in protein, such as tubers and starchy roots, is the principal reason for the greater occurrence of protein calorie malnutrition among the children. Southerners, who in addition to other foods also have fish as a resource, seem to do best.

Although Ghana produces, in the aggregate, enough food for its total population, the geographic distribution of the foods, in conjunction with the economic situation of various regions and the poor development of transportation and storage facilities, leads to a situation where food may bypass precisely those areas most in need. There may be relatively large amounts of food in the big market towns of Accra, Kumasi, Sekondi, and Takoradi, while there are relative shortages in other parts of the country. Davey found that among Fanti villages in the Central Region, distance from the road was related to the incidence of malnutrition. Peasant farmers may find themselves so far away from main roads, with no feeder roads to carry their produce, that in good years, they must watch some of the food go to waste. Postharvest losses of cereals are high: 10 to 30%. Recently, in some parts of the North and along the coast, land which was previously in food production is now being used for the production of tobacco because there is a better market for that crop and because collection and sale are very much easier for the farmer. This trend must be discouraged.

Recent important developments in the food field include the emphasis on rice production, irrigation schemes for food, and the fertilizer program for maize. There is also an effort to introduce intermediate-scale technology in order to ensure that the food that is produced is rapidly harvested and stored. Although this is currently experimental, it holds promise for the future.

Price fluctuations in food are a very serious phenomenon. Fluctuation is most dramatic in the case of high-protein foods such as fish, meat, and legumes. With legumes, price changes by a factor of four or five are common in a year. Currently, legumes, which used to form a substantial part of the rural diet, are now lagging in production to such an extent that serious problems with rural protein supplies should be envisaged. Government has increased its attention to food production recently, and base pricing is now in effect for staples; government subsidies are provided as well. But, on the whole, Ghana has been quite a heavy importer of foods in the last few years (tables 6, 7).

FOOD CONSUMPTION

Apart from the national patterns of food consumption, there is a food consumption pattern within homes which ensures that those in the vulnerable groups get even less food then the nonvulnerable. The "pecking order" within

Table 6
Value of imports by classes, 1968-73 (₡ millions)

Class	1968	1969	1970	1971	1972	1973
Food and live animals	51.0	55.2	79.5	62.6	72.2	91.8
Beverages and tobacco	5.0	1.6	3.9	4.6	2.3	4.4
Crude materials (except fuels), inedible	6.3	5.4	9.4	12.4	13.2	20.6
Mineral fuels, lubricants, and related materials	21.5	22.9	24.4	27.0	45.3	36.0
Animal and vegetable oils and fats	4.0	5.9	3.8	5.2	5.2	5.2
Chemicals	22.1	55.0	66.9	71.6	63.9	78.0
Manufactured goods	76.3	97.4	100.8	99.4	68.2	81.9
Machinery and transport equipment	86.0	94.5	108.1	131.5	104.3	89.7
Misc. manufactured articles	14.0	14.6	16.4	19.2	11.3	11.2
Other	1.7	1.8	5.8	9.6	7.3	8.6
Totals	314.0	354.4	419.0	443.1	393.3	427.5

Source: Ghana Central Bureau of Statistics, External Trade Statistics of Ghana, vols. 18-22, nos. 12, and vol. 23, no. 10

the home is such that the older male members of the household get first pick and get their full share of food, while the young children and women come last. The true physiological needs of children and women are least understood by the population. Many people feel that children need only the staple diet to fulfill growth needs.

There are also restrictions imposed by economic realities, which make it impossible for poor families to feed their children well. For instance, there has been an effort to get families to produce eggs and poultry for meat, but such efforts, even if they improve production, do not necessarily lead to better feeding of children. The eggs and poultry are sold and the amounts recovered used for buying more staple.

There have been very few studies of the amounts and types of food consumed by the vulnerable groups. One of the most significant is Davey's National Food and Nutrition Survey.[3] He showed the deficiencies in both calories and proteins which occur in the diet of the vulnerable groups. Children between the ages of 1 and 4 had between 69 and 111% of their calorie requirements satisfied, and between 46 and 102% of their protein requirements (table 8). Women also were unable to meet the requirements for both calories and proteins, but with smaller deficits.

Table 7
Amounts and values of annual food imports, 1968-73

Commodity	1968 Amount[b]	Value[c]	1969 Amount	Value	1970 Amount	Value	1971 Amount	Value	1972 Amount	Value	1973[a] Amount	Value
Sugar	86.4	8.3	66.8	8.3	129.3	16.4	59.6	10.2	44.3	14.0	48.6	18.5
Fish	10.2	4.5	10.4	4.9	11.6	13.7	14.5	11.7	16.1 (74.9)[d]	11.8 (23.4)[d]	18.5 (74.5)[d]	10.8 (25.5)[d]
Wheat and wheat products	63.2	8.6	66.4	7.6	76.8	7.4	43.7	3.9	86.5	8.8	88.8	13.5
Total dairy products	21.7	6.6	23.2	8.3	22.8	9.3	27.1	11.2	9.3	7.6	6.6	6.8
Live animals[e]	47.7	6.3	66.9	8.5	61.9	7.6	55.7	6.1	37.0	5.0	27.1	3.9
Rice	30.1	6.9	27.6	6.0	52.3	10.2	34.6	6.0	23.9	3.6	38.8	12.0
Total red meat	5.2	2.8	6.1	3.4	8.3	5.1	6.1	3.7	2.3	2.7	1.5	1.1
Total food imports	—	51.0	—	55.2	—	79.5	—	62.6	—	60.7 (72.2)[d]	—	77.1 (91.8)[d]
Total imports	—	314.0	—	354.4	—	419.0	—	443.1	—	393.3	—	427.5
Value of the cedi relative to 1968	—	1.00	—	1.00	—	1.00	—	1.00	—	0.79	—	0.79

[a] 1973 data are from January to October only.
[b] All amounts in tons with the exception of "Live animals" which are noted in numbers.
[c] Values in ₵ millions.
[d] Beginning in 1972, fish imports include imports from the high seas, not shown in previous years. The values in parentheses include these imports from the high seas.
[e] Amounts (i.e., number of animals) in the "Live animal" category are for cattle only.
Source: As table 6

Table 8
Nutrient value of children's diets

Area	Age (years)	Number of Children	kcal	Protein (gm)
Forest	1-2	4	828	18.2
Forest	2-3	7	964	21.8
Forest	3-4	15	941	19.7
Savanna (dry)	1-2	2	804	20.7
Savanna (dry)	2-3	5	778	24.9
Savanna (dry)	3-4	18	1,192	42.5
Savanna (moist)	2-4	2	1,509	53.8

Source: National Food and Nutrition Survey 1961-62 (Mimeographed Report of National Food and Nutrition Board)

Table 9
Proportion of young persons, number of consumers per family cooking unit, food selections in Danfa and James Town, 1968 (grams of food/person/day)

Locality	Danfa		James Town	
% of total population under 14 years old	48.3		44.5	
Household size	2	7	3	7
Foodstuff				
1 Cereals	484	186	367	239
2 Starchy roots and fruits	366	455	170	149
3 Sugars	8	4	16	11
4 Legumes and other seeds	33	11	11	42
5 Fruits and vegetables	114	112	97	75
6 Meats	9	8	21	11
7 Eggs	—	—	8	2
8 Fish	72	40	120	58
9 Milk	—	—	14	111
10 Oils and fats	6	3	39	19
11 Miscellaneous	—	—	1	—
Energy (kcal)	2,455	1,527	2,193	1,562
Protein (gm)	84.5	51.4	69.3	49.9
Protein calories as % of total calories	13.7	13.4	12.6	12.8

Source: Report of Nutrition Studies in Accra area, Ghana, London/Ibadan Nutrition Course, Ibadan 1967

Studies conducted in Accra and Danfa also support these findings, showing clearly that the nutrient content per capita in a family is inversely related to the size of the family. The larger the number of young children in the family, the poorer the nutrient intake per capita. This was the case both in the city of Accra and in Danfa, which is rural. However, the study showed that in extremely large families this rule did not seem to apply. One possible explanation would be that large families have more contributing adults than medium-sized families.

Unfortunately, there have been no studies to investigate the consumption of various nutrients by pregnant and lactating women to date.

Trends in nutrition and food purchasing by the vulnerable groups cannot be considered to be very encouraging. Ghana, like the majority of countries in the world, has been caught in the grip of severe and continuing inflation. Even before the oil crisis, the economy was heading for a rapid inflation. The nutritionally vulnerable in towns and peri-urban areas, who have to use money in order to purchase all their food, are finding it increasingly difficult to buy enough to meet their nutritional requirements. Studies in Ghana have shown that with increments to salary the first additive food purchase was the staple. Only when adequate quantities of staple were obtained was more nutritious and expensive food, such as milk or eggs, included in the diet. Many town workers have such low wages that after meeting fixed commitments they can only afford the simplest and cheapest of foods.

With the decline of breast feeding in the towns, money has to be used for purchasing infant-formula feeds. These, of course, are always increasing in price, and this has led to a situation where very young children are often inadequately fed. There is thus an increasing incidence of marasmus in very young children, which has become a large problem in many Ghanaian towns. Jelliffe has noted that formula feeds have caused severe undernutrition in children in many parts of the developing world.[8]

General government policies of economic growth and development, although supposedly geared towards helping vulnerable groups, do not seem to have much impact. Price controls for the distribution of foods as well as supplementation of foods have all been tried at one stage or another. Price controls have tended to take off the open market many foods that might be used for the vulnerable groups. Milk is an example of a food which periodically runs short on the Ghanaian market. Bymers and Sai[9] have discussed the limitations of price controls in Ghana's economy. The effect of price controls on nutrition can at this time only be surmised.

GOVERNMENT ACTIVITY AND THE NUTRITIONALLY VULNERABLE GROUPS

Successive governments in Ghana have recognized nutrition as a problem since 1939. Just before World War II, the colonial government had a survey made of nutrition in the empire. This showed clearly that the nutritional state of people in Ghana was not satisfactory. The study confirmed previous findings, among which was Williams' report on kwashiorkor in Ghanaian children.[3] Nothing could be done about the situation described in 1939 because of the war. After that period, other pressing concerns diverted attention from nutrition.

In the early 1950s, however, the new Ghanian government decided that nutrition was a problem and asked the Ministry of Health to include a nutrition officer on its staff in order to help define the problem more succinctly. At the same time, a small council of ministries and departments related to nutrition was formed, headed by the Principal Secretary of the Ministry of Agriculture. The council was charged with the responsibility of analyzing the findings and suggesting methods for improvement. The government also recognized that the information available was inadequate and asked for consultant help from UN agencies in 1958. Platt and Mayer undertook a survey in Ghana, which revealed gross undernutrition as a major problem in the Northern Region, as well as childhood malnutrition in various parts of the country.

From this survey and previous ones, the government understood that the Ministry of Health was in a position to help diagnose nutrition as a difficulty only after the difficulty had arisen. Another, and possibly better, method of dealing with the problem would be to watch for nutritional problems through nutrition surveys. Thus, household food consumption surveys and budget surveys of various kinds were made. All of these helped the government to identify malnutrition as a problem, and in the late 1950s, plans for solutions were made. As recently as March 1974, a national food and nutrition congress was held in Accra to reassess the situation and make new proposals. The conclusions of this meeting have been compiled in a report.

PROPOSED SOLUTIONS TO THE NUTRITION PROBLEM

Intervention Schemes

The most direct actions, aimed at the nutritionally needy, have been food supplementation schemes, run either through the government with the support of UNICEF and USAID; or through the church-related relief services, where milk products have been used as part of an education campaign for the children. In the main, however, the nutrition activities have not been coordinated and the lack of coordination of such activities has been one major reason why success has not been achieved.

The Catholic Relief Services, under US PL 480, run one of the most extensive food distribution schemes in Ghana. The activities, started in 1959, are comprised of a preschool program, school feeding programs, and food for work programs. In addition, some food is used for health institutions and in special cases, such as for tuberculosis and leprosy patients. The preschool program is the most important and consists of the following:

a Monthly assessment of weight, using Morley charts (85,000 charts have been supplied to various institutions as of March 1974).

b Interpretation of the weight to the mother.

c Physical examination of the child by a nurse.

d Group shared experience in cooking and discussion of child care and nutrition. These are aimed at teaching the mother how to use the supplements and how to prepare toddler meals, as well as to promote new and better methods of preparing familiar foods and to encourage the use of available nutritious foods.

The foods distributed include bulgur wheat, corn-soya-milk mix, and some oil. A small fee is charged for the monthly service (less than 10¢ US). The amounts supplied contribute to the feeding of most of the immediate family. In 1974 the preschool program was being run in 67 centers.

The Ministry of Health runs clinical hospitals for treating malnutrition, but these are quite expensive and, without proper follow-up, their impact on the total malnutrition situation must remain small.

Education

Another suggestion for improving the identification, as well as the solution, of nutrition problems was to emphasize nutrition education. The plan for nutrition education was to include university-level education, so that graduates could help with programs in human nutrition. The University of Ghana at Legon was assisted by the Food and Agricultural Organization (FAO) and UNICEF in establishing courses, and these continue to the present. In addition, a Home Science Degree Course was established into which nutrition teaching would be integrated. Through the Food and Nutrition Board (FNB), low-level training in nutrition was to be undertaken as well as middle-level training for nutrition-program management personnel and nutrition-education personnel.

Unfortunately, these programs have not been too well coordinated, and success cannot therefore be assessed; but the total number of graduates trained domestically in nutrition and home science is over 100. In addition, there are many overseas-trained nutrition and home-science graduates. When the FNB functioned properly, it tried to set out plans for food and nutrition activities so that programs could then be isolated for implementation by various government and nongovernment agencies. In addition to advice on general agricultural and food-production plans, there have been specific plans for nutritional activities and improvement. These include nutrition education, establishment of health-related nutrition activities (including rehabilitation centers for children suffering from malnutrition), emphasis on clinical nutrition activities, and the use of such activities for training of health personnel.

The Council

The first overall solution proposed was the formation of a coordinating authority for all nutrition activity in the country. This suggestion, made by successive advisors, both from outside and inside Ghana, was accepted. Unhappily, the board—or council, as it later came to be known—instead of working as a coordinating body, tried to encompass all nutrition activities under its wings, with the result that it did not generate the support it needed from the major agencies responsible for different facets of nutrition programs.

[Editor's note: The following has been excerpted from Dr. Sai's insightful, impromptu recollections of his personal involvement with nutrition planning in Ghana.]

As is known, Ghana gave the word "kwashiorkor" to the world. Despite the fact that it has been slowly withdrawn from the international medical literature, it was a very nice emotional word for those of us who wanted to get government commitment to nutrition programs. I entered the nutrition scene in my country in 1957, and, by luck, that very year, WHO elected to use malnutrition as the subject matter for its World Health Day. I was asked to make the major national broadcast on malnutrition as a national issue. The word "kwashiorkor" came in very handily because it was known in the capital, and it was used on radio to explain what malnutrition really meant in emotional terms. Before the end of the day, I had been hauled before the prime minister to help find out how to go about attacking the problem.

We decided to get two experts, Professor Platt and Professor Mayer, to come to Ghana and evaluate the problem. Among their recommendations was the formation of a policy group at the highest possible level, preferably within the president's office. The country was newly independent, and the prime minister wanted some subject that would have popular appeal so that he could say that he was doing something important. Nutrition lent itself to that kind of approach; so it was agreed that the National Food and Nutrition Council would be formed.

Although there had been a small nutrition committee chaired by the permanent secretary of the Ministry of Agriculture in the early 1950s, it was not until 1959 that the statutory Food and Nutrition Board was formed in Ghana. The executive secretary's post was left vacant until I could return, but the appointment of assistant executive was made politically, without reference to any of the agencies that were going to be involved in the operations of the National Food and Nutrition Board. Despite that, the effort was taken quite seriously in the beginning.

The board was chaired by the most senior medical person in the Ministry of Health responsible for public health, and the other members were representatives from the ministries of Agriculture, Education, Social Welfare, and Trade. Some of the individuals were invited simply because of their interest. When I looked at the minutes last month in Accra, I was impressed by the consistency with which the permanent secretaries or the heads of the ministries themselves attended the meetings in those early days. However, their deliberations unfortunately concerned administrative and staff matters and lacked real substance. This was not surprising as there was no one trained in nutrition available to the board and the scientific secretariat had not yet been organized. If you don't have a good scientific secretariat to service a nutrition commission, then the commission cannot function.

Unfortunately, this early period for the nutrition committee was also a period of tremendous change in Ghana. The government had come into power on a wave of popularity and there was a need to satisfy some of the constituents with jobs. The first place they turned to was the quasigovernment sector, such as the Nutrition Commission, and once people are established on a commission, even if they are not the best choice for the job, it is very difficult to change. Those of you who know the British system know that you can overthrow a government very much more readily than you can change members of the civil service.

In the beginning, the board was supposed to operate partially through the Ministry of Health, with direct responsibility to the president. After the country became a republic in 1960, the responsible area of the board was moved from the Ministry of Health to the Ministry of Agriculture. This was in fact the point at which I took over as executive secretary for the board. We had, at that time, a very knowledgeable and highly interested Minister of Agriculture and, therefore, the board was fully into partnership with the ministry when it dealt with food and nutrition problems at both the international and national levels.

At a FAO conference, Ghana gave a position paper calling on the UN agencies to make a special effort on nutrition in sub-Saharan Africa. That effort had several prongs. One was the establishment of the London-Ibadan Nutrition Course, of which there are two products at this conference. The other was nutrition literature production for middle Africa, for which Michael Latham and others helped produce quite a lot of useful material.

While this was happening on the regional scale, on the national scale the Minister of Agriculture and the principal secretary took great interest, and plans were made to have the board function as a planning, coordinating, and evaluating body. In 1961, a trained nutritionist was made available to the board. In addition, committees were established for various sectors of nutrition: clinical nutrition, food production, and nutrition information and education, each chaired by the representative of the ministry most directly concerned. It appeared for a short time that this arrangement would work well.

These committees groped but did not have too much success. One lesson we learned is that if you form a council, even if only to coordinate activities, there has also to be some funding available to be fed through the various agencies that carry out the activities. Without that, then, despite agreement on various programs at the council level, each agency is going to reassess its own priorities, in terms of what was agreed, before allocating its budget. It would have been better, with hindsight, if there had been a set target budget agreed to and then fed into the agencies' own budget without their having permission to alter that budget.

Soon the question of where the Food and Nutrition Board would be located became a political tussle. Unfortunately, when a previous Minister of Agriculture, who had lost his position in the cabinet, came up for an appointment, he was made executive responsible for the Food and Nutrition Board. This man (I'm quoting from one discussion I had with him) said, "I did biology in school. I know all about nutrition." This gives you an idea of what happened from that point on. *He* was the nutrition chief for the country, and *his* group was to do nutrition.

Thus, when funds were made directly available, this minister, with no other responsibilities, found it necessary to create a food and nutrition empire. He decided that he wouldn't filter the funds through various agencies, but, rather, he would employ people, put them on the road, and have his own nutrition show going. Without advice and with little concern for procedures, he recruited well over 100 officers in a few weeks with no job specifications. Titles ranged from Nutrition Officer to Field Assistant. Cars were purchased in curious circumstances. Before this show got on the road, the president found out about it and the new recruits were sacked, the cars impounded. The minister was removed. From then on, however, the board had lost irrevocably the confidence of ministries and agencies.

An effort at resuscitation was made in 1963 with the passage of a new act. The Nutrition Board was then given back to the Ministry of Agriculture. But the rot had already set in. This act also had little impact because the new executive secretary had no training in nutrition other than what he had acquired as a medical student. The ambitious recruitment programs shrank, but, again, the board tried to go it alone. It went into catering, into direct nutrition education, and even attempted to plant vegetables.

With the change of government in 1966, a new decree was issued which converted the board into a National Food and Nutrition Advisory Council. The idea was reinforced that this agency should be a planning, coordinating and evaluating agency, not an executive agency. For a short while, there was a serious effort made along those lines. The committees were revitalized and the slow process of rebuilding a sense of coordination and planning was started. The new council consisted not only of the heads of relevant ministries, but of the university departments concerned and the Food Research Institute as well. It did some good thinking and some progress was made, but gradually more and more ministries were being represented by the junior staff and the meetings became rarer and rarer.

Then a new civilian government came in and said that it wanted to emphasize nutrition. It also tried to reformulate the program by appointing political personnel to the board, and it lost even more ground. Since the 1972 change in government, it appears that the council has died. The nutrition staff, who have been treated as Ministry of Health staff since 1966, still function, but there is no coordinating body. The board is supposed to cooperate, but it has not, to my mind. From the minutes I was reading last month, the actual council or board has not met in the last two or three years!

A new national development plan is now being written and this document includes a nutrition-sector plan. This has been developed since the National Nutrition Congress, held last year. The congress recommended that, within the Ministry of Economic Development, there should be a nutrition planner responsible for coordination of all the nutrition activities following the advice of the Food and Nutrition Advisory Council. The planner would then formulate this into a part of the total national development plan. To date, this plan has not been completed.

There probably is a time in the life of a nation when such advisory or coordinating boards can be formed with a reasonable chance for their success. Before that time has arrived, however, perhaps other approaches might be examined. I would, myself, put forward the approach which is being planned now in Ghana; perhaps the best thing would be to have nutritionists who have also learned planning and put them within the Ministry of Economic Planning. That ministry handles the allocation of development funds. If this plan is accepted, it should be possible to allocate funds specifically for direct nutrition interventions by putting those funds into the various agencies.

I would go further and add that to make that particular secretariat or office a valuable one, and not one subject to interagency fights, the leader of the secretariat should have a small group of top executives from the different agencies as his advisors and active helpers for preparing the plans. Whether or not they use ministerial, commissioner, or other advice, I would say it should be geographically oriented rather than nationally oriented. If you wanted to improve the nutritional state of northern Ghana, this small group should seek the advice of the chiefs and some of the senior officials in the northern Ghana administrations and not sit in Accra and expect to work from there.

Operation Feed Yourself: Food Protection and Research

Ghana had been importing increasing quantities of food over a long time. Two of the major imports have been wheat and rice. In the Central Region, nutritional problems, which were greater than for the North and South, were basically due to the fact that the bulk of the staple is calorie-poor and pro-tein-poor starchy roots and fruit. In 1963, we advised that an effort be made to convert this area to a cereal crop staple. This was accepted and included in the 1963-70 development plan, and efforts were to be made to increase the production of rice and maize, as well as their harvesting and distribution. This particular suggestion has been put into operation, and it is beginning to yield quite visible results.

Aside from the establishment of the Food and Nutrition Council, the agreement by the government to help implement Operation Feed Yourself has probably been the policy with the most significant potential for an impact on nutrition. The OFY program, which has been going on for about 2 years now, awakened the whole country to the need for self-sufficiency and self-reliance in food production. It has been relatively successful, and the national food figures recently released show that the program has definitely made an impact on the availability of food within the country. Whether this availability can be translated into consumption remains to be seen.

Operation Feed Yourself was launched on February 17, 1972. The program had the following objectives:

a   Production of abundant and better food to feed the nation and thereby eliminate the present food shortages.

b   Production of industrial raw materials to supply industrial needs both for import substitution and self-reliance.

c   Promotion of export crops to earn foreign exchange to make Ghana solvent and enable it to purchase those essential items which must necessarily be imported.

First priority is on increasing production of cereals, maize, and rice specifically; but there has also been an effort to get a better distribution of the foods through the normal market system by opening up feeder roads so that the foods can move.

According to the government's description,[10] OFY "was an emergency operation aimed at using all available resources to reduce the country's crippling and largely slavish dependence on food imports." 1972-74 were declared years for intensified production of selected crops and livestock as a short-term measure. This would provide a springboard for long-term agricultural development.

Organization: The program is under the control of the National Operations Committee (NOPC) which, through a Program Control Executive (PROCONEX), composed of the Principal Secretary of the Ministry of Agriculture, the Director of Agriculture, the Principal Coordinator, the Divisional Heads of the Extension Services, Seed Multiplication, Fisheries, and Economics and Marketing, coordinates efforts and gives technical and financial directions. Regional committees have been formed to provide operational-level leadership and supervision. The program provides inputs such as land, seed, animal feed, fertilizers, and insecticides as needed. Credit facilities and agricultural equipment are also to be provided on selective bases. The operation was launched with all the resources for public education available to the government. The imagination of the public was captured and enthusiasm generated. Though it is rather early, the indications are that OFY is a successful venture.

One major recent change in the pattern of food consumption in the country is the increased use of prepared foods. With rapid industrialization and urbanization this is inevitable, but it raises the possibility that family feeding will be even more seriously jeopardized. Increased consumption of flour and flour-based products is another change in the food consumption pattern of the country. In addition, rice has started to become a very important food item in the national diet.

The development strategy of the government is currently based on self-reliance. Ghanaians are urged to produce as much as possible of their own needs, both manufactured and agricultural. This goal, in turn, has stimulated the government to help sort out problems related to food production, processing, and marketing. In this field, therefore, the government is inclined to help with investment, encouraging poor families to go into relatively large-scale production.

It is too early to attempt a detailed evaluation of the impact of Operation Feed Yourself; however, certain facts are emerging. Ghanaians have been made conscious of the importance of farming: it is no longer considered a lowly job. A new awareness of the problems of food-crop farming has led to increased efforts to find solutions.

Some foods are clearly being produced in greater quantities now. The country is almost self-sufficient in rice and it is expected to start exporting. Small maize exports have already started. Cassava exportation is to be increased. Attention is now being directed to oil seeds and legumes which will influence nutrition. Among industrial crops, cotton is receiving very high priority and a target date has been set for stopping importation of cotton.

Operation Feed Yourself is probably the most important economic program Ghana has had for some time. Its first emphasis on food production has eased the strain on foreign currency reserves for easily produced foods. Its second emphasis, on production of raw materials for Ghana's own industries, also releases foreign exchange for capital goods. The inclusion of agribased small industries will ensure more diversified activity in rural areas. The whole approach materially assists with employment, and therefore, both directly and indirectly with the problems of food and nutrition.

While production and problems related to distribution have received attention, both direct nutrition activities and important indirect ones, such as the immunization of children, have not been included in the OFY campaign. The inclusion of these would help to make the program more complete.

Research and investigation have also been emphasized. This has concentrated largely on the development of new foods for vulnerable groups. Some of this has been undertaken in the University of Ghana's research laboratories by Oracca Tetteh and his colleagues. Other research activity has been supported by FAO and the UN through the Food Research Institute. This aims to devise methods of processing and protecting foods both for commerce and for use by nutritionally vulnerable groups.

Among the research activities of the University of Ghana and the Food Research Institute, the weanling foods program is the one of most direct relevance to the problems of the most nutritionally vulnerable. Oracca Tetteh is developing various mixes of a cereal with a legume or an oil seed. The idea is to prepare a "flour" which can be used for making the gruels or staple pastes which are the bases of a child's diet. Tests so far have been encouraging. What is needed now is a coordinated venture to test acceptability and commercial feasibility. The Food Research Institute and the Ministry of Health also cooperated in testing the value of the winged bean (*Psophcarpus palustris* Desu) in young-child nutrition. It was found to be excellent even for treatment of PCM. The bean has been grown on an experimental scale and large scale propagation is to be encouraged.

The Operation Feed Yourself type of program has always been the wish of some of us in nutrition in Ghana. The country was declining in food production because of mismanagement and lack of political decision. This new government, using regional structures, providing seed and fertilizer services, a minimum price for maize, and rapid collection through the national food distribution system, is making some effort to redistribute the wealth more equitably and to get people to produce a lot more food.

I'm quite convinced that, within Ghana, self-sufficiency does not mean only "effective demand." When we say self-sufficiency, we are not saying that every single consuming unit is getting a sufficient quantity. What we are saying is that sufficiency is being produced within the borders of the country so that, if other blocks were not in the way between production and the mouth of the consumer, the consumer *would* be getting enough. The next stage is the identification of the blocks and their removal. Whether the identification of the blocks points to feeder roads, storage, intermediate technology, or nutrition education, that's an exercise that should be undertaken as an integrated effort.

At this stage OFY is being supported enthusiastically. Time alone will tell whether the momentum can be maintained for long enough to achieve the desired ends.

CONCLUSION AND RECOMMENDATIONS

Many authorities have pointed out with conviction that malnutrition is usually the result of poverty, but the conclusion that the only way to end malnutrition is through its automatic disappearance with the eradication of poverty remains questionable.

Instances can be quoted where the growth in national community or even individual or family wealth has not necessarily led to the eradication of malnutrition. In Africa, for example, one can quote the figures of malnutrition for children of coffee and cocoa farmers. It is therefore necessary to attack the problems of malnutrition from two major angles:

1 There must be programs for alleviating poverty based on human, social, health, and welfare goals.
2 There must also be specific nutrition programs aimed at target groups (be they geographic communities such as northern Ghana or physiological groups such as the preschool child).

Ghana has enough facts on which to base realistic nutrition plans and programs. Although high-level nutrition personnel with experience in program planning, implementation, and evaluation are in short supply, that, in itself, should not be an excuse for inaction. The first and most important need right now is an inventory of those activities, both direct and indirect, which influence the nutrition of the people. A national coordinating body of some kind should then be formed to help rationalize, integrate where necessary, and give direction to the activities.

Organization

Specifically, therefore, there is a need to appoint an individual with skills in nutrition *and* planning to the Ministry of Economic Development. This individual will be responsible for working with other sector planners as well as with the ministries and agencies responsible for the nutrition plans to be included in the national development plan. It will be necessary for this nutrition-planning officer to have a small group of experts in food and nutrition as assistants on an ad hoc basis. The team should include the officer responsible for human nutrition in the Ministry of Health, the Chief Community Development Officer, the director of the food-crops section of Operation Feed Yourself, and the head of the Department of Food Science and Nutrition in the University of Ghana. Other executives might be included as appropriate for specific issues. If a group of this nature can operate together on a continuing basis, then the role of an overall national nutrition advisory council can be more easily defined.

The national nutrition advisory body should be a top-level policy body meeting once or twice a year to take stock and give guidance on future orientation of plans and programs. Its members should also have an advocacy role with colleagues and the nation at large on the importance of food and nutrition. In actual fact its political role of maintaining the interest of the government in food and nutrition policies and programs and canvassing for funds from both the public and private sector for activities in the field will be much more important than any specific technical role it may perform. Its structure and composition should therefore reflect this basic concept.

Each ministry and agency with food and nutrition activities should appoint an officer to be responsible for coordinating those activities within the agency and to link with counterparts in other agencies, either directly or through the nutrition planning officer. This concept would apply to the ministries of Health, Agriculture, Community Development, and Education, as well as the Council for Scientific and Industrial Research, the universities, the Catholic Relief Services, and the Ghana Women's Council.

Content

Programs for priority consideration should include the following:

1 Massive attack on PCM in children through
   a immunization schemes;
   b development, production, and subsidized distribution of cereal/legume mixes which will form a base for weaning diets in various cultural situations;
   c health education programs which emphasize breast feeding and child spacing;
   d family planning education, information, and services close enough to the people; this activity to be a joint effort between the National Family Planning Program and the Ministry of Health.
2 Concentration on some basic food technology to help in the postharvest storage of cereals and legumes, and in the preservation and distribution of fruits and vegetables.
3 Food technology requires separate emphasis within the Operation Feed Yourself program. Unless methods for collection and preservation of the foods produced are found, the impetus of the program may be lost. There are some traditional food industries such as the river prawn and clam industry

along the Volta which may be enlarged.

4 Genetic studies and selection of satisfactory species of the major food crops as well as fruits and vegetables.

5 Massive public education campaigns on a continuing scale for better feeding practices.

6 Training should continue to be given high priority. Specialists in food science and technology are needed, but perhaps the most important categories needed are home scientists—community extension workers of various kinds with a good background training in nutrition.

7 In some areas school feeding programs may be valuable.

8 Competence in program evaluation needs to be developed as part of the planning process to ensure good management.

Some of the program lines mentioned above are general enough to form components of the overall attack on poverty. Others are specifically target-group oriented. The government must be kept constantly alert to the fact that any gains made through target group programs can only be consolidated with improvement of the overall situation of individuals and families among whom malnutrition is a problem.

The discussion for Ghana is given together with that for Nigeria, beginning on p. 123.

5 NIGERIA

Ade Omololu

Ade Omololu, perhaps Nigeria's preeminent nutritionist, is deeply involved in government, academic, and international activities. Currently, Dr. Omololu serves as Professor of Nutrition and Director of the Food Science and Applied Nutrition Unit, University of Ibadan, Ibadan, Nigeria. He is a pediatrician who received his medical training in Ireland, Nigeria, and England, and later did postgraduate training in child health and in nutrition. Omololu has served as consultant to many international organizations and was recently elected Vice-Chairman of the United Nations University's World Hunger Program Advisory Committee.

BACKGROUND

Who Suffers

The nutritionally vulnerable in Nigeria consist of:

1 99% of the 80% of the total population who dwell in the rural areas;

2 the peri-urban dwellers (another 3% of the total population);

3 the infants, children, and pregnant and lactating women of the lower 30% of the socioeconomic scale of the rest of the population.

In all, over 85% of the country's population is vulnerable nutritionally for calories and protein.

In the rural sector, average income is around ₦200 a year (Naira; exchange rate US$1,= ₦0.63); while the peri-urban dwellers may average even less than this for most parts of the year. Thus, low purchasing power is one of the factors making for malnutrition.

The relatively high cost of local foods is due to a food supply inadequate to meet the demands of everyone, as well as to the relative affluence of a small elite whose members buy from the same markets. Lack of knowledge of food is also a factor. Staple foods and foods that are culturally known but less nutritious are bought at high prices while more nutritious foods, inexpensive and easily available, are disdained.

Changes in traditional child-rearing practices due to increased "sophistication," mass-media advertising, movements to towns, the absence of a nutritionally balanced weaning food for infants and children, and infections and infestations all make for increased nutritional requirements. During the first 3 or 4 months of life, the child is usually breast fed and its nutrition and growth are excellent. From the 4th month on, the increasing nutritional requirements of the child, the lack of a good weaning diet, and infections combine to retard growth and development, often leading to marasmus.

Pregnant and lactating women in the rural areas and in the lower socioeconomic strata in urban areas often do not increase their prepregnancy nutritional intakes. Food-consumption studies have shown that the average nonpregnant woman has an average intake of 1,850 kcal and 48 grams of protein per day, which is below the normal requirement. The extra needs of pregnancy make the unmet requirement even larger. The needs of lactation are also not met and if lactation continues over a long period, the deficit becomes more pronounced. Frequent pregnancies and infections also play a large role in the malnutrition of this group.

In the rural and peri-urban areas, the effect of infections, poor water supply, and poor environmental sanitation increase the malnutrition of the entire population. Even the men are affected by these factors and overt malnutrition is shown by increased absenteeism from work and low output, apparent in most of the factories and work places.

Relationship of the Health System to the Nutritionally Vulnerable

The availability of immunization services to children all over the country is very low. Of all the immunizable diseases, only in the case of smallpox is immunization effective throughout the country. Measles immunization is so thinly spread and sporadic as to be useless. Triple antigen (DPT) is only available in certain hospitals and centers in the main towns, and even here, very few children complete the inoculation series. BCG vaccine is rarely available in the rural areas.

Prenatal visits are fairly frequent in most urban areas where there are maternity hospitals, maternity centers, and health centers. Most pregnant women attend from the fourth month of pregnancy. Over 50% of deliveries, however, take place at home. In the rural areas, where health centers and maternity centers are few, most pregnant women attempt to attend a prenatal clinic at least once. Over 90% of deliveries, however, are at home with no professional supervision. Complications are usually brought to the centers or hospitals later.

According to the government, the present health services cover only 25% of the population. In view of the lack of accurate statistics, this figure must be accepted on good faith. There is no doubt, however, that this 25% consists mostly of the people in the big towns. Hospitals and health services as well as personnel are concentrated in the big towns. During the 1975-80 development period there are plans to extend health services to 60% of the population by improving delivery to rural areas using mobile clinics and health centers.

The nutritionally vulnerable are the last to be affected by and the last to utilize the present health services. Those in the rural areas are so far away from the available services that they are not served at all. Even those in towns have to wait their turns, along with patients with various diseases, in the scramble for attention and beds. Theoretically, infants and children are treated free in all government hospitals, but there are so few pediatric beds and physicians that these patients, too, have to join the long line to be seen by the one doctor in each of the government hospitals. The Maternal-Child Health (MCH) services exist only in name, and most of the ones that do exist concentrate on antenatal care and well-baby clinics. No patient—adult or child—can be given special diets or food supplements in government hospitals except as an inpatient. As hospital beds are few, this means that the nutritionally vulnerable have to be in a very bad state before qualifying for treatment.

The health budget includes all monies for salaries, curative and preventive medicine, and hospital maintenance, with no specific budget lines for each. The state governments contribute ₦186 million, and the federal contribution is ₦486 million. The money for new hospital and health center construction comes from the 5-year development plan, for which the state governments have allocated ₦487 million and the federal governments ₦750 million for the period 1975-80.

There are, in the country, the following health personnel:

doctors	3,672 (1,400 foreigners)
dentists	142
nurses and midwives	38,000
pharmacists, medical technicians, and radiographers	1,580

Eighty percent of the doctors are based in 6 or 7 big towns and at teaching hospitals with a total population of 5 million, while the remaining 20% are scattered around the country in the government and missionary hospitals trying to reach and serve over 65 million people. This distribution is also true, to a large extent, of dentists and nurses and midwives and other paramedical staff.

Food and Agriculture System

One cannot talk of an average family consumption figure for the country. Wide variations occur not only in diets and intakes but also in the composition of the family.

Average per capita daily allowance for the whole country is 2,470 kcal and 35 grams of reference protein. At the calculated average net protein utilization (NPU) of 65, the amount of crude protein required would be 53.8 grams/day. While hard-working adults will need more and children will need less, the figures above (2,470 kcal and 53.8 grams protein) reflect the demographic composition of the country, with 47% of the population under 15 years.

From actual measurement, based on weighing for 7 days, it has been found that the daily consumption figures for the rural areas are:

North	1,778 kcal	43.7 grams
West	1,613	41.7
Midwest	1,545	49.2
East Central	2,470	66.8
Southeast	2,111	58.0

The intakes of children also vary from state to state. Results of surveys show that they do not receive enough of either calories or proteins—in some seasons of the year, as little as 50% of the requirements.

Diet patterns and staple foods vary from state to state, from season to season. The country can best be divided nutritionally into 3 parts:

1 North
2 Southeast, including Rivers, Southeast and East Central states
3 Southwest, including Lagos, West, Kwara, and Midwest states

North: Staple foods in this area are cereals, such as sorghum and pennisitum (millet). Not many detailed food consumption studies have been carried out in this area. The average dietary intake is about 70% of the requirement of the adult rural population.

Children are fed on gruels of cereals and water supplemented by breastmilk and slowly weaned onto the adult diet. Protein-calorie malnutrition is regularly seen in the hospitals in this area.

Southeast: Staple foods here are cassava, yams, plantain and corn. The main bulk of the diet and a large source of energy is yams. The caloric requirement of this group is usually fulfilled, though during the "hunger season," from March to June, intake may fall by 40% or more.

Southwest: The diet is based on cassava, although some yam and maize are also eaten. The calorie intake in this area is very low, as is the protein intake. The intakes, as percentages of the requirements, are as follows:

	Calories	Protein
Children 2-12 yrs.	50-80%	50-70%
Adolescents (both sexes)	52-73	44-50
Adults	84	90
Pregnant and		
Lactating Women	57-73	48-65

In all these figures, the effect of the hunger season is masked in the per capita per day averages.

The intake of women is 1,860 kcal/day. This is not increased during pregnancy or subsequent lactation, which may last up to 21 months.

Infants are breast fed for a long period, but supplements are usually added to their diets from the 6th month: gruels of maize and water, yam mashes, and so on.

Purchasing System   The purchasing system of the vulnerable groups differs but little from that of the elite. In towns, all foods are purchased from the daily markets and both the rich and poor compete for the same types of foods. In the rural areas, the farmers too have to purchase a large percentage of the food they eat. In the midwest state, studies in the villages show that between 16% and 75% of the food eaten by the villagers is bought. In the Western state, between 25% and 75% of food consumed in the rural areas is purchased.

Exports and Imports of Food   For 1972, imports of food totalled ₦48,082,812, including beef and meat products, live animals, milk and milk products, fish (canned, fresh, and smoked), wheat, rice, maize and other cereals, coffee, cocoa and other beverages, animal feeds, and wines and other alcoholic drinks.

Food exports totalled ₦71,224,654 for the same year and included shellfish and crustacea, coconuts and kola nuts, cocoa, edible nuts, spices and ginger, and groundnut cake and other feeds.

Food Transport and Storage   There is a great problem in the transportation and storage of food. It has been estimated that at least 30% of foods harvested never reach the table. In the case of soft fruits, like tomatoes and oranges, at least 70% must be wasted. The problem starts with improper harvesting and packing on the farms. Harvesting is often done when it suits the farmer, to meet a "market day," or to beat the market, and not at the best time for the crops. Due to the absence of insecticides and pesticides, crops are often infested before harvesting. All produce is harvested into baskets. This practice causes bruising of soft fruits and breaking of hard tubers. These baskets are then carried to market either on the head or in overpacked vehicles. By the time the crops get to the market, they are bruised, broken, and weeping.

There are very few storage facilities on the farms. Yams may be kept for 3 to 6 months on racks. Cassava is left in the ground until needed. Spoilage is great for all stored products, whether on the farms or in the market stores. A few silos are now being constructed and small storage facilities are also being developed.

Land Tenure   The pattern of land tenure differs in the North and South. In the North, the land belongs to the government and local councils; thus it is relatively easy to control its disposition, sale, and use. Unfortunately, most of the land in this area needs irrigation for proper yields and this is only now being developed.

In the South, land tenure is more rigid and traditional. Land belongs to families and the heads of families can sell or dispose of the land. At the death of the owner, the land is usually divided up by the sons amongst themselves. This continuous fragmentation of land has resulted in the small plots of land presently available to peasant farmers. The average area per farmer is 1.2 hectares. Farmers may have to travel 10 miles or more from their homes to find larger tracts of land to borrow or lease in other villages.

Subsidies and Price Controls   There has been no attempt at price control or subsidy of food commodities in Nigeria until very recently. At all times, government policies have been directed to the production of "cash crops": cocoa, groundnuts, and palm oil and kernels. These have all been subsidized or had prices fixed by the government. Most imported foods are subject to some price control, as well as to a policy to increase imports whenever prices rise beyond a certain level. Until recently, however, production of food crops has been left largely to the peasant farmers with the hope that supply will meet the demand and thus result in stable prices. Within the past year, the government has realized that this has not happened and is now trying to subsidize fertilizer purchases through cooperative societies. This practice is very recent and very limited.

Agrarian Reform   No agrarian reform is taking place or envisaged for the country. Peasant farmers with their small holdings are being exhorted by the government to produce more food. The government is trying to encourage cooperative farming, so that farmers will pool their land for better use. Model and demonstration farms are also being developed so that peasant farmers may see what can be done even on their own small farms.

New Technologies   The government also had stations which carry out research on food crops and the use of agricultural machines. New faster-growing and pest-resistant varieties, as well as better cultivation techniques, are being developed. At present, the bottleneck is in the transmission of these new technologies to the farmers themselves. Unfortunately, due to small acreage, poor agricultural-credit facilities, and illiteracy, most peasant farmers are at present making little use of these advances. The government is making tractors available on hire and more money is made available for agricultural-credit lending, but the illiterate poor farmers cannot benefit fully. The few literate and relatively rich farmers are at present benefiting most from these government programs. In addition there is a great shortage of extension workers, and those that are available have been used traditionally to encourage cash crops. The shortage is acute and the Ministry of Agriculture is aware of the need for an effective extension service. One hopes that as more extension workers reach the present farmers and more cooperatives are formed, all farmers will begin to benefit from the government's help.

Income Distribution

Income distribution in the country is lopsided. There is a relatively rich 1% made up of private entrepreneurs, government senior servants, and the elite. This is followed by a small middle class; finally, there is the 80% or more of the population that lives at subsistence level.

   The minimum expenditure necessary, per person, to support the *present* average dietary level is about ₦90.00 a year (US$144.00). Most of the 80% of the population in rural areas cannot afford to purchase this amount of food, but are able to grow some of their own food. The urban slum dwellers, who have to buy all their food as well as housing, clothes, and so on, are even worse off.

   There is at present no conscious policy to change income distribution. It is hoped that as more money becomes available, rural dwellers and the urban poor will receive a greater share of the country's income. In addition, it is hoped that the present farmers, by increasing production, will receive more income from their crops.

GOVERNMENT POLICY

The government does not at present recognize a nutrition problem, but concentrates its energies on a *food* problem: the relative shortage of commodities with resultant high prices. One is often left with the impression that the government does not differentiate between *food* and *nutrition.* The food problem was noticed because of the agitation of workers for increased wages necessitated by the high prices of food. Statistics from health and agriculture are, in fact, so inaccurate that they do not show the nutritional problems accurately.

The main solution being pursued by the government is that of making more food available on the market. It plans to do this in the long run by increased food production. In the short run, the government plans to alleviate the problem by increasing wages, thus expanding the money supply, and by increasing food imports.

These solutions were evolved because of the perspective of the problem as a food problem and not a nutrition one. Since most advisors and senior officials equate food with nutrition, it is probable that no other solutions of the problem were discussed or proposed before the provision of more food was accepted as the answer.

The government identified the following as major blocks to the program of increased food availability:

1 difficulty of stimulation of peasant farmers to increase food production;
2 problems in the development of seeds, elaboration of better cultivation techniques, provision of fertilizers, credit facilities, and so on to the peasant farmers.

To overcome these blocks, an expenditure of ₦2,291,000,000 on agriculture is planned over the next five years. The federal government will spend ₦1,013,000,000 and the state governments ₦1,189,000,000. There is an "Accelerated Food Production Program" to work on better seeds, better varieties of maize, yam, and cassava, and improved cultivation techniques so as to ensure increased production by the farmers. Agricultural research will be intensified on food crops. At present 5 research centers exist and a new one on fruits and vegetables will be developed. In addition, more agricultural extension workers will be employed by the state governments.

Agricultural credit for farmers will be liberalized by setting up state regional credit boards and banks. Cooperatives will be built so that farmers may be easily reached and may make use of credit facilities, subsidized fertilizers, and so on.

Even with the achievement of increased food production proposed by the government and the vast sums of money being spent to achieve this goal, there are problems still unrecognized by the government:

1 Statistics on food production in the country are very inadequate. The results achieved by the vast sums of money now being spent cannot be evalu-

ated in 5 years' time, as there are no definite production targets for any of
the food items.
2 The food policy is directed at all food items. There are no specific plans for
encouraging production of nutritionally desirable foods. Thus cassava production may be trebled with no improvement in legumes or animal protein. On
the other hand, a lot of money may be spent on dairy cattle to increase the
production of cows' milk while other important items of the diet may be
neglected.

The federal and state ministries of health occasionally have nutrition units,
but have these as mere appendages and never expect much from them. Most
of the staff of these units are relatively junior, and they are not consulted
about policy and planning. Furthermore, most have no budgets. Thus the
ministries of health do not and cannot use these nutrition units for policy and
planning.

The thirteen ministries of agriculture—one federal and one in each of the
twelve states—have been wholly responsible for dealing with the problem.
These ministries decide on and are able to present cogent and coherent policies to the economic planners, based on their aforementioned orientation
toward food rather than nutrition. The economists, having no nutrition advisers or planners on their own staffs, have no choice but to accept the agricultural policies. Other groups, outside the government circle, can be effective
only indirectly. Nutrition groups are found in the universities, and there is a
Nutrition Society of Nigeria. Members of these groups can serve on "advisory" committees and pass resolutions, but they have no guaranteed influence
on the government.

There is no national nutrition council or committee. There are only advisory committees on nutrition to the national councils of Agriculture and
Health. The National Council of Agriculture is made up of the federal and
state commissioners of agriculture and their senior staff officials. The advisory committees on nutrition are established by the respective national councils
to advise on the nutrition matters which arise in these national councils. The
advisory committees cannot initiate action nor make new proposals and thus
have little impact. For example, the advisory committee to the National
Council on Agriculture has been called together only once in the past 4 years.
The advisory committee on nutrition to the National Council on Health is
called together about once a year. This committee is working on a food and
nutrition policy for the country and has invited representatives from the
ministries of Economic Planning, Agriculture, Education, Statistics, Labor
and Social Welfare, and the Nutrition Society to contribute.

Although government plans are intended solely to increase food production, there are other governmental programs that will have effects on nutrition.

Nutrition Education

The federal government is planning a universal primary education program for the whole country starting in 1976. It has been possible to put some nutrition education into the curriculum by working through the national Ministry of Education. Teachers in the teacher training colleges are now taught some nutrition, to be included in the home economics section of the primary school curriculum. Also, by working with the Ministry of Education, it has been possible to use nutrition materials in the textbooks being prepared for teaching English in the program.

Soyi-Ogi

This is a food developed from maize and soya beans nearly 10 years ago by the Federal Institute of Industrial Research, a government organization. Soyi-ogi has a high protein content (10-20%) and can be used either as an infant or an adult food. Ogi, or maize gruel, is the main weaning food in most parts of the country. It is also eaten by adults about once a day. In the traditional form, its protein content is around 1%. The new high-protein food is being produced in a pilot plant with a daily capacity of 3 tons. It is hoped that an industrial plant, partly or wholly funded by the government, will be in operation before the end of the 1975-80 development period.

Road Development

Large sums of money are being spent by federal and state governments on road building and development. New feeder roads from farms to towns are being built, and parts of the roads in towns are being enlarged. There is no doubt that these roads will allow for easier movement of food and thus affect nutrition, not only in towns but also in the small villages.

Water Supply

Dams   At least three big dams are being constructed in the country for irrigation and power, as well as many smaller dams for local irrigation. These dams will supply irrigation water throughout the year and ensure higher yields.

Potable Water   Less than 20% of the population currently enjoys a good water supply. During the dry seasons, most villagers have to trek 6 or more kilometers to collect dirty water from stagnant pools. Waterborne diseases are rife in these areas. Guinea-worm incapacitates farmers, reducing productivity; diarrheal diseases and waterborne infections work synergistically to make malnutrition worse. The federal and state governments plan, within the next 5 years, to provide pipe-borne water to 50% of the population. This program will be a great step forward in the fight against malnutrition.

All these programs are in the 1975-80 Development Plan and thus still in the early stages. Results cannot now be evaluated, though there is no doubt that they will all have direct and indirect effects on malnutrition.

Legislation

The government has never passed any legislation relating to nutrition. The first Federal Adviser in Nutrition, a medical officer, was appointed for the term 1947-50 because of the insistence of the British government on the improvement of nutrition in the colonies. The post has been maintained in the national Ministry of Health ever since, but has lost its importance, and the present incumbent is known as Consultant Nutritionist. He is but one of many consultants in the medical service, with many senior and chief consultants above him.

Recently, laws were promulgated concerning food manufacture, standards, and contents. Food inspection officers are now being trained to effect this legislation. There is also a Food Standards Committee which works on standards along with the Codex Alimentarius Committee.

The Food and Drugs Act was promulgated in 1974. Enforcement will start as soon as enough inspectors are trained.

Policy Toward the Private Sector

Government policy with respect to the private sector in industry and agriculture is tied into the government program of increasing food production and food availability. Support for this sector is given in many ways: help in setting up factories and farms, and by making possible the importation of fertilizers and equipment. In many cases, state governments are ready to go into partnership with private industry to ensure the success of projects.

Nonprofit Sector

Charities have played very little part in nutrition in the country since the end of the civil war in 1970. The local voluntary organizations concentrate their nutrition work in helping orphanages, the sick, and the distressed with gifts of food whenever they can do so. Although their activities are officially encouraged, the impact is localized and sporadic.

Churches and religious groups tend to concentrate their nutritional programs on affiliated organizations. Foods, nutrition education, etc., are given to needy members. Nigeria has many religious organizations, and the various governments find it difficult to give strong support to them due to their parochial activities.

Communications

The federal and state governments have no direct policy regarding the mass media, although all the radio and television stations are government owned as are at least 8 of the 12 daily national newspapers. In spite of this, government control of the mass media is very loose. There is no direct interference or control apart from choice of personnel. The general policy of the mass media seem to be to (1) remain viable and a commercial success, and (2) entertain and educate. As the government has no policy on nutrition, each station editor has a free hand in giving news. Thus, talks on the radio and television can be arranged with directors and producers of special programs. Also, by personal contact, it is easy to get articles on nutrition published in any newspaper regardless of whether the article is for or against government policy. During the 1st African Nutrition Congress held at Ibadan in March 1975, all the national newspapers reported the daily proceedings; talks were given by participants on the broadcasting service; and panels, made up of participants, appeared on television to discuss the themes of the congress. The recommendations of the congress were also widely publicized by the media. This, however, was not because of government support or acceptance of the recommendations of the congress.

INTERNATIONAL AID

The developing world, and especially Nigeria, had high expectations for the efficacy of international agencies in solving nutrition problems. Unfortunately, these expectations have not materialized. The reasons, although sometimes not obvious, are many times extremely obvious.

The UN agencies have had very little impact because of the many restrictions they have imposed on themselves and their advisers. The government of Nigeria does make use of UN agencies; however, UN advisers and consultants are enjoined by their agencies only to concern themselves with what they are asked specifically to do. But nutrition problems are interdisciplinary, both in causation and erradication. Most UN consultants are constrained to offer advice only in their specific field of expertise, but not on the prerequisites that are lacking, personnel that must be trained, easier and cheaper ways of managing programs, and so on.

In addition, nutrition is part and parcel of life: part of the culture, the traditional economy and the education of the people. Without knowing something of these aspects of the life of the people, it is always difficult to advise or plan for better nutrition. Yet, the UN agencies prohibit the use of nationals as consultants and instead bring people from outside who have little or no idea of the background or way of life of the people. Thus, their advice is very superficial and frequently fails to get to the root of the problem.

Bilateral international agencies and advisers are much worse. Apart from little knowledge of Nigeria and its nutritional problems, they try to promote their country's products or to solve Nigeria's problems the way their home country has approached its own nutritional problems. For an example, agencies and advisers from the United States may be more interested in pushing soya beans or high lysine maize as panaceas to Nigeria's nutrition problems, while agencies from Scandinavian countries see stockfish or fish powders as the answer. Yet Nigeria itself has a lot of foods much better than any of these for which no new technique or education would be required.

Milk and milk products, soya beans or soya powder, stockfish or fish powders alone cannot make an impact on nutrition in the country. What is needed is a compact package of nutrition education, increased food production with emphasis on high protein foods, food subsidies, research on and use of better storage facilities, improved health services with immunization, a good water supply, basic family health and family planning, and a judicious redistribution of money.

International agencies can make an impact in the country by repeatedly putting indirect pressure on the government to realize that there is a nutrition problem. This can be effective if the consultants invited to advise on agricultural technique, seeds, technology, nutrition training, clinical nutrition, and development planning, seize the opportunities to help their local counterparts realize that there is a nutrition problem as distinct from the food problem.

FUTURE DIRECTIONS OF GOVERNMENT POLICY

In January and February of 1975 ₦300-400 million were added to circulation as the result of a minimum 30% pay rise plus arrears for government workers. Most workers in industry received comparable increases. About 5% of the *working* population benefited from this salary increase, but the self-employed and the farmers did not. One of the direct results of this policy has been an enormous increase (30-50%) in the cost of local foods and a higher rise in the cost of imported foods. How this will affect nutrition cannot be forecast.

The main developmental strategies of the government for the future are (1) quick industrial growth, (2) strengthening of the infrastructure, and (3) an egalitarian society.

Industrial growth includes the development of new industries and the strengthening of existing ones. In the next 5 years, an iron and steel complex, petrochemical complex, 3 vehicle assembly plants, and enlargement of cement, textiles, and plastics industries are envisioned. This section receives the first government priority.

The government, however, realizes that the proper development and growth of the industrial sector depends upon good infrastructure. This is currently lacking in the country, so a lot of money will be spent on infrastructure during the next 5 years. Projects will include roads and feeder roads, telecommunications, energy and power, education, housing, and food production. A low priority in this sector is health, which is thought of mostly as a social service.

It is in the provision of an egalitarian society that the best hope for the nutrition of the people lies. If the government can be made to realize that increasing the availability of food does not guarantee that the poor and needy will get enough and that special steps and policies need to be followed to ensure adequate and balanced diet for all, then the battle will be won. Another aspect that must be looked into in the fight for an egalitarian society is the need for a redistribution of income and wealth. At the present time, little action is being taken to redistribute income and wealth. The elite and rich seem to be getting richer while the poor are getting relatively poorer. A general food subsidy/control could go a long way toward ensuring the poor and nutritionally vulnerable a fair share of the available foods.

DISCUSSION (GHANA AND NIGERIA)

Winikoff

Unfortunately, at the last moment Dr. Omololu found that he could not travel to Bellagio, so Fred Sai is standing in for him and will discuss both the Ghana and Nigeria cases.

Sai

We have been groping in the economic field, the agricultural field, and so on, and wondering how to get a proper mix which will ultimately help to influence the nutritional status of people. There is also the other side of the question: *is* it possible, by some more direct approaches, to influence, in a short-term period, the nutritional status of identifiable needy groups?

To help identify the "vulnerable groups," in the nutritional sense, I put a graph on the board. In developing countries, now, there is what is called the camel-back mortality phenomenon. In Europe, there is a relatively high mortality in the very early days and months of life, but, by the age of two to three, there is practically no mortality among children. We also have a very high initial mortality rate—probably ten times as high—in developing countries, but we also have, at the time when European rates are low, an additional hump. It is not as high as the first-year peak, but it certainly is high. It is in this area of mortality that direct nutrition intervention, properly conceived and properly supported, ought to be able to achieve some rather rapid results.

A second target group would be pregnant women and nursing mothers. You will find, again, when you compare Western mortality patterns to those of the less developed countries, that the mortality rates of women from about 15 to about 40 in our countries is relatively high. Indeed, it it almost the only mortality rate in the world in which the female rate exceeds the male, and it is partly a result of poor nutritional status. To a certain extent, the approaches that were taken in Ghana to deal with the nutrition problem, however unsuccessfully, did have an identifiable input into addressing these problems.

In dealing with both Ghana and Nigeria, I would like to note the truism that a mouse and an elephant are both animals, but that's all they have in common. Nigeria and Ghana are two countries in West Africa. One country has taken good cognizance of its size and, therefore, does a reasonably good census. It thinks of itself in more coherent terms, despite occasional outbursts. The other country, because of the political implications of each new citizen in a one-man/one-vote situation, and because of the distribution of national wealth by state, has been finding it very difficult to count heads officially, although it has spent a lot of money on at least two censuses. The most recent government in Nigeria has officially cancelled the census that was done in 1973, and therefore, a new census will be undertaken.

We do have, however, some indicators which are of crucial importance in the nutritional sense. Between 45 and 50% of the population of both countries is under 15 years of age; about 20% of the population of both countries is under 5 years of age. This under-5 population in both countries contributes something like 50% of the total mortality of the countries. This is where nutritional status contributes considerably. Despite Giorgio's doubts as to whether this has an identifiable influence on the national economy, it cannot be good for a national economy to make women go through a nine-month pregnancy, one-and-a-half years of breast feeding, and then lose the product without its growing up to produce anything at all for the population. I'm no economist, but, in my simple-minded way, this is how it sounds to me. There are aspects, of course, in which the two countries are significantly different. Ghana, unfortunately, unlike Nigeria, has no oil and therefore, with the current economic crisis, Ghana has had to pay a very high price for petroleum. Despite the recent rise in the price of cocoa, the country may try to get itself put into the MSA (most seriously affected) category.

In his paper, Dr. Omololu makes the clear point, by contrasting sharply with Ghana, that there has really been no serious national awareness of nutrition as a problem in Nigeria, although recently a lot of noise has been made about food. There are reasons for this. In a country which is still importing a large quantity of food, which is agricultural, which has a huge territory, and, therefore, distribution problems, it is a good thing for that country to emphasize local-level production and variation of the food production pattern. What Dr. Omololu should emphasize, I think, is that this in itself will not solve the nutrition problem and that other things have to go with it.

There is no nutrition board or nutrition council in Nigeria. They tried to form a national nutrition association, but I don't think it is doing very much right now. Despite this, they have done some marvelous studies in nutrition with surveys and research on the growth of schoolchildren and experiments with school feeding programs. Dr. Omololu himself has been handling the London-Ibadan nutrition training course for the last three years. The emphasis of this whole course has now shifted so that it has become a nutrition training course run for people from developing countries, handled by the University of Ibadan entirely. It not only has a theoretical part to it, but it has quite a large element of practical training.

I think that if we're trying to get at things which have happened and how they have happened, the people who have been involved actively ought to identify themselves and let you know their inputs and their feelings. I was very glad when the field work of the London-Ibadan course was handled in my laboratory in the Danfa area and in Accra. This type of training might be studied by countries or regions which are still trying to develop nutrition training to see whether it can be replicated for other areas.

Vamoer
The experience of the Ghanaian board was that it shifted from health to agriculture, gradually becoming an independent organization. Now, you are advocating that probably the best way to handle the nutrition situation in Ghana is by introducing a combined economist and nutrition planner into the

Ministry of Planning. What is the best way of accomplishing this—organizing the Ministry of Planning and doing nutrition for the whole country?

Sai

I wouldn't see that person as doing nutrition for the whole country, just as you wouldn't see any other member of the Ministry of Planning as doing any of the sectors for the whole country. I see him helping the executive agencies' senior personnel to identify their needs in solving the nutrition problem. Then he would get these needs into a tidy package to be included as one of the sectors of the overall plans which are being formulated. Having done that, he and some of the others help to interpret, at the operational level, the decisions that are required, backed up by the fact that they have the control of the release of the funds for those agencies.

I would expect that that particular person as well as his colleagues in the planning secretariat would be able to put their fingers on methods for the overall evaluation of how their plan is being implemented and whether it is succeeding. For each person, there might also be a need to have direct links with the agencies carrying out different sections of the plan.

Vamoer

Are you saying that this planner should be a link between units within the different ministries and plan through them? Then success also would depend on the effectiveness of those units within each ministry.

Sai

Exactly. For example, here we have within the Ministry of Agriculture, the Operation Feed Yourself program. Now, this has captured the imagination of the whole country. As I said, they are emphasizing cereal. With the present level of laboratory work on the winged bean and the possibility of mixing it into a basic flour, which can then be used for preparing all the usual foods, there is absolutely no reason why Operation Feed Yourself, which has no money for intermediate level technology, cannot include this food source. This person should be able to encourage Operation Feed Yourself, Oracca Tetteh, and the Food Research Institute to come together and move on that item. If increased bean production succeeds and the beans get distributed properly, it would literally make available an additional 10-20% in the protein consumption of the young child.

Vamoer

In Zambia, we are thinking along the same lines: we should have a nutrition planner. But where should we put the planner? Should he be with the commission? Should he be with the Ministry of Health? Should he deal with Agriculture and Rural Development? Should he be with Planning? The first choice was to put him in Planning. The reaction of Planning was, "We don't plan nutrition. If you want a planner, put him in Agriculture and Development." This was despite all our arguments that this has nothing to do with production but has something to do with planning.

Finally we had to locate him in Rural Development. Rural Development said, "Okay, if you want us to have this additional cost, we will have to have a say in the plans." So, it was reluctantly accepted. Then they said, "Since we have been associated with the Ministry of Health, let's first have the support of Health." What that means is someone who is doing nutrition is forced into Rural Development. So Health puts its foot down and says, "We must have power on the National Food and Nutrition Commission although we have no individual there."

Sai

This has been said over and over again: This is how political decisions work. There are many ways of tying the animal, but the point is that there should be some place high enough for the planning and integration of a minimum package which will constitute nutrition.

If you put the Nutrition Planning Commission in the Health Ministry right now, there is the problem that Health and the National Family Planning Program view each other with daggers drawn; but if you put it in Agriculture, Operation Feed Yourself is the blue-eyed boy. A new program somewhere else in the Ministry of Agriculture right now is therefore unlikely to have high visibility, even within the Ministry. It so happens that in Ghana they have started strengthening the Economic Planning Ministry. They have identified the sectors of the planning procedure, and they are trying to pull together the proper kind of people, so that the Ministry can perform its actual planning functions.

You see, nutrition is really, finally, a function: it is the product of many inputs, such as food production, immunization programs, etc. When you are planning by function, like nutrition, if you don't have a special person within the planning secretariat, you get involved in the problems you describe. For Ghana, I think the nutrition planner is the right approach. I wouldn't go beyond that.

Solimano

I couldn't agree more. I think that experience currently is demonstrating that these Food and Nutrition boards are unable, in some way, to tackle the whole problem. There is no specific location for the programs, and, wherever it is put, it will be biased toward that sector.

We must also remember that planning is just the beginning of the game. The next step is how the program is going to be developed and how the activities are going to be performed and what is it we are going to say to the people in the field. Sometimes we do not give enough attention to doing because we are so concerned with planning!

How are you going to do education? Only through the educational system. To do anything else, to duplicate functions, is dangerous. So how do you sell nutrition to the educational system, to the Ministry of Education? I would like to try to come out with some specific recommendations for new approaches to this problem of planning with other areas of government. I think programming and activities are suffering because we are too concerned with high-level planning, and we are not giving enough consideration to implementation.

Antrobus

It seems, in any of the food and nutrition planning, inevitably some specialized programs lodged in particular ministries will result. As an example, you mentioned. Operation Feed Yourself. Bear in mind both the manpower situation in the countries that we are speaking about and also the fact that there is a strong political drive to set up these special programs. Is the manpower situation becoming more critical because these specialized programs skim off the best people? Are the day-to-day, run-of-the-mill programs in agriculture or education or health, in fact, suffering as a result?

Sai

Ghana, despite the usual statement of manpower shortages in LDCs, is not even in the lower half of the developing countries in terms of manpower resources available. In fact, one of the problems in the public sector has been overstaffing and bad deployment of the human resources. There is a lack of a definition of activities for individuals within various agencies, although there is some effort at change. People who had collapsed in their chairs and were passing paper from place to place are now getting out into the field to see what is happening and do the work that they are trained for. I am quite convinced that, even in medicine, despite the ratios that you see, doctors can be made to do a lot more work if they are moved around and placed with other types of personnel. I wouldn't give the same answer if I were talking about Chad or the Central African Republic, but we are, here, dealing with two of Africa's countries which, in terms of human trained resources, cannot say they really are lacking.

Antrobus

Are you saying that these specialized programs, then, can be executed purely by effective redistribution?

Sai

Yes, because, if you look at the objectives of Operation Feed Yourself, which we are calling a specialized program, it is only reorienting the Ministry of Agriculture's objectives. It puts the emphasis on food crops, whereas the emphasis before had been on cash crops. Second priority is on cash crops which produce raw material for local agriculture, and last on crops for export. So it is a reorientation and reorganization of the group with much clearer objectives and much clearer tasks.

Montgomery

The last three country studies, in contrast to the first, do not give us a completed program which has had impact on a target group, but that does not mean we cannot learn from this experience. On the contrary, we have to recognize that food and nutrition policies are constantly in a state of birth, infant mortality, survival, malnutrition, and then obesity.

What you need to do in order to learn from these experiences, in my opinion, is to start with a target group, look back at the three decision orders, and then see what stages they go through. We can evaluate the performance of the government in stages even before a program starts. For example, the first stage has to be the stage of data gathering, finding out what the problem is. So we have all the questions about census-taking and nutrition data. You can look and see how well this has been done.

The next thing that has to be done is that this information has to reach the people who get ideas about what to do. This is what we call the promotion stage. Now you have different actors who begin to get involved once the data become available. These people begin to see possible solutions. They offer different proposals, and they begin to fight with each other and the different bureaucracies which stand to benefit from each of the different proposals.

Finally somebody says, "Well, we are going to do it this way." And this is the next stage, which we call the prescription stage, in which the president uses power and says, "I am going to do it this way. I'm going to have this kind of organization."

The next thing that happens is the stage we call the invocation, in which the president (or his surrogate) says something like: "Should we do it with the Ministry of Health? No, we tried them; now let's try the Ministry of Agriculture." Such a decision is a very important element in policy history. Why switch from the Ministry of Health to the Ministry of Agriculture? If the program switched from Health to Agriculture, what did Health continue to do that had relevance? What was the connection between the bureaucracies?

The point I'm making is that we can learn even from programs that are just getting started because other countries that are getting ready to make a change in their existing policy may be even further behind in the birth cycle. Even before the birth of a policy we can learn about gestation. I think Ken's question, for instance, is perfectly appropriate for us to consider: "What is the muscle that is going to be behind this thing?" Now that it is getting started, what are the prospects? Why do you think it's going to work in Colombia when it didn't work in Nigeria?

6 INDONESIA   Soekirman

Soekirman was born in a rural area of Bojonegoro Regency, East Java, Indonesia. He earned his Bachelor's Degree in Nutrition from the Academy of Nutrition, Bogor, Indonesia; his MPH degree from the Graduate School of Public Health, University of Indonesia, Jakarta; and his MPS (Master of Professional Studies) degree in International Development from the Graduate School of Nutrition, Cornell University, Ithaca, New York. The author was a public health nutritionist in Aceh Province, northern Sumatra, from 1960 to 1966. Since 1966 he has been Head of the Division of Community Extension Service, Academy of Nutrition, Jakarta. In 1975, Soekirman was assigned to the staff of the National Development Planning Agency (BAPPENAS) to deal with nutrition planning, policy, and programing at the national as well as regional levels. This high level responsibility is a new type of post in developing countries, and gives Soekirman the kind of front-row seat that few nutrition advocates have had previously in the process of government planning of national development policy.

INTRODUCTION

As a developing country with a population of over 130 million, consisting of thousands of islands, and inhabited by many ethnic groups, Indonesia faces at present multidimensional development problems. With a population growth rate of 2.1% annually, the problems have become more and more complex.

Not until 1966 were the social and economic problems of the country properly approached. In 1969/70-1973/74 a first Five Year Development Plan (PELITA-I) was launched, and at present the government is implementing the second Five Year Development Plan (REPELITA-II, begun in 1974/75).

The national development program is based on the state's Basic Policies, *Garis Besar Haluan Negara* (GBHN) promulgated by the People's Consultation Assembly *(Majelis Permusyawaratan Rakyat)*. This states that the ultimate aim of national development is to achieve a just and prosperous society, in a material as well as in a spiritual sense based on "Pancasila," the country's basic philosophy of Five Principles. It emphasizes that national development will, in essence, be the development of the Indonesian Man as an individual and of the Indonesian Community as an entity.

The development of the Indonesian Man and Community includes the development and improvement of the human environment. Consequently the problems of the human environment, such as food and nutrition, are receiving more attention in REPELITA-II.

This paper attempts to delineate the nutrition problems in Indonesia, the role of the various factors which might affect the nutrition status of people and the Indonesian government's policy and programs in dealing with these problems.

NUTRITION PROBLEMS IN INDONESIA

Indonesia is the fifth most populous country in the world, and population growth is the real problem in Indonesia, specifically in Java, the crowded main island. The nutrition problem, the development problem, and the poverty problem are all centered in Java as well, because it is so densely populated.

Protein-Calorie Malnutrition

Since malnutrition and infection are synergistic, it is worthwhile to note here the overall picture of child health problems in Indonesia. As shown in table 1, in almost all age groups, acute respiratory infection and infections of the skin and subcutaneous tissues are the most prevalent diseases. It is also significant that the prevalence rate of diarrheal diseases is high in under-five children. All these infections result in increased nitrogen loss and diarrhea reduces the absorption of nutrients from the intestinal tract as well. The infant and under-five mortality rate is still high: 125-150 per thousand or 50% of total deaths. This reflects the poor nutritional status of under-five children in Indonesia.

In other words, the overall picture of child health in Indonesia suggests that malnutrition, particularly mild and moderate PCM, is widespread. An average of 28% of all the children under five in Indonesia are suspected to suffer from mild and moderate PCM, as defined by Gomez, with about three percent suffering severe PCM (table 2). This means that more than seven million under-five-year-old children must be protected from the immediate danger of severe malnutrition, and more than 600,000 children who are already suffering from severe malnutrition should be treated in order to prevent premature death.

Vitamin A Deficiency

The data on vitamin A deficiency is probably more widely available than information on any other nutritional disease. This is because of the extensive surveys carried out over many years, starting before World War II (table 3). Currently the prevalence rate of xerophthalmia (1972-73) is found to be 3.1-4.7%.[1] Unfortunately, because of the variations in criteria used in each survey, it is impossible to see whether any decrease has occurred in the last decades in the incidence of xerophthalmia. From the data available, however,

Table 1
Household survey, Indonesia, 1972. Disease pattern in preschool children

Rank	Disease	Number of cases	Percent
1	Acute upper respiratory infections	284	25.1
2	Infections and inflammations of the skin and subcutaneous tissues	265	23.4
3	Diarrheal diseases	129	11.4
4	Acute lower respiratory infections	96	8.5
5	Nutritional deficiencies	59	5.2
6	Infections of the eye	53	4.7
7	Other infections and parasitic diseases	40	3.5
8	Infections of the ear and mastoid	32	2.8
9	Malaria	25	2.2
10	Measles	20	1.8
11	Others[a]	129	11.4
Total		1,132	100.0

Note: Total 14,177 children, between the ages of 1 and 4 years.
[a]"Others": diseases other than those listed here.
Source: See ref. 3

Table 2
Prevalence of PCM in children 0-5 years, using Gomez classification

Country and Region	Year	n	Moderate PCM (Percent)	Severe PCM (Percent)	Note
Indonesia					
Jakarta	1953	415	7.3	2.7	squatter area
Bogor	1959	110	44.0	3.6	squatter area
Jakarta	1967	118,631	29.6	1.6	hospital
North Sumatra	1972	103	22.0	2.0	villages
8 Provinces	1973	699	27.0[a]	4.8[a]	villages
Philippines	1972	57,703	?	3.86	hospital
Asia	1966-69	?	16-43.1	1.4-2.9	from 4 countries
Latin America	1966-69	?	4.4-32.0	0.5-4.1	from 12 countries
Africa	1966-69	?	5.6-27.2	0.5-7.6	from 8 countries

[a]The standards of classification used in this survey vary somewhat from the traditional Gomez groups. Severe PCM is here defined as weight less than 80% of standard and moderate is weight between 80-85% of the standard reference weight. (For traditional Gomez classifications, see footnote, p. 2.)
Source: See ref. 4

it appears that the prevalence remains essentially unchanged from studies done in 1938 up through the latest, done in 1973.

Data from the Eye Hospital of Bandung indicate that there was a trend of increasing numbers of cases of xerophthalmia among children aged 0-15 years. In 1967-71 the prevalence in this group was 12.9%. It increased to 15.9% in 1972-74. This is probably due to seasonal variation or because more attention was given to the problem.

Factors contributing to vitamin A deficiency are as complex as with PCM. However, massive oral doses of 200,000 IU vitamin A plus 20 IU vitamin E have demonstrated effectiveness in reducing the incidence of xerophthalmia in pilot areas of rural Java[2] and in other countries.

This massive dose program is not the answer, however; it is only an "emergency" measure. In the Indonesian nutrition program it is called a "special measure." A rural development program which includes nutritional inputs is probably the correct long-term solution.

Goiter and Endemic Cretinism

Although goiter is relatively easy to prevent, it is still a serious problem in some parts of the world, including Indonesia. Goiter and endemic cretinism in

Table 3
Prevalence of xerophthalmia from hospitals and communities

Country and Region	Year	n	Xeroph-thalmia (Percent)	Note
Indonesia				
1 Pacet, West Java	1937	487	5.0	village
2 Kemayoran, Jakarta	1953	415	22.0	squatter area
3 Jogyakarta and Semarang	1953	7,000	4.0	hospital
4 Semarang	1955-59	5,699	6.0	hospital
5 Bogor	1959	156	12.8	squatter area
6 Pondok Pinang, Jakarta	1960-66	877	13.0	semirural village
7 Bogor	1967	2,487	7.1	nutrition clinic
8 Central Java rural	1963	867	4.0	village
9 Central Java rural	1973	1,374	5.2	village
urban	1973	1,438	4.3	squatter area
10 Jakarta	1968	118,631 35,048[a]	1.64 5.56[a]	hospital
Philippines	1961	29,746	8.9	hospital
Ceylon I	1955-58	5,245	8.4	north hospital
Ceylon II	1955-58	16,124	0.5	child hospital
East Pakistan	1962	537	18.6[b]	hospital

[a]Number of those classified as malnourished, and the percentage of these suffering from xerophthalmia.
[b]Recorded as xerosis and keratomalacia.
Source: See ref. 4

Indonesia were originally reported in the studies done before World War II. Eighty to 90% of the population in the mountainous areas is afflicted by goiter. Salt iodization was, therefore, introduced by the Dutch government in the 1930s. At that time, salt production was a government monopoly, so the legislation was relatively easy to enforce. However, after independence, salt production ceased to be a government enterprise.

In the first two decades after independence, goiter was a neglected problem. It was only in 1960 that several studies on goiter were started in West Irian, Central Java,[5] East Java, North Sumatra, East Java, and Bali. Data from these studies demonstrated that the prevalence rate of goiter was as high as in the preindependence period. Sixty to 90% of the children in rural areas of Sumatra, Java, and Bali, were found to have goiter (table 4).

The problem was demonstrated even more strikingly when Djokomoeljono[5] mapped the widespread prevalance of goiter in Indonesia (figure 1). He confirmed the existence of endemic cretinism (defined as two or more of the following in children born in an endemic goiter area: mental retardation, permanent hearing disability, or permanent neuromotor abnormality) as anticipated by the preindependence document on goiter. In one goitrous village of Central Java, he found that 17% of the people were cretins: the highest prevalence found in the world.

Djokomoeljono estimated that at present there are about 10 million people in Indonesia afflicted by mild and moderate goiter with 100,000 suffering from cretinism.

It is urgent, therefore, that a program to alleviate goiter be given priority. Resources required to implement this program are minimal compared to what is required to alleviate other nutrition problems, and, in addition, the probability of success is high. In 1976/77 ten small units of iodization equipment will be installed throughout Java and Sumatra. About 120,000 metric tons of

Table 4
Prevalence of goiter among schoolchildren, by sex

Country and Region	Year	Boys		Girls	
		n	Percent	n	Percent
Indonesia					
1 Kediri (E. Java)	1966	182	54.3	173	58.9
2 North Sumatra	1972	874	59.8	909	65.2
3 West Sumatra	1972	1,080	85.2	1,143	93.4
4 East Java	1972	950	82.6	763	85.2
5 Bali	1972	586	79.5	398	79.4
6 Jogyakarta					
Kulon Progo	1973	1,585	31.0	1,450	37.9
Bantul	1973	503	46.9	524	55.7
Gunung Kidul	1973	967	47.8	810	50.4
Sleman	1973	1,366	75.6	1,252	81.5
Total Indonesia		8,093	61.9	7,422	67.3
Ukinga, Tanzania	1965	1,676	74.0	869	81.4
West Pakistan[a]	1955	–	41.3	–	72.3
Thailand	1958	2,856	32.3	2,816	40.6
Brazil	1943	850	38.6	712	44.8
United States[b] Michigan, Wisconsin	1924	–	40.0	–	60.0

[a]Total children examined = 319.

[b]Before iodized salt was introduced. After iodization, the rate dropped; it was 1.4% in 1951, among 53,785 school children examined.

Source: See p. 45 of ref. 4

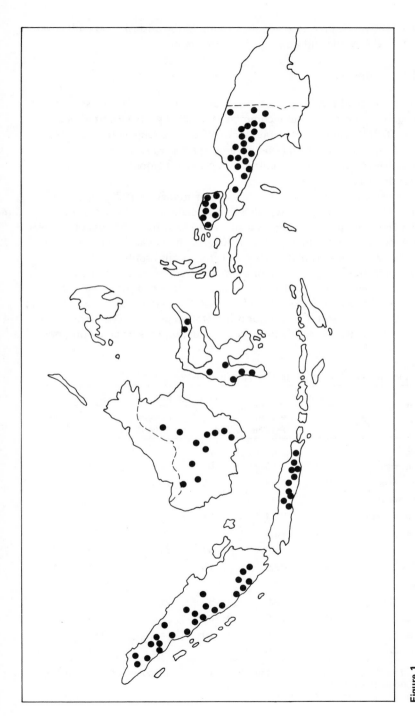

Figure 1
Goiter in Indonesia. Source: See ref. 5

iodized salt will be produced and distributed to the critical areas with government subsidy for the additional cost of production.

Nutritional Anemia

Although detailed studies on nutritional anemia in Indonesia are scanty, it is
recognized as one of the more common nutritional problems. Studies carried
out in 1972/73 demonstrate a prevalence of anemia ranging from 50-92%
among pregnant women, and 35-85% among nonpregnant women in rural
areas (table 5). Nutritional anemia is also prevalent among construction and
plantation workers (table 6).

Of a sample of 573 Indonesia male workers studied in 1972, 28-52% were
anemic. Most of this anemia was due to iron deficiency. The prevalence rate
among 398 plantation workers studied was 45%; of this, 60% was due to iron
deficiency. The epidemiology of nutritional anemia in adult males suggests
that income constraints play a dominant role in this problem.

The public health significance of anemia, including lower productivity, poor
work habits, and high maternal death rate, was partly confirmed in the
studies by Karyadi[6] in 1974. No definite solution has yet been formulated to
deal with this problem. Iron pill supplementation proved to be effective in
correcting nutritional anemia for experimental purposes. It could not, how-

Table 5
Prevalence of anemia based on the hemoglobin level, WHO standard

Country and Region	Pregnant		Nonpregnant		Males	
	n	Percent Anemic	n	Percent Anemic	n	Percent Anemic
Indonesia						
Bandungan	40	92.5	84	84.6	34	35.2
Bogor area	109	68.8	75	35.1	—	—
Indramayu-						
Purwakarta	51	78.4	21	56.0	10	50.0
Gunung Kidul	54	50.9	34	44.1	53	28.3
Bali	57	54.6	31	38.7	25	36.0
Bali	46	46.9	19	47.3	31	16.1
India						
New Delhi	100	80.0	95	64.3	—	—
Vellore	100	56.0	100	35.0	99	6.0
Mexico	124	26.6	110	11.7	111	0.9
Venezuela	95	37.0	107	14.9	52	1.9

Note: The WHO standard is: Less than 11g/100 ml for pregnant women, and 12g/100
ml for nonpregnant women.
Source: See p. 27 of ref. 4

Table 6
Distribution of hemoglobin for tappers and weeders at plantations

	Weeders		Tappers	
	n	%	n	%
Hemoglobin (g/100 ml)				
above 14.9	7	4.7	12	4.8
13.0 - 14.9	76	51.3	122	48.8
11.0 - 12.9	53	35.8	103	41.2
9.0 - 10.9	10	6.8	12	4.8
below 9.0	2	1.4	1	0.4
Number examined	148		250	
Mean	13.0		13.0	
Standard Deviation	1.4		1.4	

Source: See p. 31 of ref. 4

ever, be adopted for a larger program, let alone a national program.

Iron fortification is being considered in Indonesia. The difficulty lies in finding the right carrier to reach the target group. The technology for iron-fortified salt is not yet available in Indonesia, but experimental work being carried out in India raises hope for the future.

FACTORS AFFECTING THE NUTRITION PROBLEMS IN INDONESIA

It is well recognized that the ecology of malnutrition involves many variables: (1) food availability, (2) adequacy of family income, (3) food habits and education level, and (4) prevalence rate of infection.

There is no systematic study of the relative importance of these various factors in Indonesia. In practice, the four factors merge and it is most likely that all are important factors in the nutrition problems of Indonesia, with the exception of goiter.

Food Availability

Total food availability is determined by food production, import, export, and waste.

Food Production   Table 7 shows food production in PELITA-I (1969-74) and the first year of REPELITA-II (1974). During this period, production kept pace with population increases. There was some success in promoting the production of rice, meat, eggs, and milk. Unfortunately, this was not the case for corn, tubers and legumes, yet these latter are actually the commodities most likely to be accessible to low income groups in rural areas, mainly in

Table 7
Food Production, 1968-73 (thousands of tons)

Food	PELITA-I						Average Increase, Percent, 1968-73	REPELITA-II
	1968	1969	1970	1971	1972	1973		1974
Rice	11,666	12,249	13,140	13,724	13,183	14,607	4.8	15,452
Corn	3,165	2,292	2,825	2,606	2,254	3,600	0.7	3,239
Cassava	11,356	10,917	10,478	10,685	10,385	11,186	-3.6	13,775
Sweet Potato	2,364	2,260	2,175	2,211	2,066	2,387	-2.5	2,916
Soybean	420	389	498	516	518	541	3.6	550
Groundnut	287	267	281	284	282	290	1.2	315
Sea Fish	723	785	808	820	836	860	3.6	893
Land Fish	437	429	421	424	433	440	0.1	449
Meat	305	309	314	332	366	403	5.7	394
Egg[a]	1,162	1,300	1,319	1,503	78	81	10.4	101
Milk	28,600	28,923	29,306	35,797	38	35	7.0	57

[a]1968-71, number of eggs; 1972-74, kg of eggs.
Source: Presidential Address to the Congress, August 16, 1974 and 1975, Annex

Java, South Sumatra (Lampung), and Irian Jaya.

As indicated in table 8, 24% of the calorie and 30% of the protein intake of the rural poor are derived from corn; while for better-off rural groups only 13% of both calories and protein are derived from corn. On the other hand, urban people, even the poor, rely mainly on rice. The urban poor appear to have a food intake level even worse than that of the rural poor.

Rice has been the focus of the food production scheme in PELITA-I and REPELITA-II. As shown in table 9, rice production is projected to increase from 15,032,000 tons to 18,183,000 tons in 1978. Meanwhile, the demand for rice accelerated from 14,810,000 to 17,180,000 tons. Output from intensification schemes (BIMAS/INMAS) is projected to rise from 70.6% of consumption demand in 1974 to 87.4% of demand in 1978.[8] It is unlikely that rice demand can be met by total domestic production in this period.

Based on the trend of rice production and demand in 1968-74, Sugyanto and Tedjokoesoemo (1975) projected the production and demand of rice in 1978-98. If rice production increases at the rate of 5-6% annually, they projected that the demand for rice could be met after REPELITA-II, assuming achievement of the goal of a 25% decrease in the fertility rate by the family planning program in Indonesia. Without reduction in fertility rate, rice demand will not be met by the year 2000.

Aside from rice, the production of some animal protein sources (meat, eggs, and milk) was also increased considerably by 1973. It is probable that increased production was partly due to the impact of a poultry-raising campaign launched by ANP-Indonesia, particularly in 8 provinces of Java, Bali, West Nusa Tenggara, and Sumatra.* The agricultural people feel that the increased production of animal protein must be an important improvement in the nutrition of the people; but nutritionists must explain that people who are most affected by malnutrition don't drink milk, and they don't eat eggs. The improvement is for hotels because tourism is increasing, which, of course, is a good thing economically. In addition, there is a rising demand for animal protein because many incomes are getting higher. But, if one looks at the protein sources of the poor rural people, there is no progress at all. By examining these figures, we can show that what has been done in the last five years is *not* a *nutrition* policy but a *food* policy, mainly for rice and some animal foods.

"Not by rice alone" is a message which is being actively delivered to people as part of the new nutrition education process. The government of Indonesia became fully aware of the drawback of the "rice policy" in PELITA-I. Therefore, in September 1974, a presidential decree (INPRES No. 14/1974) on "The Improvement of People's Menu" was issued. This is in line with the food production policy in REPELITA-II. In this plan, the food production scheme will not be concentrated on rice only, but on secondary crops as well.

*The fallacy of this "campaign" to meet a "protein gap" in Indonesia was presented by Sajogyo in his recent paper.[20]

Table 8
Food intake of rural and urban households in Java, by income levels, October-December, 1969

	Rural Households (59.3 million)			Urban Households (11.9 million)		
	Poor (52%)	Better Off (48%)	Mean	Poor (54%)	Better Off (46%)	Mean
I. Calories (kcal)						
1 Rice, corn, tubers	1,143	1,778	1,455	1,009	1,325	1,182
2 Pulses, coconut	40	66	54	45	77	61
3 Fish, meat, eggs	24	84	52	30	121	77
4 Sugar, oil	76	244	157	107	280	193
Total calories	1,283	2,172	1,718	1,191	1,820	1,513
Calories from rice (%)	47	60	55	76	70	71
Calories from rice and corn (%)	71	73	71	79	71	73
II. Protein (g)						
1 Rice, corn, tubers	21.4	35.3	27.8	20.3	27.3	23.7
2 Pulses, coconut	0.8	3.4	2.2	1.5	5.1	2.9
3 Fish, meat, eggs	4.7	14.9	9.7	5.6	19.1	12.2

Total protein	26.9	53.6	39.7	27.4	51.5	38.8
Protein from rice (%)	47	51	49	69	52	58
Protein from rice and corr. (%)	77	64	68	73	53	60
Vegetable protein (%)	83	72	76	80	63	69
Protein (calorie percent)[a]	8.4	9.9	9.2	9.2	11.3	10.3

[a]Calories from protein as a percentage of total calories.
Source: See ref. 9; calculations from SUSENAS, the Central Bureau of Statistics, Jakarta. The poverty line is set at the per capita annual-income equivalent of 240 kg rice for rural households and 360 kg for urban households

Table 9
Projection of rice output and demand, Indonesia, 1973-78

Item	Unit	1974	1978	Average 1974-75	Annual Increase 1974-78 (percent)
Total population	thousands	129,082	141,578	135,260	2.3
Rice consumption demand					
Total	thousands of tons	14,810	17,180	15,988	3.8
Per capita per year	kg	114.7	121.3	118.2	1.4
Total rice output	thousands of tons	15,032	18,183	16,493	4.8
Per capita	kg	116.4	128.4	121.9	2.5
Percent of consumption demand		101.5	105.8	103.1	
Rice output from intensification	thousands of tons	10,466	15,027	12,684	9.5
Per capita per year	kg	81.0	106.1	93.7	3.1
Percent of consumption demand		70.6	87.4	79.3	

Source: See ref. 7

REPELITA-II aims to increase the production of corn from 2.6 million to 4.15 million tons, sorghum from 55,000 to 249,000 tons, cassava from 9.9 million to 1,275 million tons, soybean from 495,000 to 670,000 tons, and peanuts from 275,000 to 355,000 tons.

Food Import and Export   Calculated in calories and protein per capita per day, food imports in 1969 showed a negative balance for calories (more exports than imports) and a positive balance for protein (more imports than exports). The situation was reversed in 1973: calorie imports were double the calorie exports due to a significant increase in rice and wheat imports. However, more protein was exported, mainly from soybeans (table 10).

In 1973, soybean production increased less than 15% over 1969, while soybean exports increased fifty times.[*] Thus, a substantial amount of soybean was diverted for foreign trade. This, of course, increases the price of soybeans. Soybean is the only good protein source available for low income people, yet higher prices hinder the promotion of soybeans for domestic consumption, particularly for a weaning-food mixture to be developed in the future nutrition programs in Indonesia.

[*]Preliminary data available for 1974 showed that there was a significant drop in soybean and groundnut export: 88 and 45% lower than 1973, respectively. No information is available as to why this was the case.

Table 10
Calorie and protein import-export balance (per capita per day)

	Export							
	1969				1973			
	(midyear population = 113.63 million)				(midyear population = 124.32 million)			
	Thousands of tons	g/cap/day	kcal	Protein (g)	Thousands of tons	g/cap/day	kcal	Protein (g)
Corn	155	4	14.4	0.36	181.3	4	14.7	0.36
Groundnut	20	0.5	2.3	0.13	21.4	0.5	2.3	0.13
Soybean	0.7	0	0	0	36	7.8	25.8	2.70
Dried cassava	304	7	24	0.10	75.4	1.6	5.4	0.02
Cassava flour	0.6	0	0	0	1.3	0	0	0
Fish	10.71	0.3	0	0	26.07	0.6	1.2	0.10
Meat	10.80	0.3	0	0	11.88	0.3	0	0.06
Copra	157	4.0	14.4	0.14	44.60	0.1	0	0
Total			55.1	0.73			49.8	3.37
	Import							
	1969				1973			
Wheat and bulgur	347	8.5	31	0.76	648	15.8	6	1.4
Rice	796	19.4	7	0.13	1230	30	108	2.0
Milk powder	20.4	0.4	2	0.09	25.8	0.6	3	0.15
Fish products	–	–	–	–	6.5	0.1	0	0
Sugar	108	2.6	9	0	6.0	0.1	0	0
Total			49	0.98			117	3.55
Balance: (import-export)			–6.1	+0.25			+67.2	+0.18

Sources: Statistical Pocketbook of Indonesia 1972/73. Presidential Address to Congress, August 16, 1974, Annex; Presidential Address to Congress, August 16, 1975, Annex, Chapter VI

The policy on second crops, especially corn and soy, as envisioned in REPELITA-II, is that they should not be geared primarily for export. Efforts should be undertaken to promote more domestic consumption of corn and soy. This can be accomplished through nutrition education plus supplementary feeding using local foods (rice, corn, sorghum, soybean), as well as appropriate technology. These interventions would increase both awareness and domestic demand. Coupled with proper market institutions, this might be an incentive for farmers to produce more of these crops. In addition, a food policy is envisioned to guarantee that the increased production of soybean is not diverted for animal feed. The four lowest socioeconomic deciles, who live "below the poverty line," would benefit most by the promotion of soybean for direct human consumption.

Food Supply   Tables 11 and 12 indicate that there was no significant change in calorie and protein supply per capita per day between 1969 and 1972, during the first development plan. In this period, the mean calorie and protein supply were close to the WHO/FAO requirement (1971), namely 2,000 kcal and 40 g protein per capita per day.

The food pattern changed only slightly. In 1972 there was less consumption of root crops and fish and more of pulses and meat. It should be noted, of

Table 11
Calorie supply, Indonesia, 1969-72 (per capita per day)

| | Available Calories | | | | |
| | 1969 | | 1972 | | |
Item	kcal	%	kcal	%	Change (%)
Cereals					
Rice	1,030	52.9	1,040	52.9	—
Other	251	12.9	253	12.8	0.1
Rootcrops	251	12.9	226	11.4	−1.5
Pulses	105	5.4	114	5.7	0.3
Meat	19	1.0	23	1.2	0.2
Fish	23	1.2	21	1.1	−0.1
Milk	3	0.15	5	0.25	0.1
Egg	1	0.05	3	0.15	0.1
Fruits and vegetables	47	2.4	65	3.2	0.8
Sugar	116	5.9	123	6.2	0.3
Fats and oil	99	5.1	99	5.0	−0.1
Beverages	2	0.1	2	0.1	—
Total	1,947	100	1,974	100	

Source: See ref. 8

Table 12
Protein supply, Indonesia, 1969-72 (per capita per day)

| | Available Protein | | | | |
| | 1969 | | 1972 | | |
Item	g	%	g	%	Change (%)
Cereals					
Rice	19.5	47.6	19.8	47.5	−0.1
Other	6.8	16.6	6.4	15.6	1.0
Rootcrops	2.0	4.8	1.9	4.6	−0.2
Pulses	6.0	14.6	6.6	15.9	1.3
Meat	1.2	2.9	1.1	2.7	−0.2
Fish	3.5	8.5	3.3	7.9	−0.6
Milk	0.1	0.2	0.2	0.5	0.3
Egg	0.1	0.2	0.2	0.5	0.3
Fruits and vegetables	1.6	3.9	1.8	4.3	0.4
Fats and oil	—	—	—	—	—
Sugar	—	—	—	—	—
Beverages	0.2	0.5	0.2	0.5	0
Total	41.0	100.0	41.6	100.0	

Source: See ref. 8

course, that aggregate data on food supply is not identical to what is really consumed by the families and must therefore be interpreted with extreme caution. However, because of the supply figures above, as aggregate data, agricultural people have often felt that nutrition is not a serious problem. This attitude has created disagreement with nutrition people.

Data from a Food Balance Sheet can only be meaningful if coupled with both food consumption data on a household basis and clinical evidence. Agricultural people are proud of their success in increasing supply, but household surveys show that most of the people are still deficient in calories and protein. In Java, the problem is very acute, and there is also a problem in South Sumatra. North Sumatra and Bali are somewhat better as they have a calorie deficit but no protein problem. In Indonesia, it is most useful if data is collected on a regional or provincial basis, but the fact that there are 7 million under-five children suffering from PCM in Indonesia, and that about 40% of the low-income workers are afflicted by nutritional anemia, is evidence enough of the existing shortage of food in certain groups of the population.

Family Income

There is no argument about the importance of inadequate income as a major constraint to better nutrition, although its exact role remains to be defined. In Indonesia the anemic plantation workers consume diets very low in calories and protein, and they also belong to the lowest income group. The vicious circle of low income—inadequate food—malnutrition and/or anemia— low productivity—low income is likely to operate continuously in this group of people. One can observe that the only significant difference between the anemic and nonanemic plantation workers is income level. It is believed that increasing income, at least to the level of those who are not anemic, is the only effective and feasible alternative to improve the nutrition of this group.

About 46% of the population of Indonesia, or 55 million people, live below the poverty line, most of them in Java (table 13), and an Applied Nutrition Program (ANP) evaluation study indicated a substantial gap in calorie and protein consumption between the "poor" and "better off" people. The former consumed 30-40% less calories and had half the protein intake of the latter.[9] Cases of PCM, however, were found in the poor as well as in the better off families. A similar phenomenon was found by Lauw Tjin Giok and his co-workers in West Java in 1962.[10]

Thus, although income is important, it cannot be viewed as the panacea for malnutrition, particularly for under-five children. For them, income is likely to be effective if coupled with better education of parents and a favorable environment. For example, infant and under-five child mortality rates among medical doctors' families in Indonesia, were found to be as low as in developed countries: 15.9 per thousand and 73.5 per ten thousand, respectively.[11] The figures imply that in this relatively high income *and* well-educated group the nutritional status of the children is undoubtedly satisfactory.

Table 13
Number of people below the poverty line, Indonesia, 1969/70 (percent)

	Rural	Urban	Rural and Urban
Java	57	54	56
West Java			35
Central Java			64
Yogyakarta			67
East Java			60
Areas other than Java	28	38	
North Sumatra			21
South Sumatra			10
Bali			35
West Nusatenggara			47
Indonesia (overall)	46	49	

Note: The poverty line is set at the per capita annual-income equivalent of 240 kg rice for rural households and 360 kg for urban households.
Source: SUSENAS, 1969/70. See ref. 9.

In short, although income generation alone is probably effective in reducing malnutrition in adults, this might not be the case for under-five children. More comprehensive efforts involving the sociocultural aspects of nutrition and health must be worked out in the development plans.

Social and Cultural Constraints

Contributing to nutrition problems are lack of knowledge and education, improper food habits, and commonly held beliefs. Mothers and grandmothers, with their own concepts of what is good and bad for infants, have a special role in determining the health of children. Unfortunately, these concepts often run counter to the well-being of the child.

Indonesia has abundant resources of vitamin A in green leaves, yet vitamin A deficiency is prevalent among children under five. Most mothers do not know that green vegetables are necessary for children. In addition, they themselves are not used to eating them. Green leaves available in the villages have a low social value, and it is considered inappropriate to serve cassava leaves, *kangkung* (water cabbage) or papaya leaves in a feast.

The traditional weaning food is rice mixed with a very small amount of soya sauce, or brown sugar and banana, regardless of the economic status of the family. There is no concept that legumes, in the form of foods familiar to village people, such as *tempe* or *tahu*, are good for children.

It is hard to meet the calorie and protein needs of children with rice alone because it is so bulky. In addition, a carbohydrate diet is very bland; and this may diminish appetite. Thus, despite accelerating biological needs, the child consumes less calories and protein. This can be observed by body weights which are often level or declining after 6 months of age (figure 2). By this age, infections (particularly respiratory infections) and diarrhea often aggravate the poor nutritional status of the children.

In addition, diarrhea is often considered normal unless the loose stool is more than 6 times a day. Unfamiliar food is blamed for the condition,[12] and therefore, mothers and grandmothers are more cautious in giving food to the infants and young children, who may thus receive less than their nutritional requirements.

A "modern" cultural practice of bottle feeding, encouraged by the milk industries in Indonesia, is suspected to be influencing the breast feeding pattern. Table 14 summarizes a survey of rural weaning ages in Indonesia, carried out in 1970.[17] Fortunately, rural Indonesian mothers seem to breast feed into the second year. A nutrition survey done by the senior students at the Academy of Nutrition in August 1975, in rural Central Java, confirms this data.

In the city of Yogyakarta, however, a recent survey indicated that more than 70% of mothers weaned their infants by one year of age.[13] Early wean-

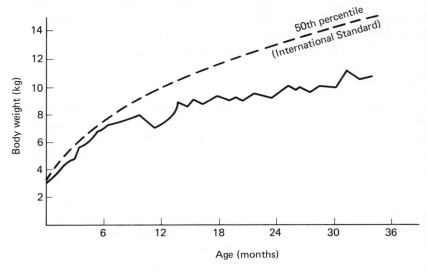

Figure 2
Body weight of children under five, rural Yogyarkarta. Source: See ref. 13

Table 14
Percent weaned, by age, various areas of Indonesia

Age (years)	W. Java	C. Java	E. Java	Bali	S. Sumatra
1	10	1	5	1	7
1 - 2	67	48	69	26	51
2	11	46	20	56	37
Not known	12	5	6	17	5

Source: See ref. 14

ing is followed by bottle feeding without any knowledge of the importance of uncontaminated water or other aspects of hygiene. This, of course, frequently leads to infections.

   The problem of intrafamily distribution of food is another cultural constraint. Children under five and pregnant or lactating women in rural areas of Indonesia are "nonprivileged" members in the family as well as in the society. Food is distributed accordingly, and as a result children and women often do not obtain an adequate share of the available food.

Infection

The high prevalence of respiratory infection and diarrhea among children under five is believed to be a significant factor in causing PCM. Subidyo and his colleagues found in 1974 that many malnourished children whose condition did not improve despite food supplementation had active pulmonary tuberculosis.[15] In another study, a wide variety of microorganisms were isolated from specimens of gastric and small-intestinal contents of 21 malnourished children in Jakarta,[16] lending support to the thesis of the synergism of infection and malnutrition. These facts also reflect the inadequacy of environmental sanitation and rural health services in Indonesia.

HEALTH SERVICES IN INDONESIA*

The components of the Indonesian health services system are: Hospitals, Health Centers, Maternal Child Health (MCH) Centers, and Polyclinics. There is a referral system linking all these components. The Health Centers are the basic component, and the MCH Centers, as well as the Polyclinics,—which function as sub-Health Centers with one auxiliary nurse—are branches of the Health Centers.

A case study in rural West Java in 1973 indicated that the utilization of health facilities in this province was low. Of all diseases in this area, 54.1% were untreated, 25.0% treated by a traditional healer (*dukun*) or self-treated, 18.8% were handled by paramedical personnel, and 1.6% by doctors. In addition, 96.2% of all obstetrical deliveries were assisted by traditional midwives and 3.3% by professional midwives.[†]

This low level of utilization of health facilities can be attributed to several factors:
- the low educational level of the people.
- the general inaccessibility of health services in the rural areas.
- the income constraint. (Health services in Indonesia are not free of charge. A fee of about $US0.60 is required for minor treatment, but the charge is waived for people who are very poor.)

The government is aware of these problems, and therefore, made plans to accelerate the program in REPELITA-II. The objective is to provide better health services more efficiently and effectively by:

- expanding health education activities;
- improving health infrastructure in quantity and quality; and
- training more health personnel, especially for rural health centers.

The budget for health, family planning, and social welfare in 1974/75 was Rp25.1 billion, or 2.2% of the total budget for development. Although the proportion of the budget for health was similar to the preceding years, the absolute amount was significantly larger.

*Unless otherwise indicated, figures cited in this chapter are drawn from these documents: (1) Department Kesehatan RI, 1975: Pelaksanaan Program Pembangunan Bidang Kesehatan Dalam Repelita-I 1969/70-1973/74; (2) Lampiran pidato Presiden RI, didepan DPR RI tgl. 16-8-'75 bab XV, p. 661.
†Unpublished data of Manpower Training Center, Department of Health, 1973.

In 1973/74 Health Centers did not cover all the subdistricts* in Indonesia. In Java, 60-70% of subdistricts had a Health Center, each of which was supposed to serve about 50,000 people. Outside of Java and Bali, the average coverage per Health Center was larger, approximately 95,000 people. Ideally, each center should serve 30,000 to 50,000, the exact number depending on the geographical situation.

The total number of Polyclinics has decreased since 1972 while the number of Health and Maternal Child Health Centers has increased (table 15). This is in part because the government is trying to increase the number of Health Centers by upgrading Polyclinics to Health Center status. The geographical distribution of these facilities has also changed somewhat (table 16). Between 1973 and 1978, the government aims to distribute health facilities equitably, according to population throughout Indonesia's 26 provinces.

In 1974 there were 512 government hospitals and 96 private hospitals[†] (table 17). Each hospital served approximately 217,000 people within a radius of 5 km. The occupancy rates averaged 55-85% of the available beds. Reasons for the low occupancy rates were: (1) frequent urban location of facilities, far from most of the people in need; (2) insufficient medicine available at the hospital; (3) inadequate facilities for good service; (4) poor delivery of services by the hospital; and (5) economic constraints. Private hospitals, also generally located in the cities, usually have better services, but these hospitals, with few exceptions, are accessible only to the higher income groups.

Medical and paramedical personnel are also unevenly distributed throughout the country. In 1974 there were 6,221 medical doctors, or about 5 doctors per 100,000 population. In Java this ratio was 4.6 and outside Java 5.6 per 100,000. There were 8,323 midwives and 7,736 nurses in 1974; most of these personnel were located in cities as well. The highest ratio of doctors to population was in Jakarta and Yogyakarta: 25.0 and 10.3 per 100,000, respectively. The lowest ratios were in East and West Nusa Tenggara (table 18).

Table 15
Total number of Health Centers, MCH Centers, and Polyclinics

	1973		1974		1975	
	Number	Population Per Unit	Total Number	Population Per Unit	Total Number	Population Per Unit
Health Centers	2,175	56,600	2,343	58,810	2,843	45,404
Maternal Child Health Centers	6,610	18,620	6,801	18,530	6,909	18,683
Polyclinics	7,418	16,596	7,124	17,690	6,975	18,507

Source: Dept. of Health, 1975

*The subdistrict is the lowest administrative echelon above the village level; subdistricts have an average population of 40,000.
†Excluding special hospitals.

Table 16
Number of Health Centers, selected provinces of Indonesia

Province	1973	1974	1975
North Sumatra	69	69	110
West Sumatra	33	40	63
South Sumatra	54	54	72
Jakarta	27	95	102
West Java	308	291	334
Central Java	263	386	442
East Java	576	576	616
Bali	50	14	29
West Nusa Tenggara	23	20	33
Central Kalimantan	26	29	46
South Sulawesi	172	124	150
Maluku	24	46	54
Total for Indonesia	2,175	2,343	2,843

Source: Dept. of Health, 1975

Table 17
Hospital facilities, Indonesia, 1973

Type	Number	Total No. of Beds	Hospital Beds Per 10,000 Population
General Hospital	608	61,241	4.85
Mental Hospital	32	7,570	0.60
Eye Hospital	7	1,035	0.08
Sanatorium	16	813	0.06
Leprosarium	70	6,256	0.49
Maternity Hospital	202	3,109	0.24
Total	935	80,024	6.35

Source: Dept. of Health, 1974

In order to improve health services for rural people, a regulation was enacted in 1974 to ensure that more health personnel, particularly doctors, work in rural health centers. By 1974/75 about 34% of all Health Centers had medical doctors, compared to 22% in 1972/73. In early 1975, even more health personnel (432 medical doctors and 2,270 paramedics) were assigned to rural Health Centers.

It is clearly understood that the present health services in Indonesia are by no means ideal, and new approaches are being studied. One of these is rural health insurance (*Dana Sehat*) initiated by Gunawan Nugroho in Central Java.[17]

The state of environmental sanitation in Indonesia is still poor. About 50% of urban people and 88% of rural people have no adequate public water supply.[18] In addition, approximately 29% of urban and 92% of rural people are not adequately covered by sewage disposal services.[19]

Since 1969/70, the urban as well as rural drinking water supply in Indonesia has expanded. In 1970-74, 2,882 hand-water pumps and 2,456 latrines were installed in those rural areas with poor water supply and a high incidence of diarrhea. It is estimated that more than 700,000 people have benefited, and the program is being continued.

GOVERNMENT NUTRITION POLICY AND PROGRAM

Historical Notes

The Awareness Period Nutrition activities in Indonesia began early, soon after Eijkman, the Dutch physician, found the connection between polished rice and beriberi. The forerunner of current nutrition activities in Indonesia was the Dutch Nutrition Research Institute in Jakarta (1935-50). Though the Institute was a part of the Ministry of Health, the interdisciplinary nature of nutrition was recognized early and staff members included biochemists, agriculturists, physicians, and statisticians. The activities of this old institute were primarily nutrition education and manpower training; nutrition research was minor.

Table 18
Distribution of health personnel per 100,000 population, Indonesia, 1972 (selected provinces)

Province	Population (thousands)	Doctors	Nurses	Midwives
North Sumatra	6,929	6.1	24.1	17.6
West Sumatra	2,815	6.4	16.9	18.2
South Sumatra	3,464	5.4	19.4	10.2
Jakarta	4,903	25.0	45.4	16.0
West Java	22,036	2.7	10.0	4.3
Central Java	22,770	2.2	9.0	5.7
East Java	26,443	3.6	7.2	5.4
Bali	2,146	4.7	20.5	14.1
West Nusa Tenggara	2,236	1.2	4.5	3.4
Central Kalimantan	726	2.1	19.3	8.0
South Sulawesi	5,386	3.2	21.2	7.1
Maluku	1,162	3.0	22.0	8.6
Total for Indonesia	123,115	4.2	14.2	7.6

Source: Department of Health, 1974

At first, the Institute was known as *Lembaga Makanan Rakyat* (The Institute of People's Menu). The words were literally translated from the Dutch, because the word "nutrition" in Indonesian had not yet been invented. *Gizi*, as a term for "nutrition," has been popular since 1960 and is now formally used for scientific as well as lay communication.

Although systems analysis was not yet known in Indonesia in 1960, its principles were used in analyzing the causes of nutrition problems. Food and nutrition policy was introduced to the policymakers even at this early date, and a National Food Board was even established once. However, since understanding of the concept of nutrition was still minimal, and the socioeconomic situation was unfavorable, a national program on nutrition was never formulated. Instead, nutrition education was implemented to create awareness, not only of the science of nutrition, but also of the complex nature of nutrition problems and the need for an interdisciplinary approach.

The Applied Nutrition Program (ANP) phase in Indonesia (1957-70) can be seen as a period of creation of public awareness through a multisectorial approach. Despite the fallacies of the Applied Nutrition Program concept, it did play a positive role in this sense, but the "mis-" and "non"-conceptions of ANP seemed to predispose the nutritionists in Indonesia to work without any conceptual scheme.[20] The period required to create awareness would have been shorter if the nutritionists themselves had had clearer overviews of their own field.

The Trial Period   Until 1965, the government was not dealing seriously with the economic or food problem but rather with politics and nationalism, trying to unify the country in the face of racial, religious, and provincial quarrels. Though there had been nutrition committees and programs, these were only lip service. Starting in 1965, the government realized that it faced a very serious economic problem. In 1968, the government initiated the first five-year development plan with food production as the main program. This program did not yet include nutrition.

In the second five-year plan, REPELITA-II, nutrition was included as part of the food policies; nutrition is now regarded as an important component of the development process. The government is thus now interested in "development nutrition,"* and the scope of nutrition is being enlarged from the traditional "health-nutrition" and "home-economics nutrition." This change resulted from the advance of the science and technology of nutrition, as well as the fact that the traditional nutrition focus did not solve the problems of malnutrition in the world.[21]

*Development nutrition is nutrition related to the overall process of economic and social development. Thus, it is a broad concept.

Health nutrition = nutrition limited to health aspects.

Home-economic nutrition = nutrition limited to agricultural extension activities.

Health and home-economics nutrition, in this paper, are together referred to as traditional nutrition.

What motivates the government at this time to adopt nutrition in the development policy? First, the change is probably the fruit of the awareness period. There has been nutrition education since 1938; though it was very traditional and poorly planned, it has had an impact in increasing awareness. Second, there is new knowledge about the reciprocal effects of nutrition and national development. Third, the role of international agencies in "persuading" the government to adopt nutrition as a part of development is undoubtedly significant. Fourth, the political, economic, and social situation in Indonesia at the present time is favorable for nutrition programs on a larger scale. With more stability, increasing incomes, and rising living standards, the government is able to attend to welfare issues, one of which is nutrition.

This analysis suggests that the enthusiasm for nutrition we are witnessing in Indonesia is the outcome of a long process with many inputs. This initiative has to be followed up with clear demonstration that development nutrition is as significant as the other development sectors. Hence, nutrition merits astute planning and programing.

This is thus a trial period for nutrition work and a critical moment for nutrition workers in Indonesia. Pilot projects in different aspects of nutrition should be tested. There is no doubt that a "success story" in nutrition has to be presented to the policymakers. As a result, capable leadership for the nutrition movement is badly needed in this period, and this is what is most likely still lacking in Indonesia.

Food and Nutrition in REPELITA-II

As mentioned, in contrast to PELITA-I, in REPELITA-II the section of the plan dealing with food is combined with nutrition concerns.

Food policy is directed toward:

A The stabilization of food prices at a level which is affordable by most of the population. At the same time, the rice price has to guarantee a reasonable income to the farmers, in order to provide the incentive to produce more rice.

B The improvement of the nutritional value of the people's food. Some steps to achieve these objectives are summarized below:

1 Improve market institutions and maintain floor and ceiling prices for rice.
2 Diversify food production and consumption, so as not to rely only on rice.
3 Promote production of vegetables, fruits, meat, eggs, milk, and so on for nutritional improvement. Couple these efforts with improved processing and marketing.
4 Improve the land tenure and land use systems, especially for the benefit of small and landless farmers. This program will be a part of the internal migration scheme.
5 Improve food storage and processing at the community level.
6 Undertake specific nutrition interventions: fortification, supplementary feeding, nutrition education, community nutrition programs, xerophthalmia

prevention programs, goiter eradication programs using Lipiodol injection or salt iodization, and caries prevention using water fluoridation.

7 Intensify nutrition research activities.

8 Enhance the development of food technology.

9 Formulate food laws which consider the nutritional aspects of food supply regulation.

10 Establish and develop nutrition units at the provincial hospitals.

11 Create an efficient and effective system of coordination, since all these activities involve different sectors of development.

What is Being Done?

A   Presidential Decree No. 14/1974, "The Improvement of People's Menu," is the most vital step in facilitating all the nutrition activities delineated in REPELITA-II. Among other things, this decree instructed the establishment of a Ten Ministers' Forum coordinated by the Minister of State for People's Welfare, and including the Minister of State for Economics and the National Development Planning Agency, and the Ministers of Health, Agriculture, Internal Affairs, Information, Education, Religion, Industry, and Finance. The word "forum" is used to indicate that this is not an institutionalized body.

This group is assisted by a Technical Commission. The membership of the commission includes a representative from each of the above ministries and is assisted by several ad hoc subcommissions on which sit technical people from different disciplines.

The subcommissions have succeeded in formulating guidelines for salt iodization, wheat fortification, nutrition education, and a revised ANP. A guideline for the promotion of breast feeding is being worked out.

B   Nutrition Task Force. Prior to the establishment of the Nutrition Technical Commission, a Nutrition Task Force was created under the National Development Planning Agency (BAPPENAS) in order to develop nutrition program plans. The members are technical experts from different professions.

The innovative concept of development nutrition was developed, and a Nutrition Intervention Pilot Project is being planned to carry out this idea. The project attempts to test the feasibility of complementary measures in preventing PCM at the village level.

Plans are also being made for developing new approaches to nutrition education, and for the development and extension of the Nutrition Research Center, the Manpower Training Center, and the Food Technology Development Center.

C   Health Nutrition activities will be continued as the routine job of the Nutrition Division of the Department of Health. This includes nutrition education, supplementary feeding, vitamin A programs, and goiter prophylaxis. Also under that department are nutrition surveys and research, assigned to the Center for the Research and Development of Nutrition, located in Bogor, as well as manpower training, continuing at the Academy of Nutrition in Jakarta. Home-economics nutrition is taught at schools under the auspices of the Departments of Education and Agriculture.

DISCUSSION

The Government's Food Policies and Their Nutritional Impact

The food production schemes in PELITA-I and REPELITA-II are directed toward:

1 Increased food production, especially rice.
2 Expansion of employment opportunities for the population.
3 Increased farmer income.
4 Increased production of export food commodities.

There is no question that the larger farmers benefited more from the increased production of rice to date. However, as demonstrated by Sajogyo,[9] malnourished under-five-year-old children can be found in both poor *and* better-off rural families. Thus, it is unlikely that increased production of rice automatically reduces the prevalence of PCM in villages of Indonesia.

Labor-intensive agriculture is the backbone of development in Indonesia. The basic purpose of the development programs is to provide enough food through increased production and to provide employment for rural people, yet for the farmers who do not produce rice, the small holders, and the landless farmers, benefits from the use of high yield rice are minimal at best. In the northern part of Central Java, use of the high yield variety (HYV) of rice reduced the need for harvest laborers because a new, more efficient method of rice harvest called *tebasan* replaced the traditional labor-intensive sickle harvesting. The old way represented a traditional form of income distribution, since the rich people, during the harvest, used every woman who had no land and then gave each a share. With the new methods, the rich people do not need large groups of workers, just a few laborers who come in a truck, harvesting and gathering for cash. So, now a lot of people have no way to get a share of the grain. Thus, the adoption of HYVs has not helped solve the problems of unemployment and income distribution in Java.[7,22]

A similar problem of new technology occurs with milling. Previously, rice was hand-pounded, but now the government has introduced small milling machines in every village. This represents a loss of work for the woman who used to get a share of the harvest for pounding the rice. When we explain this problem to planners, they say, "Everything has side effects." They want documentation of the exact extent of the problem, but we have, in fact, no data.

Thus, it is unlikely that the food policy in PELITA-I had a positive impact on the nutritional status of low income workers. In REPELITA-II there are more rural development programs being implemented, and, it may be hoped, this will mean more employment opportunities. Projects are started on labor-intensive works and agricultural development to open up opportunities for employment. In its "rural development" schemes, the government gives money to the villages, and the village decides how to spend it. One volunteer is assigned to work in the village for two years as a "change agent" who tries to motivate the people for self-development, in a way similar to that of the US Peace Corps. There is also a program for environmental health, in which the government gives money to villages for latrines, water supply, health posts, and special vaccination programs. Before the nutrition group came, there was no nutrition input at all. Now we are saying that if nutrition components are added to the program, the whole package may, indeed, lead to improved nutrition in the villages.

The Problems of Intersectorial and Interdisciplinary Approaches

The establishment of the Ten Ministers' Forum and the Nutritional Technical Commission must be commended, as such bodies are indeed necessary for coordinated and consistent nutrition policy. There had been, in fact, three similar committees in the past. The first (1952) was called the National Food Improvement Committee (*Panitia Perbaikan Makanan*). The second (1958) was the National Food Board (*Dewan Bahan Makanan*), which tried to deal with the whole nutrition problem but actually just worked on rice. Both of these first committees were chaired by the prime minister. The third committee (1970) was the Central ANP Board (*Behan Perbaikan Gizi Pusat*). In spite of the efforts exerted in establishing these committees, the results were not encouraging, a phenomenon also found in other developing countries.

In a seminar held in Bangkok in 1960, the two reasons offered to explain the lack of success of such commissions were "the absence of clearly defined functions and programs, [and] lack of trained nutrition workers to provide technical advice."[23]

More important is that these committees often failed to function as a system. Therefore, it is imperative to analyze the effectiveness of a nutritional institution, whatever it is, by looking into the factors affecting the performance of the system. Havelock's[24] summary and analysis indicates seven such factors:

1 Linkage: the degree of the interrelatedness and collaboration among members, and with outside institutions.

2 Structure: the degree of systematic organization and coordination.

3 Openness: willingness and readiness to accept outside help, willingness to listen. Readiness to consult and be consulted. A social climate favorable to innovations or new concepts or ideas.

4 Capacity: the capability of the members to analyze nutrition problems.

This is highly correlated with intelligence, professional training, educational level, experience, authority, and so on.

5 Reward: the frequency, immediacy, amount, mutuality, and structuring of positive reinforcements.

6 Proximity: nearness in time, place, and context, familiarity, similarity among members and the "outside world," particularly in the field of their concern.

7 Synergy: the willingness to support each other.

In order to have a nutrition system work efficiently and effectively, one must look not only into the organizational structure, but at the relationships of the people within this structure. The seven factors suggested by Havelock can be used as a tool to analyze the human factors affecting the system.

DISCUSSION (INDONESIA)

Soekirman

In sum, Indonesia is a new country, and the development process is going on
in all areas. But, without knowing the background provided in the paper, it is
difficult to understand why nutrition is now given priority.

My own involvement with the government's nutrition policy provides an
interesting vignette, demonstrating the interactions of many different forces
on the final shape of government organization and programs. What was done
after nutrition was written into the second five-year plan? In that document,
there was a section on agriculture and another on food and nutrition. In the
past, there had been nutrition programs in the ministries of Health and of
Agriculture, but without any clear concept of how they related to each other.

As a first step, after the announcement of REPELITA-II, a Nutrition Task
Force was established in the National Development Planning Agency
(BAPPENAS), and a senior nutritionist for nutrition planning was needed.
Fortunately, simultaneously, Cornell offered to train a practicing nutritionist
in planning and nutrition policy. So the government sent me to Cornell,
hoping that, when I returned, I would help work out planning for nutrition. I
came back to Indonesia last year and immediately was assigned to
BAPPENAS, part-time, to work on programs for the nutrition project which
will be supported by the World Bank loan.

I started by making a checklist of what is written in the five-year plan to see
what could and should be done immediately.

Planners said, "Now you have a place in the plan. Go ahead and accomplish
something. If not, the next five-year plan probably will contain no nutrition."
Then the agriculture people said, "We have done nutrition from the beginning
because we are providing food for the people. That's nutrition." The planners
were further confused because everybody claimed they knew all about nutrition and, in fact, that they had *done* nutrition.

My first difficult assignment was to demonstrate to various groups that
nutrition is not only a province of the Ministry of Health or Agriculture but is
involved in development. That's why I tried to introduce the new terminology, "development nutrition." How is "development nutrition" different
from what has happened in the past? I tried to sell the concepts elaborated by
Jim Levinson, Alan Berg, and others and to relate them to facts about mortality, morbidity, and productivity. We have some domestic data in Indonesia as
well as international data. So I made a matrix to relate each sector, each activity, to the total input for the development process.

It was hard work, but gratifying, because, when I finished, they believed
me. But then, because I had a diploma in public health, and they were short
of manpower, my boss said, "I assign you, not to nutrition, but to health.
You deal with health. Nutrition is part of health." But my nutrition colleagues and I resisted, because my time would be absorbed with the Health
Centers, hospitals, and so forth. Finally, my colleagues said, "If you can show

them that nutrition is something to be dealt with specially, you will most probably be assigned to nutrition." So I worked on the program to be supported by the World Bank, an innovative nutrition intervention project. We tried to show the connections between agricultural development, family planning, rural development, and then fit the nutrition input into that. Afterwards, they agreed to assign me to nutrition. I got much support from the World Bank team, including Dr. Latham and Mr. Thomson, in convincing the policymakers of the planning agency of my concept.

Now the challenge, after we work out the planning, is to implement it next year. We have to show a success story on our projects; otherwise the policymakers will not continue to trust us. With the idea of "development nutrition," nutrition is not an isolated program but an input in all development programs. So it will not be like the ANP, previously the kingpin of the village program. We never go to the village without our friends, the other rural development components. My assignment now is always to talk about what we are going to do in a village or an area as a whole. Which water supply, education, and nutrition inputs can you add?

Within the planning agency communication is now made physically easier because representatives of all sectors of development are represented in each room and there are also weekly staff meetings. At last, we are hoping we can make progress on nutrition in the context of development.

Levinson

Perhaps the first thing I would like to say is, that is a sad story. When we were in Indonesia, there seemed to be more optimism in the air, maybe because the increased oil revenues were so significant that there was talk of a budgetary surplus. There was pressure from the students, and officials were concerned that they not repeat Thailand's experience of student unrest in Indonesia. In addition, there seemed to be a certain amount of genuine interest in greater efforts directed toward social-sector programs. This isn't the sense that I get from your comments now.

My question is: What would happen to nutrition, and what would happen to you specifically in your role in BAPPENAS if you developed an index number similar in concept to per capita GNP, but meant to measure the welfare of the poor, weighted heavily with nutrition and health parameters, and, then, rather than having to prove that nutrition was important to development, you challenged the planners in BAPPENAS to find ways, in their development planning, to improve that number? You could then indicate that the programs for which nutrition people have a responsibility can, at best, supplement broader development patterns but can't substitute for them in solving the problem of malnutrition.

Maletnlema

The difficulty is that you have to have power to challenge the planners. Soekirman isn't given that power.

Levinson
Yes. It may, in fact, be impossible.

Soekirman
Are you talking about social indicators as a measurement of development?

Levinson
Not necessarily. Michael Latham talked about measures of development that would include social indices, but I'm thinking of some number that would gauge the welfare of the poor, per se, and the parameters that would go into such a number. Perhaps one could use level of housing, level of clothing, and so on. Health and nutrition indicators are obvious ones as well, so I don't think it would be at all misleading to weight such an index heavily with those indicators. If some of the most important components of welfare are health and nutrition, why not use those indicators in an index number and then continually challenge the development planners to raise that number? Nutrition people would agree wholeheartedly to be part of that effort, but, at the same time, would make it clear that their efforts alone can only supplement a larger effort.

Soekirman
Planners always want us to prove that nutrition has a role as a separate input, so we need research to back it up!

Antrobus
May I be facetious and ask, do you really have to prove what role nutrition has in this? Do you have to prove what role housing has in the situation? Do you really have to prove it? It's a component. Do you have to prove that, as an isolated input, it has a special impact here?

Soekirman
Yes, because the planners don't always believe it. But, if we don't have success in isolating it—showing that, without nutritional input, you have *this* result, and with nutritional input, we have *that* result—there won't be a national program.

Latham
Haven't you already included social indicators in Indonesia even if you have not derived a new index number?

Soekirman
Yes. What is emphasized in Indonesia now is income distribution. The welfare of the poor is the express concern of the president.

Caloric intake is used as one indicator of welfare, as well as average weight gain of children. So, some nutritional indicators have been chosen as measures of the success of welfare programs.

In the five-year plan it states that the government will provide supplementary feeding for poor children who are undernourished. But planners want to know if it can be guaranteed that that kind of program will have a direct impact. We are hypothesizing that, without other inputs, it is impossible to guarantee success, and we told them so. That's why we will not go alone. We have to be supported by the overall program as a separate component, similar to agriculture or family planning, not only as a part of health. As long as nutrition is only *part* of *health,* that means it is still in the traditional mold and will not solve the problem.

Now, we plan to develop projects, and the government will get the data to show that, in fact, if you relate agricultural development to nutrition and food, if you help the poor farmers generate income while giving supplementary feeding to their children and nutrition education, you will get results. We hypothesize that the impact of the development programs will be greater with a nutrition input than without a nutrition input.

Sai

When we talk about development geared to the poor people, we sometimes give the impression that these poor are gathered together in one locale within the community. One of the major problems is that governments in the uncontrolled, nondictatorial economies must appear to give a governmental "developmental presence" in all corners of the community. Thus, the chances of a government permitting you to make several inputs into one geographic area, all at a given moment, or even allocate resources region by region, are pretty thin. This effort gets diluted by government saying, "Well, we can only afford six major inputs in MCH this year; then we can put three into this and four into that and so on."

One of the important questions is how you obviate the political reasoning of giving somebody the icing on the top of the cake, giving somebody else the raisin from within the cake, giving another person a bit of cake itself, and hope that everybody will feel reasonably happy.

Maletnlema

In addition, national planning, especially when there are few nutrition workers, often becomes the plan of a small group. It is then very difficult to carry it out to the population as a whole. I would like to hear more about how your national plan is developed, whether there is regional planning, and how the regional planner, if there is one, plans for his nutrition activities in the region. These regional people are the ones who are going to apply all your ideas and theories if it is every going to get down to the people who need it.

Soekirman

For Indonesia, it's extremely difficult to make a national plan for nutrition because it doesn't work for every region. In developing the project with the World Bank, for instance, our approach is at the grass roots. In some Indonesian provinces, there is a province nutrition board called BPGD and also a regional planning board, BAPPEDA. We give our concept of the World Bank-assisted project to the regional planners. They work on it, and then, if they predict it is applicable to their area, it is approved. But, if at any time they refuse the plan, it does not go forward. Not only nutrition, but most regional planning and rural development is done this way in Indonesia.

Levinson
As I recall, in Indonesia, one of the most promising and exciting development programs was the Kabupaten program of employment. It basically involved funds allocated to specific rural areas to develop broadly participatory employment efforts. BAPPENAS itself has already decided where these are going to be placed. It might, then, be reasonable to put your nutrition and health resources in those areas which have already been decided upon.

Soekirman
That's my assignment now: to look at the regional development planning. Indonesia is so diverse that every program has its own characteristics, and that's why mapping nutrition problems is important. We must have a clear target group. To avoid wasting budget funds for vitamin A and goiter, we have to know where the problems are concentrated.

The traditional program is supplementary feeding, through MCH, that has been there for years but without integration. It is an activity of the Ministry of Health, mounted without considering whether people are poor, whether there is a clean water supply, or whether food is available. They just give food as routine work. This has gone on for years.

Now the planning board is asking, "Is this nutrition? Can you show that there will be an impact?" We realized, looking at new data, that this approach doesn't work. Activities at village level in family planning and sanitation must be coordinated with "development nutrition" projects. We must identify those who are in need: the poor, the malnourished, and we give to those direct nutrition inputs, health inputs, and income-gathering activity such as the Kabupaten employment program. We give priority to certain villages because the problems are severe. This can only be done through the planning agency, and it is possible because in Indonesia all activities—central and provincial—in the country come out of the planning agency, which also decides the budget for these activities.

Thomson
Jim said that this was rather a pessimistic presentation, but I think it has not been possible to explain the breadth of what has happened since he was there. The Ten Ministers' Forum described by Soekirman is in charge of the whole nutrition program in Indonesia, known as Improvement of the People's Menu. Under the forum, there is a technical committee in charge of policy. It has a series of subcommittees, dealing with iodization of salt, vitamin A problems, nutrition education, and so on. This is all part of the organization in addition to what is happening in BAPPENAS, the development ministry.

Soekirman

There is also a coordinating commission, established last year. Again, however, we have a phenomenon in which many people are appointed to sit there
who know little about nutrition and have little contact with nutrition people.
Fortunately the basic policy was mandated by the president and so has power
behind it.

Barnes

This Indonesia story does contain one giant step backwards, and I'd like to
know why it was taken historically, in case there are lessons for us. Under the
Dutch, salt was iodized. Now you have surveys for goiter and are discussing
putting iodine into salt. Why did you take it out in the first place? Was there
economic pressure from the manufacturers? Was it some political maneuver?
How could there be a political maneuver to re-create goiter?

Soekirman

During the Dutch regime, salt production was a monopoly of the government.
There was only one factory, so it was easy to iodize salt. When independence
came, salt was not monopolized anymore.

Barnes

But you still had a law?

Latham

But how do you enforce it if you have 1,000 salt manufacturers?

Soekirman

Salt is produced now by individuals along the coasts, and it's impossible to
control. Most of the nutritionists, in fact, even forgot about the possibility of
goiter because of iodization under the Dutch. One reason that goiter is not
such an attractive problem for medical doctors is that goiter is a problem of
rural people, and most of the doctors don't go to the rural areas. Interest in
goiter just revived a few years ago with the new, increased budget for nutrition.

Barnes

Has a mechanism of enforcement appeared now that wasn't there five or six
years ago?

Soekirman

Now the administration is better, with better coordination. In fact, the Minister of Industry has worked out a project under which salt will be iodized and
will be distributed through the cooperative agencies. This is a difficult problem because we have to distribute this salt to isolated mountain areas.

Schlossberg

Just by way of historical fact: When we ran a nutrition survey several years
ago in the United States, we found that there was a recurrence of goiter and

that it was related to the marketing of noniodized salt in the United States.
So it happens in the United States, as well as in Indonesia. Since then, a regulation was promulgated to require that noniodized salt be labeled as "noniodized."

Mellor

I think that we have had presented a very genuine concern with problems of
leadership at rather high levels. On the other hand, I don't think it terribly
simplistic to say that, with the exception of a defunct Chilean government,
and with the possible exception of Tanzania ("possible" because I think there
was an unfortunately heavy emphasis on cash crops and underemphasis on
food crops in Tanzania), every country that has representatives at this conference has national allocative approaches to development which are simply
inconsistent with improving the diet of low income people in those countries.

I have a feeling that Indonesia is a prime case in point. It is my understanding that the big oil operation has pulled in vast quantities of money and,
added to that, has made large borrowings abroad to achieve a multiplier effect
with that oil money. But then it has gone into extremely capital-intensive
types of investment and has not funneled money into massive rural development, road systems, electrification, improvement of irrigation, the whole
process involved in massive expansion of the food supply. Therefore, it is an
approach to development which is inconsistent with making a major impact
on the nutrition of low income people. It seems to me that that then presents
a very unfavorable background for the actual programs. I would say that we
are talking about specifics which cannot work within the environments in
which they are set forth.

Now, there are not many countries which are providing what I consider a
favorable environment. On the right of the political spectrum, Taiwan probably is and, quite possibly, South Korea. In the middle, Ceylon probably is
providing it. India, first on one side and then the other side of the spectrum,
probably is, in some areas, e.g., Kerala, and perhaps in some time periods.

India, in fact, has a very rich literature on why these kinds of programs fail.
They fail fairly consistently because people just do not get enough income
and basic food supplies to make the specific target-oriented type of program
successful. I make these statements not to be nasty, but because I think that
we are creating a lot of heartsickness among many people in the world who
try to operate the specific programs in a context in which they *cannot* operate. I think we are being very irresponsible in this respect.

Latham

I think John's point is very well taken and very important, but, as he said,
there are only a handful of countries that would satisfy his requirements and
are really fertile for doing the things he thinks necessary. Then the question
is: Should a conference like this ignore nineteen out of twenty countries because there is only one country in twenty that's got a genuine and a complete

commitment?

If a country is not totally committed to sharing its resources and to doing everything it can to raise the level of the poor, is there then nothing it can do to improve the general nutrition or specific nutritional problems like goiter and vitamin A deficiency? I think there are places where you can make some progress. Indonesia has not used all its money to the extent that it could have for rural development and for solving the problems of poverty. I don't think Nigeria has either. But I still think that what's going on in Indonesia is not something one need be pessimistic about in terms of nutrition now versus what was going on in nutrition some years ago.

One can, I suppose, legitimately take the view that treating the symptoms and not the underlying causes is reprehensible and that it is better to do nothing. I don't take that view, but it is an important issue that deserves discussion.

López

In fact, it cannot really be very constructive to presume that all people in certain political systems cannot do anything to improve their lot. It is better to examine the information, see how one can make things work faster and better, not just simply leave some places out of the ball game because they don't meet a preconceived description.

Mellor

In general, I do favor working with countries, but the critical question is: Do you make some effort to get at the underlying factors or not? To what extent do you pour people down the drain by putting them in circumstances where they are not going to have any significant impact? It seems to me that would be cruel.

Schlossberg

To the more optimistic view, I would like to add that it seems to me that the establishment of a high-level body to deal with nutrition as a national issue is in itself a step forward. If the president has put himself out on a limb, and if he's serious about it, he must expect to receive some political benefit from it. He must think that if he can deliver, it will redound to his benefit in terms of support. So the question does remain: Why is there not a connection being made with the revenues generated by oil so that some percentage of that revenue is directed into the nutrition effort as opposed to capital-intensive efforts?

Soekirman

Actually we can see that that economic structure of Indonesia until 1985 will be basically agricultural, although oil revenue may become more important. As stated in my paper, Repelita-II contains more room for rural development. The money for social welfare, including nutrition, is there. For instance, in fiscal 1976/77, the government will allocate more than a billion rupiahs (approx. US$2.5 million) for nutrition activities. This is, comparatively, a lot of money given to nutrition, something which would never have happened in the past. In fact, the capital-intensive investment is simply to develop the oil itself, and I don't see room for labor-intensive activity in the oil business.

7 NUTRITION AND GOVERNMENT POLICY IN JAMAICA   A. C. Kenneth Antrobus

A.C. Kenneth Antrobus is currently PAHO/WHO Adviser in Family Health
for the Caribbean Area. Until recently, he was Medical Nutritionist and Acting Director, Caribbean Food and Nutrition Institute (a Pan American Health
Organization-sponsored institute, located in Jamaica but not an organ of the
government of that island) and editor of CFNI's bimonthly nutrition magazine, *Cajanus.* In his capacity as a CFNI employee, Dr. Antrobus has spent
many years as a resident of Jamaica although he was born and raised in
St. Vincent. As a non-Jamaican working in a nongovernment institution but constantly in touch with official Jamaican activities in nutrition, he is in an ideal
situation to observe the Jamaican nutrition scene objectively. Dr. Antrobus is
a medical graduate of London University, University (College) of the West
Indies, with training in pediatrics and public health at the Universities of
Birmingham (UK), and London. Dr. Antrobus has had extensive clinical and
field experience in child health and nutrition programs throughout the Caribbean, and is Associate Lecturer, Department of Social and Preventive Medicine, University of the West Indies.

This paper does not necessarily reflect the views of the Caribbean Food and Nutrition
Institute.

INTRODUCTION

The entire Caribbean region includes about seventeen different countries, some independent, some not. Collectively, these are smaller than any of the other countries represented here. But this is not an apology: nutrition problems are not made any less significant because of smaller area or smaller population. Indeed, the strategies and the solutions that are required can be just as difficult to develop and implement.

The recent Jamaican experience in relation to nutrition and government policy merits some attention because the government has focused on such fundamental issues as land tenure and land use, food production, literacy, and skill training within an overall national development strategy. Also, this period has seen increased governmental concern for nutrition, to the point where a national food and nutrition policy was developed, articulated, and adopted, and is now in the process of implementation.

Jamaica, the largest of the Commonwealth Caribbean islands, is situated to the south of Cuba and west of Haiti and geographically stands in relative isolation from her English-speaking sisters clustered together in the eastern part of the Caribbean Sea. The population of the 4,000-square-mile island, estimated at 2,030,400 in 1974, is of predominantly African origin but includes Europeans, Syrians, Chinese, and East Indians as well. In 1974, there was a natural increase in population of 1.7% over 1973, with the birth rate at its lowest recorded level of 30.6 per thousand. Other vital statistics for the year 1974 show an infant mortality rate of 25.9 per thousand and an overall mortality rate of 7.2 per thousand. Of special interest, however, is the 1-4 year mortality rate of 4.5 per thousand, the leading cause of death being protein calorie malnutrition.

With 43% of its people under fourteen years of age, Jamaica's population structure resembles that of other developing countries. In a labor force of over 800,000 there is an unemployment rate of 20% (12% among men and 30% among women) amounting to 166,000 persons (greater than the population of any one of the smaller Caribbean states).

Agriculture, forestry, fishing, and mining accounted for 30% of employment, manufacture 11.7%, and public administration and commerce 11% and 10.5%, respectively. The labor force was made up of 33% self-employed and in independent occupations, 15% craftsmen and in operation occupations, 14% service, and less in unskilled and clerical occupations. The sugar industry remains the largest single employer, with 4½ times the number of people involved in the tourist industry and 7 times the number in bauxite and aluminum.

MALNUTRITION

While poverty is unquestionably at the core of the problem of childhood malnutrition, there are other forces which contribute significantly:

1 Large family size, associated with short birth intervals, and early parenthood, particularly very young mothers.

2 Reduced practice and shorter duration of breast feeding than previously known and a high incidence of infection, especially gastroenteritis associated with early supplementary feeding.

3 Poor environmental sanitation, especially water and waste disposal, in association with very inadequate housing.

4 High rate of illiteracy associated with ignorance of desirable child feeding practices. Inadequate use of child health services and, possibly, resistance to change in nutrition behavior.

5 Inadequate services in nutrition, especially within the framework of maternal and child health.

6 Occasional cultural influences and taboos which run counter to acceptable child-rearing practices.

7 Domestic instability often created by irresponsibility and desertion on the part of fathers.

The prevalence rate for all forms of protein-calorie malnutrition in children under five is about 35% with a peak of severe malnutrition in the second year of life. Schoolchildren aged 5 to 15 years from low income families suffer from a mild or moderate degree of malnutrition reflected in the stunting of their heights and weights. Undernutrition in childbearing women exists, but no exact figures are available. It is estimated that about 45% have iron deficiency anemia. We do not have vitamin A deficiency or goiter.

The extent of the problem of malnutrition may be further ascertained from the fact that, combined with the diarrheal diseases, it ranked third among specific causes of death for the entire population. Moreover, malnutrition was responsible for the longest average length of stay in hospital in 1974: 32 days, compared with 24 days for all forms of tuberculosis and 20 days for diabetes.

INCOME

The per capita income in 1974 was J$857. The gross national product increased by 31% in current dollars to J$2,055.2* million; real growth, adjustive for inflation, was of the order of 4.5%. Although the country is mainly agricultural, bauxite and aluminum dominate the export market and, in fact, accounted for 74% of the total value of exports in 1974. In third place was sugar (12%), with bananas taking a lower place than usual. The value of other exports from the agricultural sector showed citrus, pimento, coffee, rum, and ginger as important supplementary crops to sugar and bananas. As an earner of. foreign exchange, however, the island's non-export industry, tourism, ranks second only to bauxite.

*J$1.00 = US$1.10.

When one examines the statistics more closely, it can be seen that there is marked maldistribution of income: 40% of the employed labor force earns less than $700 per year, and 80% less than $2,000 per year. 70% of households make up the lower income group, and in the majority of these more than 60% of income is spent on food. It should be no surprise, therefore, to find that children, pregnant and nursing mothers, the indigent, and laborers doing heavy work often do not get enough food. Easily the most vulnerable are the children under five years of age, among whom there is a prevalence rate of about 30% for all types of malnutrition (mild, moderate, and severe), with a peak of severe malnutrition at 3% in the second year of life.

LAND TENURE AND LAND USE

Land ownership, in a predominantly agricultural economy, not surprisingly, shows a maldistribution pattern similar to that reflected in income. According to the Agricultural Census of 1968, 1.5 million acres of land, slightly more than half the land area, were taken up by 193,400 farms at an average farm size of 7.7 acres. But, as table 1 illustrates, 78% of farms were under five acres in size and accounted for only 15% of the land in farms, while farms over 500 acres in size, and representing only 0.15% of the number of farms, occupied 43% of the land. It should be noted also that several thousand of the small farms were located on steep lands of low fertility.

Most agricultural land is worked on a freehold basis, although there remains a small proportion of it that is occupied free of charge by squatters, a practice which started on the plantations even before emancipation. Evidently the leasehold system of land tenure never attained significant popularity in Jamaica.

Land settlement schemes have had a long history in Jamaica but, for a number of reasons, have never proved completely satisfactory as a method of land reform. Problems included the poor quality of land, the small size of parcels, the inadequacy of support for developing and protecting the land, and, sometimes, overhasty settlement brought about by the pressing demand for land and worsening unemployment.

It is somewhat paradoxical that there should be "idle" land in a small agricultural country like Jamaica, but it was estimated in 1974 that some 83,000 acres of land on farms larger than 100 acres were idle, and a large but unestimated acreage on smaller farms.

HEALTH SERVICES

The Government Health Services are intended to serve the entire population. It is known that this goal has not yet been achieved, but no precise and meaningful data are available of the extent of coverage actually provided by these services.

Table 1
Farms and acreage in Jamaica

	Under 5 acres		5 - 25 acres		25 - 100 acres		100 - 500 acres		500 and over		Total	
	No. of Farms	Acres	No. of Farms	Acres	No. of Farms	Acres	No. of Farms	Acres	No. of Farms	Acres	No. of Farms	Acres
	51,700	229,200	37,600	340,800	3,100	127,200	699	148,000	293	644,000	193,400	1,489,000
	(78.5%)	(15.4%)	(19.5%)	(22.9%)	(1.6%)	(8.5%)	(0.4%)	(9.9%)	(0.2%)	(43.2%)	(100%)	(100%)

Source: Adapted from Agricultural Census, Department of Statistics, 1968-69

In 1973, there were 706,635 recorded attendances at health centers, a rate of 356 per 1,000 population. 44% of children paid a visit to the child welfare clinic during their first year of life, but more than half of these did not pay their first visit until age 6 months or older. It is, therefore, not surprising that immunization coverage among preschool children is at the low level of 40-50%. Immunization services for school children, such as for tuberculosis and poliomyelitis, are thought to achieve a somewhat higher coverage.

Antenatal services, recently integrated with family planning services, are also very underutilized, especially in the first two trimesters of pregnancy. Some 25,000 deliveries (40% of total births) took place in government hospitals in 1974, while in the nine new rural maternity centers brought into operation during that year there were only 270 deliveries.

The budget for the health sector in 1974/75 was J$65.19 million, of which $4.99 million was for capital expenditures. The remaining $60.20 million represented 11.8% of the national recurrent budget. The emphasis has been shifting noticeably towards preventive medicine and primary medical care, and nearly half of the capital budget is devoted to the construction of new health centers in the fiscal year 1975-76.

In 1974 there were 570 doctors practicing in Jamaica—120 in private practice and the remaining 450 in the Government Medical Service. Three hundred sixty doctors (63% of the total) were in the capital, Kingston, and its environs—which contains less than 40% of the population.

One hundred thirty public health nurses and approximately 2,600 nurses and midwives are employed in hospitals and health centers and for district field work. They are supported by 83 public health inspectors and a new type of nursing auxiliary called the Community Health Aide, of whom 350 have already been trained and another 850 are currently undergoing training.

The entire population is served by 106 dentists, a ratio of 1 to 20,000, but their distribution between the capital and the rest of the country is even more disproportionate than is physician distribution. There is a small, active training program for dental nurses aimed at alleviating some of the deficiencies in the service.

FOOD CONSUMPTION

As an aid to understanding the food consumption and dietary patterns of the population, it would be useful to examine the situation with respect to food availability. Existing data, derived principally from food balance sheets, indicate that in 1972 available energy was 30% and available protein 70% higher than needed (based on recommended dietary allowances). Indeed, table 2 shows that between 1960 and 1972 there was an upward trend in the availability of both energy and protein.

It is estimated from food consumption and food expenditure data that, while there may be an inordinately high quantity of energy and protein available (probably as much as 200% of RDA for protein) in the highest income

Table 2
Trends in adequacy of energy and protein supplies, Jamaica, 1960-72

	1960-62		1965-67		1970-72	
	Average Amount (per capita per day)	% RDA[a]	Average Amount (per capita per day)	% RDA	Average Amount (per capita per day)	% RDA
Energy	2,188 kcal	97	2,444 kcal	109	2,820 kcal	125
Protein	54 g	126	58 g	136	71 g	164
Animal Protein	22 g		24 g		30 g	
Protein-Calories %[b]	9.9		9.5		10.1	

[a]Recommended Dietary Allowance.
[b]Calories from protein on a percentage of total calories.
Source: I. E. Johnson and H. Fox (unpublished data)

group, the low income group, to which 70% of the population belongs, has a shortfall of 27% and 14% respectively in its energy and protein consumption.

It is of further interest to look at the relative importance of different foods as suppliers of energy and protein for the various income groups. In the lowest income group, sugar provides more calories than any other single food. It is replaced as the prime source of energy by flour in the middle group and rice in the upper group. Butter, which ranks twelfth in the upper group, is not among the first twenty foods in the lowest group.

With regard to protein sources, the first three foods for the low income group are all cereals (flour, rice, bread), while beef, chicken, and bread are, in that order, the top protein sources for the highest income group (tables 3 and 4).

These differences in food consumption and expenditure patterns have clear implications for the development of a food and nutrition policy for the country. In 1972, the lowest weekly per capita food expenditure was put at J\$1.19 with a median of \$2.38 in the lowest income group. In February 1975, the Nutrition Division of the Scientific Research Council estimated that for a family of five (2 adults and 3 children) to meet their minimum dietary requirements and at the same time have a palatable diet, they would need to spend at least J\$14.00 per week,* or \$700.00 per year, the upper

Table 3
Sources of energy by importance to families in various food expenditure groups

Food	Low	2nd	3rd	Upper
Dark Sugar	1	3	6	11
Flour	2	1	3	5
Rice	3	4	1	1
Oil	4	2	2	2
Green Bananas	5	7	7	6
Bread	6	5	5	4
Yam	7	8	8	9
Condensed Milk	8	6	4	3
Cornmeal	9	10	9	13
Coconut	10	9	17	14
Margarine	11	16	14	15
Sweet Potatoes	12	15	19	—
Granulated Sugar	—	13	10	—
Butter	—	17	13	12
Beef	20	12	12	8

Source: See ref. 1

*In July, the estimate was revised to approximately J\$18.00 per week.

income limit of 40% of the country's wage earners and more than $2 greater than the average weekly expenditure of 5-member families in the lowest income group.

As in most other parts of the world, the Consumer Price Index for all items rose very sharply in 1973 and again in 1974. The average increases in the capital city, Kingston, and the rural area for 1974 were 27.2% and 32.9% respectively (table 5).

These price increases were particularly marked in the case of food and drink. For example, there was a 44% increase in the price of pork in the Kingston area and a 65% increase in the rural area between December 1973 and December 1974. Early evidence for 1975 indicates only marginal declines in the rate of increase of the index. This situation has been particularly grave for the poor of the country who must spend a disproportionately high percentage of their income to provide themselves and their families with food.

FOOD PURCHASING AND MARKETING

While the supermarket has very largely displaced other traditional food sales

Table 4
Sources of protein by importance to families in various food expenditure groups

Food	Low	2nd	3rd	Upper
Flour	1	1	3	7
Rice	2	5	2	4
Bread	3	2	4	3
Salted Cod	4	6	7	6
Yam	5	10	10	10
Condensed Milk	6	3	5	5
Green Bananas	7	11	14	14
Cornmeal	8	12	12	16
Canned Mackerel	9	16	16	15
Chicken	10	4	1	2
Red Peas	11	9	11	12
Congo Peas	12	15	—	—
Beef	13	8	6	1
Chicken Neck and Back	14	16	—	—
Salt Beef	15	7	9	8
Lamb	—	18	18	9
Egg	—	20	13	13
Pork	17	13	8	11

Source: See ref. 1

Table 5
Percentage change in average annual consumer price index for all items

	1970 / 1969	1971 / 1970	1972 / 1971	1973 / 1972	1974 / 1973
Kingston area	9.7	6.7	5.9	19.2	27.2
Rural area	10.5	7.1	5.5	20.4	32.9

Source: See ref. 2

outlets in the commercial centers of the larger cities, the small shop remains a well-established part of the purchasing system of the poor. This system is one of small daily cash purchases of food, with a diminishing element of credit, once a common feature of the system. Also important to the low income purchaser is the *higgler.* This is a person (usually a woman) who buys produce, local foods in particular, for resale to the public either in markets or at roadside stalls. This activity is a source of income for some 20,000 Jamaican women.

In 1974 Jamaica imported J$120.00 million worth of food, an increase of 42% in cost over the previous year, with only a 14% increase in *volume,* a reflection of inflationary trends. Cereals, particularly wheat, were the main foods imported, followed by meat, fish, and dairy products. In fact, 95% of all cereal consumed is imported. On the food export side, sugar led by a long way, with bananas next, then rum, coffee, ginger, and citrus.

Within the food marketing system, transportation and storage stand out as important problems—particularly for the small farmer. While there is no exact estimate of losses from spoilage, especially of fresh fruit and vegetables, it is known that the losses are considerable. This situation is aggravated by the seasonality of several food crops and a tendency for gluts to occur where marketing intelligence and communication are faulty. Thus, there is obviously room for adjustment in the system at the level of producer, distributor, and consumer.

Price control exists as a legislative instrument restricted to a selected range of commodities. Included among them are a large number of staple foods, although some meats have recently been removed from the list because of unrealistically low prices. There were more than 1,200 complaints about over-pricing to the Price Control Authority in 1974, and a substantial number of successful prosecutions, but there still is no useful way of determining the efficacy of price control as an anti-inflationary measure.

Until two years ago, the government granted direct subsidies on several foods, including condensed milk, cornmeal, rice, and sugar for the benefit of the whole population at a cost which was fast approaching $20 million a year. These subsidies were withdrawn because of the excessive cost, and a new approach was adopted. Indirect food subsidies were introduced by way of fuel subsidy for electricity and a fertilizer subsidy that reached 33 1/3% (or J$105 per ton) in 1974. Production subsidies or guaranteed prices for sugar and bananas, the principal export crops, were also introduced. Direct subsidies on foods are now more selectively applied for the benefit of the low income consumers (see below).

GOVERNMENT POLICY

There is no doubt that the present government came into power in February 1972 with a clear recognition that Jamaica had a nutrition problem. What cannot be so readily determined is how well the magnitude and scope of the problem were understood at that time. The prime minister in his book, *The Politics of Change*, states that "one of the great problems in the development of poor countries like Jamaica arises in the field of nutrition," and goes on to refer to "the apparent paradox of widespread malnutrition being found in an agricultural country." Thus, in the view of the prime minister, the problem of malnutrition was first perceived within the context of economic development and social justice.

It became increasingly apparent that, in spite of the creditable rate of economic growth experienced by Jamaica during its first decade of Independence (1962-72), there were large sections of the population which were relatively untouched by this growth and, in fact, remained "impoverished and unemployed." It was, therefore, imperative that alongside the goals of economic and social development, the goals of better nutrition and education should be given places of prominence. In this way, the government has given formal recognition to the significance of good nutrition in the development of the people, not only as an end in itself but also as a means of attaining greater national goals, important among which is an improved quality of life.

Nutrition Advisory Council

One of the earliest steps taken to help guide government policy specifically in the field of nutrition was the creation of a Nutrition Committee by the Minister of Health and Environmental Control. Within a short time, this body gave way to the more formally constituted Nutrition Advisory Council (NAC) which was inaugurated in October 1973.

The NAC draws its membership from relevant government ministries such as agriculture, health, and education, and from other agencies which can provide extra technical inputs, such as the Caribbean Food and Nutrition Institute, the Tropical Metabolism Research Unit of the University of the West Indies, and the Scientific Research Council.

In addition to carrying out its prime function of advising the cabinet through the responsible minister on all aspects of food and nutrition, the NAC has also been charged with:

a   coordinating the work of and maintaining liaison with agencies concerned in the field of food and nutrition b   reviewing all nutrition programs

c   reviewing the nutritional implications of legislative measures

d   preparing and, later, monitoring the national food and nutrition policy

The council meets once a month, but maintains activities through a number of subcommittees for select purposes, such as social interventions, educational matters, evaluation. In this way the NAC fully exploits the wide range of expertise which its members represent.

While the present structure of the NAC has enabled it to fill a much needed role in government, there are a number of problems associated with this structure:

1   The NAC has not so far taken firm root in any one ministry. After an initial period of eighteen months in the Ministry of Health, it was placed under the aegis of the Ministry of Marketing and Commerce, which takes care of some other important nutrition activities. The NAC has thus been denied the continued and total commitment of any one minister of government during its short life of less than three years. While its new location may prove advantageous, no firm forecast can be made at this time.

2   There is lack of uniformity in the level of representation of the various government ministries and departments. In some instances, this level has not been sufficiently senior to ensure the effective transmittal of decisions and ideas accompanied by appropriate action in the concerned ministry.

3   There remains some reservation about the efficacy of the inter-ministerial approach required for the effective functioning of such a council. The concern is that the specific sectoral interests of individual ministries more often than not tend to receive greater attention and, indeed, priority.

4   The purely advisory nature of the council and the absence of any executive authority—for the implementation of programs, for example—imposes considerable limitation on the expected or desired rate of progress in the development of nutrition activities.

5   The administrative and secretarial staff are not of sufficient strength for the NAC to carry out fully and effectively all those functions that fall within its mandate. In addition, the staff lacks experts in the disciplines of sociology and economics.

6   It is open to question whether this Council may be operating too much within a traditional bureaucratic framework of Government and may not, therefore, benefit from an infusion of some more modern style of operation.

It is not possible to say to what extent these deficiencies in structure and function have influenced the work of the NAC. There have, however, been clear-cut and very creditable achievements, most notable among them being the construction of a Food and Nutrition Policy for Jamaica in 1974 with help from a number of supporting agencies. After a period of intensive review and some modification, the policy was accepted by the Cabinet in 1975.

In the context of this new policy, the NAC influenced the government to pinpoint particular aspects of the nutrition problem most deserving of attention:

1 *in population terms*—young children and pregnant and lactating women
2 *in geographical terms*—selected rural areas with high prevalence rates of childhood malnutrition, e.g., the western parishes of Jamaica
3 *in nutrient terms*—deficiency primarily in energy, but also in protein intake; also deficiency of iron

It is already apparent that much of the advice of the NAC has infiltrated policy decisions relating to food and nutrition during the past months. Nearly all of the programs and activities, implemented or planned, described below are derived either directly or indirectly from the Food and Nutrition Policy.

Health System and Nutrition Policy

The approach to the nutritional problems of the most vulnerable group of mothers and children has been primarily through the Maternal and Child Health (MCH) services of the Ministry of Health.

Within the last year there have been important steps made towards the integration of family planning and nutrition into MCH programs by the Ministry of Health, with the objective of improving the overall health of this group of population. The means by which it is hoped to attain this objective are:

1 Improvement in the staff structure and training of personnel for health centers.

2 Expansion and physical improvement of health and maternity centers.

3 Increased and improved nutritional surveillance of young children, and better coverage of mothers and children by clinic services.

4 More intense teaching of basic nutrition through demonstration techniques to community groups at health centers and other suitable locations.

5 Introduction of a supplementary feeding program for mothers and children. The first stage of this program is scheduled to begin shortly, and it is planned to reach some 82,000 young children and over 30,000 pregnant and nursing mothers in the western parishes of Jamaica with an appropriate food supplement.

6 The distribution of iron and folic acid supplements to all pregnant women through the MCH centers and district clinics.

Complementary to these approaches are:

1 The development of family planning education and services within the context of a family life education program designed to reach the public as well as schools. Recently also, there has been a more open position taken regarding the sales of contraceptives and they are now available in shops and bars, as well as in the special sales outlets through which subsidized food is sold to the poor.

2 There has been a powerful government thrust in the field of day care,

also within the last twelve months. Though still embryonic, this program holds promise for the improved nutrition of children of working mothers and, also, enhances the job opportunities for the unemployed mothers of young children.

Agriculture and Nutrition

Operation GROW   Mindful of the prevailing patterns of land ownership and land use, Prime Minister Michael Manley, on assuming office in 1972, launched a program of agrarian reform aimed primarily at a revitalization of the agricultural sector. This was put into a framework succinctly and very aptly entitled Operation GROW (Growing and Reaping Our Wealth).

The basic objectives of this program are to:

a   achieve the fuller use of two of the country's most important resources: land and people
b   ensure that the agricultural sector increases substantially its contribution to the economic development of the country
c   produce locally as much of the national food and raw material requirements as is economically feasible, thus reducing dependence on imports
d   achieve the widest possible distribution of opportunity for access to the use of agricultural land among *bona fide* farmers
e   assist in removing the stigma attached to agricultural work by ensuring that the farmer reaps his due share of improved living standards
f   achieve better health standards for the population through the production of foods of higher nutritional value

As a subsidiary undertaking, Project Land Lease was established to provide supplemental tenancies to small farmers who genuinely needed more land for the increased production of traditional food crops. By the end of 1974, more than 10,000 farmers had been placed on nearly 20,000 acres of land and reaped crops worth between $4-5 million. It is projected that within three years there should be 75,000 acres occupied by about 30,000 farmers.

Also associated with the above objectives is Project Food Farms, aimed at utilizing 50,000 acres of government land to produce a wide range of food crops such as vegetables, pulses, tubers, and tree crops. This approach is being encouraged to a large extent as a group or cooperative activity.

The total operation seeks to be more all-embracing than previous types of land settlement programs. Moreover, it takes into account a number of aspects of development which are of critical importance to the viability of the small farmer, viz., infrastructure, fertilizer subsidy, technical support, and credit facilities, as well as liaison with the Agricultural Marketing Corporation—a statutory government organization. Thus, Jamaica has chosen to take what David Hopper* refers to as "the political risks inherent in implementing

*W. David Hopper, President, International Development Research Center, in "To Conquer Hunger: Opportunity and Political Will," a lecture in the John A. Hannah International Development Lecture Series.

policies of economic incentive for food production" and face the immense
task of balancing this and other related aspects of development "within the
push and pull of nationhood."

Nutrition Holdings Nutrition Holdings has been one of the more imaginative
and successful steps taken by the present government in its pursuit of practical measures for the improvement of nutrition in the country. As a wholly
owned government undertaking, Nutrition Holdings was set up because of the
need to protect the Jamaican economy from wide and rapid fluctuations in
commodity prices, particularly of grain, and also because Jamaica had been
experiencing some shortages in staple foods. Nutrition Holdings is the principal importer of certain staple foods, such as wheat, corn, salt fish, canned
milk, and soya for the livestock industry. Nutrition Holdings functions by
finding the cheapest markets and, by bulk purchasing, further reducing costs.
Moreover, by channeling surplus revenue into a price stabilization fund, Nutrition Holdings has ensured that the retail prices of selected foods can be
maintained, or even cut back from time to time. The most recent example has
been the reduction in the price of corned beef by approximately 20%.

Low Income Shops Another innovative component of government policy
with the same objectives as Nutrition Holdings is the low-income retail outlets, established under the Agricultural Marketing Corporation.

Since 1974, 25 special shops and 26 mobile units for the sale of food and
other basic household items have been established in carefully chosen areas
for the benefit of the poorer sections of the population, both urban and rural.
All products are sold at 20% below the price in the regular shops of the Agricultural Marketing Corporation, and, so far, it is estimated that more than
150,000 people benefit from these retail outlets. A government survey has
shown that 88% of the shoppers are satisfied with the scheme while 12% wish
that certain other types of food were made available. In light of the unequivocal success of the program of selectively subsidizing food for the poor, the
government has undertaken to increase the number of shops to 60 and mobil
units to 50 so that 300,000 people should have been benefited by the end of
1975.

In this type of program there is always concern about the potential abuse of
special services by the persons who are entitled to use them and about illegal
patronage by persons ineligible because of higher income level or place of
residence. To deal with these possibilities, a number of safeguards and monitoring systems have been built into the program. Although it is not certain
how effective these measures have been, available reports suggest that misuse
has been minimal.

In the meantime, the government has continued to maintain tight controls
on a select list of food items. The monitoring of this pricing system, however,
is not an easy exercise, especially in the face of the widespread practice of

hoarding and "marrying" of goods. (The latter practice refers to shopkeepers compelling purchase of a nonessential item along with an item that is in short supply.)

Partly because of this problem, and also because of the basic importance of wise buying, a program of consumer education has been launched. So far, this has been on a small scale and it may be a number of years before there is any significant national impact.

Agricultural Development for the Future Agricultural development has taken a significant turn in the direction of greater self-sufficiency in food by maximizing the use of available land. The Food and Nutrition Policy calls for:

• "Change in policy of land use to ensure that adequate suitable land is made available for growing domestic food crops."
• "Change in policy of crop investment and management so that export and domestic markets are considered together."
• "Improvement in efficiency of food production, e.g., increased yields, improved varieties, use of crop rotation, etc."

The most important developments have been:

1 The increased production of root crops, especially yams and sweet potatoes, as part of Project Land Lease. This program is progressing towards the acreage and production targets set for 1980.

2 6,000 acres of land, out of a 10,000 acre target for 1980, are currently being developed for rice production as a project of the Agricultural Development Corporation.

Other programs identified but not yet in full operation are:

• rotation of red peas, maize, and soy beans on 2,500 acres of new land
• rotation of maize and cow peas on 6,000 acres of new land
• rotation of maize and peanuts on 8,000 acres of new land

These programs will be accompanied by other specific action aimed at the improvement of storage facilities to reduce food loss.

The above programs are geared primarily toward increasing the availability of food to make up the shortfall in calories and protein of the low income 70% of the population. In addition, these and other development programs are being promoted with the closely related objective of reducing by 20% the proportion of energy and protein supplied from imported foods by 1980. Programs include plans for increased livestock production, ranging from small stock based on goats and rabbits to beef and dairy cattle. The NAC has taken care, however, to advise that these latter projects should receive lower priority than the preceding food production schemes.

Because these agricultural programs have been put forward against a background of import substitution, the importation of certain foods with high nutrient cost and doubtful nutritional value has either ceased or been severely curtailed. Foods in this category include ready to eat breakfast cereals, apples, preserves and jams, and fancy canned meats and vegetables. It can be deduced that it is the better-off section of the society that has been "deprived," and not the low income purchaser. At the same time, this policy, along with other previously described measures, has undoubtedly created greater opportunities for the production of local substitutes, thereby reinforcing the stimulus to Jamaican farmers to produce more food.

New Food Development

Experience has been limited largely to gift foods such as WSB (wheat-soya blend), CSM (corn-soya mixture) and bulgur supplied through international agencies for use in young child and school feeding programs.

The success of these foods has not been formally evaluated but several problems have been readily apparent during the years of their use:

1 Supplies and distribution within the country have often been irregular and unreliable; and there is an unknown amount of spoilage.

2 New foods have never attained the high level of acceptability of indigenous foods. This leads to a good deal of additional waste.

3 The cost of handling the new products probably makes these types of feeding schemes more expensive than they are usually assumed to be.

While there has been some work in Jamaica on the development of a weaning food based on local products (e.g., corn, rice, soya, banana, cassava) this has not yet been transformed into a manufacturing enterprise to meet the needs of the population but is now being pursued with renewed urgency.

Quite interestingly, however, as part of the overall food and nutrition policy, the government has been seeking "new sources for old foods" through its recently established Nutrition Holdings. A typical example of this has been the use of a new source of salt fish (salted cod), a food of great cultural significance: instead of buying from the traditional, but now relatively expensive, Canadian market, Jamaicans now use the cheaper "Bacalao d'Espana" from Spain. More recently, arising from the same economic and nutritional considerations, "La Crema" condensed milk has been imported from Cuba for sale in the low income shops.

Education Campaigns

Education campaigns have not been a feature of nutrition programs at the national level. The only nationwide effort on record is the Food for Family Fitness (3F) Campaign carried out more than twenty years ago, of which there is very little evaluation. In fact, nutrition education as it has taken place in schools and clinics, has been done by a staff that is usually overburdened, inadequate in training and numbers, built on a weak and, in some cases, inappropriate structure, with insufficient outreach to the target population. It is hoped that the revised concept of Family Life Education with nutrition as an integral component will ensure that these deficiencies are overcome.

The chief organs of mass media available in Jamaica are one government-owned television station, one government and one private radio station, and two privately owned daily newspapers. There appears to be no policy laid down by the government in regard to nutrition and the media: neither positive direction or incentive, nor obstruction to the wider promotion of nutrition through the media. The present picture suggests that the mass media are underexploited in this regard and that there is need for the formulation of a policy and programs to correct this.

In the meantime, under the auspices of the NAC and the Government Nutrition Unit, a Breast-Feeding Campaign of nationwide dimensions is being planned with the emphasis on educating women in particular, but also all health professionals, schoolchildren, and the general public, using all the media resources and educational techniques available. The major objective is to correct what has been identified as a dangerous trend in the pattern of infant feeding in Jamaica insofar as it adversely affects the nutritional status, morbidity, and mortality of children under one year of age.

School Feeding

School-age children represent 30% of the population (about twice the number of preschool children), yet their nutritional problems are comparatively mild and they are, therefore, given a lower priority. For the most part, the school feeding programs, which have been in operation for several years, are poorly organized, inadequately financed, and badly executed. Many have been based on "gift foods" from overseas and depend also on small, sporadic harvests from school gardens. Added to this is the indifferent and unimaginative role played by school staff in many of the island's schools. This program is badly in need of upgrading to ensure a greater regularity and a higher standard of meals.

Two years ago a modern concept of school feeding was put into action by the government in collaboration with the US Agency for International Development. Today, a centrally located plant produces patties (a traditional Jamaican vegetable meat pie) and milk as a midday meal for 65,000 schoolchildren in the Kingston area. It is understood that there are plans for establishing other plants throughout the island so that more children will benefit from this scheme.

THE OBSTACLES

It is clear that a variety of approaches and strategies have been conceived to improve the nation's food and nutrition situation. Equally clear is that they cannot, and certainly will not, all be put into action, at least in the anticipated sequence and stated time frame. What then, are the obstacles to effective action and purposeful implementation?

1 The first, and perhaps the most important, factor must be the depth of commitment on the part of the government to a whole-hearted pursuit of nutrition objectives as part of total national policy. It is possible that a centrally enunciated policy may not be clearly grasped or interpreted as part of a coherently structured approach to development by key political, administrative, and technical officials in concerned ministries and departments of government. This may be attributable either to inadequate orientation to the problem or to lack of conviction that nutrition is a priority in development. Particularly germane is the well-known poverty of communication and understanding that still, to some extent, characterizes the relationship between economic planners and nutritionists.

2 The dominance of sectorial and traditional interests within individual ministries still occurs. This is of real significance in relation to nutrition, a subject requiring interdisciplinary inputs for effective implementation. There are, however, signs that the vitally important Ministry of Agriculture is growing more sensitive to the value of nutrition-oriented policies and programs.

3 Inadequacies in infrastructure have created delays and caused other problems in program implementation. Outstanding examples are the lack of roadways, necessary for more farm land to be brought into production, and lack of water supply for the irrigation of crops and maintenance of livestock.

4 There are deficiencies in the numbers of trained technical staff and extension workers. Thus it is impossible to staff adequately both the special development program in agriculture and land reform as well as the regular posts in the agricultural establishment. In fact, a situation has arisen where one group can benefit only by recruiting staff from the other. Optimal progress cannot be made by both these agricultural sectors in the face of such shortages.

5 Together these factors contribute to the failure of synchronization of nutrition-related activities, because progress within one sector is not always matched by that in other sectors when simultaneous intersectorial action is required.

6 Lack of preparedness among the potential beneficiaries of some of these schemes may make for inefficiency or low productivity. As one national newspaper commented editorially on the subject of financial help for farmers: "The truth is that there is available credit at the disposal of the farmer. But much of this credit is unused because the farmer is unable to take advantage of it."* Evidence of weakness in the area of management by small producers points to the need for considerable strengthening in the teaching of management skills in a way that will benefit the smaller farmers in the country.

7 Above all, a major and prevailing constraint to effective action is the lack of financial resources, further aggravated by the recent burdensome inflationary trends. This has already led to the deferment or modification of some key

*Jamaica Daily News, July 20, 1975.

projects outlined in the national food and nutrition policy.

8 Because of the urgency with which the government views its whole development strategy, it may have in some cases rushed to the implementation stages of projects without adequate thoroughness of consultation or forward planning. Thus, the imposition of political will or, conversely, the absence of political will, may be a more significant determinant of what is done than any professional or technical rationale.

CHANGING PATTERNS IN NUTRITION

In spite of the continued existence of substantial malnutrition in preschool children and lesser degrees of undernutrition in schoolchildren and adults, there is unequivocal evidence to show that, taken as a whole, the nutritional status of the Jamaican people has improved along with such indices as the crude death rate and the infant mortality rate. The average calorie and protein intake of the population has also improved, while obesity is being recognized more and more as a nutritional problem.

As the duration and incidence of breast feeding have declined, the commercial milk and baby food markets have been booming. Parallel to this has been a persistent shift towards convenience foods such as frozen pizzas and precooked fried chicken. Inevitably, also, small pockets of food faddists have been emerging, principally in the form of vegetarians and "natural foods" fanatics.

Among the more plausible reasons for these changing patterns are:

• dominance of North American influences on eating habits brought about by geographical proximity, frequent two-way travel, tourism, television, and other forms of exposure to the American way of life, many aspects of which are emulated by Jamaicans
• there is an increasing proportion of households in which both parents work full-time outside the home and are thus eager to use the precooked, ready-to-serve foods
• intensive advertising of commercial baby foods and the infiltration (recently discontinued) of health centers and hospitals by commercial "milk nurses"
• the steady wave of rural-urban migration of people, coupled with the increased cost of domestic help, which has contributed to reduction in home food production

NUTRITION IN DEVELOPMENT

Nutrition as a specific thrust in the field of national development represents a relatively new area of government awareness and an additional dimension in its thinking and planning for the future. This has, however, occurred at a time when there are also strong needs for the accelerated development of infrastructure in education, health, social welfare, defense, and housing, among other areas.

Nutrition has found itself in a curious dilemma: it bridges a number of front-line ministries, but in none of them does it have first claim on budgetary resources. For the most part, nutrition is left to compete individually with many different issues in a number of ministerial arenas. Nutrition does not yet have the appeal that would ensure the same level of financial commitment given to a national literacy program or a national youth service, programs of the greatest ideological significance. It has, however, won commendable government recognition in a relatively short period of time.

Outside of government, other groups within the society that assume some responsibility for solving the nutrition problems include churches and voluntary agencies. Most of the programs they execute are in the area of group feeding, or food distribution and day care, in some cases backed up by nutrition education. Theirs has been an important and steadfast contribution over a long period of time.

The involvement of the private and business sectors has been far less significant and has usually been in the form of direct grants or food gifts for specific nutrition projects. It appears that subsidized canteen services for workers are not common, but business has made an initial foray into the field of day care services.

International agencies have also contributed materially and technically to the solution of Jamaica's nutrition problems. Among the agencies which have given food during the last two decades are UNICEF, Catholic Relief Services and the World Food Program; and helping at the technical level have been the Caribbean Food and Nutrition Institute and the Food and Agriculture Organization and other UN agencies. While it cannot be denied that food donated for the feeding of young children has been an invaluable supplement, the failure to accompany its distribution with adequate nutrition education has limited the potential impact of these programs, some of which have come to an end.

ECONOMIC POLICY: A MIXED ECONOMY

The last years have seen the steady evolution of a government policy based on a mixed economy in which government ownership, participation, and direction in industry, the utilities, and the distributive sector have increased progressively. Nowhere is this more evident than in agriculture. The government has rapidly acquired, by purchase or lease, a large number of properties as a prerequisite to the implementation of its land lease and land use policies which are intimately bound to its stated goal of increased food production. The right of the government to acquire "idle lands" has in itself been an incentive to the increased use and productivity of such lands.

Sugar, bananas, and citrus—the three most important crops in economic terms—are all subject to quasigovernment control through statutory bodies.

The government provides the producers of these crops with a number of incentives, including a minimum guaranteed price. More recently, in the sugar industry, steps have been taken to make worker participation in management and ownership a reality.

The government's intervention in industry follows lines similar to its intervention in agriculture. Through its own Food Technology Institute and food processing unit, new processed foods are developed and brought onto the market.

Government policy aims to stimulate the food industry through restriction on the importation of a wide range of processed foods, from tomato ketchup to frankfurters. This has opened the way for a number of thriving food industries for both local and Caribbean Community (Caricom) markets. Additional incentives are provided through duty-free entry of food processing equipment and essential raw materials. Additional advantages accrue from these ventures in the form of savings in foreign exchange and an increase in local employment.

OTHER PROGRAMS WHICH AFFECT NUTRITION

The Government of Jamaica is totally committed to the development of an egalitarian society through an equitable distribution of income, agrarian reform, and other measures, described earlier in this paper. In line with this policy is the government's recent Impact Program to create employment. At present, nearly 30,000 previously unemployed persons (some of whom have been described as unemployable) are in regular employment as unskilled laborers, mainly in road construction and cleaning programs. It is significant that more than half of this number are women, who are predominantly the heads of households and primary breadwinners for their families, especially in low income groups. It can be assumed that the income of these 30,000 workers, 30%-40% above the per capita figure for the country, substantially increases the amount of food available to their dependents, estimated at 60,000-80,000 persons. In addition, legislation has been passed to assure equal pay for equal work for men and women. On the other hand, it is not possible to say what the implications of this employment of mothers is for young children who may be deprived of adequate day care. It is hoped that some relevant evaluation of the impact of this program on nutritional status will be done.

Another recent development has been the introduction of a minimum wage bill* in parliament. It is already known that strongly divergent views will have to be accommodated in arriving at the "magic figure" for a minimum wage. A delicate balance is being sought between a wage that is socially just on the one hand and economically bearable on the other, so that there will be mini-

---

*The bill, passed in 1975, stipulates a minimum wage of J$20.00 weekly for all but a few special categories of workers.

mal disruption in the socioeconomic life of the country in the course of raising the living standards of the working class.

Of a somewhat different nature are the national literacy and skill-training programs which, between them, reach tens of thousands of Jamaican adults. This upgrading of individual skills inevitably equips people to become better wage earners, thereby enabling them to break out of the basic economic constraints to better nutrition.

One of the more distressing aspects of poverty in Jamaica is the frequently substandard quality of housing and the attendant inadequacy of such amenities as water and waste disposal. The government's emphasis on low income housing development will create healthier social and environmental conditions vital to the improvement of nutritional status. So widespread is the demand for housing, however, that the development schemes, imaginative as they are, will almost certainly continue to lag behind the need for some time to come.

In pursuing a policy of social legislative reform, the government has instituted a family court combined with a number of related advisory services. This system aims to restore stability to family life and safeguard the rights of the child, among them adequate financial support from the father. The social aspects of the epidemiology of childhood malnutrition, including the role of paternal irresponsibility and the inadequacy of measures to correct it, give reason to welcome this new approach with some optimism.

EPILOGUE

The present Government of Jamaica is now in its fourth year in office. Over two years ago, it very firmly enunciated a policy of democratic socialism in which state ownership and private enterprise are perceived as compatible partners in building a nation of equal opportunity and social justice for all. The government has traveled a far way along the road of its declared policy: the remodeling of education and health care systems, reform in land use and land tenure, the national youth service, special employment programs, and rural development projects are all reflections of this new direction. Throughout, the target of the changing systems has been a better life for each individual member of society.

The implementation of this concept is relatively new for Jamaica, despite some similar political postures several decades ago. Today, the direction seems more in tune with the times, and fully in accord with trends in other developing nations.

The economy is the central force that maintains the life of the country, hence the continuing emphasis on economic development strategies. These, however, need to be accompanied by capital inputs, management, technical expertise, and the virtues of dedication and discipline. For these reasons, it is not possible for a young, small developing nation to coast toward its goals.

Jamaica does not possess all the development requisites in sufficient quantity to meet its needs: there must be constant acceleration in their acquisition if all the national ambitions are to be realized.

It may be as much in the achievement of general economic and social well-being, as in the programs of direct nutritional intervention, that nutritional improvement will ultimately be realized. Not only, therefore, is there room for these two approaches, direct and indirect, but they are clearly complementary and should be simultaneously and harmoniously pursued.

Jamaica possesses a nutrition-conscious development strategy in which increased food output and supplementary feeding programs can find a place alongside day care services and low income shops, all perceived in the context of an overall plan of national development. In nutritional terms, Jamaica has thus embarked on an exciting national adventure.

DISCUSSION (JAMAICA)

Montgomery

I'd like to ask two questions. One is how Prime Minister Manley used nutrition programs to mobilize political support, which seems to have happened about the same time you were carrying out this very ingenious strategy of mobilizing technical support from the different ministries. Is this another case like the Colombia experience with political leadership in nutrition?

The second question is whether this NAC, which, you say, has very weak links to the program implementation side, has worked out methods for using the contacts with ministries to monitor their performance in nutrition terms so that, even without having implementing power, they can make their advice relevant to the perception of the ministries.

Antrobus

First, it is true that Prime Minister Manley came into government with certain clear notions as to how he was going to achieve economic development and social justice. Programs, particularly in the agricultural and land reform séctor, were in motion before a nutrition policy was even thought of as a separate entity. I think it was simply that, when specifics in nutrition came up, these dovetailed very well with the prime minister's own concept of development.

The monitoring through ministries is a very difficult part of the whole exercise of the role of the council. Frankly, maybe because of the relatively small size of the country, much of this depends on the strength of the individual members. So that where there is a strong and *interested* ministry representative on the council, one can see action in that sector. In the case of agriculture, this strong and interested representation on the NAC is showing some returns, whereas, in other sectors this may be less evident. However, there is very little one can do about it. The council hasn't really got any teeth. That's the problem. The structure of the council has undergone some revolution in its short history. Whether all the changes have been for the better is not clear.

Levinson

I think one should add here that Ken is very modest, and the CFNI had no small role in this development. In the context of a receptive atmosphere, CFNI made some very important inputs. This could be contrasted, I think, with the inability of INCAP in Guatemala to make virtually any inroads at all with a government that is not the same.

Antrobus

In Jamaica the idea of planning a food and nutrition policy gained ground by a diffusion process from the Caribbean Food and Nutrition Institute to the Nutrition Division of the Ministry of Health. The council, originally set up as an advisory body, was charged with the formulation of such a policy.

A small committee from the Nutrition Division of the Ministry of Health, in collaboration with CFNI, planned the approach to policy development. They decided to hold a five-day workshop with participants from all the relevant ministries: education, health, agriculture, trade, and so on. The representatives decided on certain topics which should be presented at the meetings. Data and critiques were prepared by these representatives from within their own ministries. Then, they met in one or two plenary sessions and afterwards in about six different workshop sessions, thrashing out the various issues arising from the papers. Each group devised a series of recommendations which were then channeled back to a committee and put together as the flesh and bones of a food and nutrition policy. In other words, the exercise was carried out by technical personnel from within the ministries to provide the basis for writing a policy. The result was a document which set out objectives, specifying target dates and responsible agencies, as well as a series of programs, each of which had associated projects.

Solimano
Could you illustrate a bit more the evidence you cited which shows that, "taken as a whole, the nutritional status of the Jamaican people has improved"? Do you have figures on those changes to show what is possible wii ' this particular pattern of development?

Antrobus
It certainly cannot be stated that nutrition has improved only since these programs started. It is simply too short a period of time to monitor outcomes carefully. What I refer to is that, over the last decade, there is evidence, from food availability data, food consumption data, and data on nutritional status in different surveys, all pointing to an improvement over the period.

Solimano
Have you devised some sort of tool to monitor the changes that are going to occur due to your new approach?

Antrobus
Within the NAC, there are several subcommittees and task forces and a built-in evaluation mechanism. Already, policy has been revised as a result of a review of what is taking place, and it is the intention to have a constant on-going evaluation. I don't know whether evaluation is planned in such a way that it will be able to determine what impact each segment has had on the outcome.

Solimano
I keep emphasizing this point because I think it would be one of the ways, in the future, to know exactly the impact of the different policies in different settings. A lot more needs to be worked out in the methodology of evaluating the impact of these policies. If we do not concern ourselves with this, in ten years we will be asking again, "What happened in Jamaica when they implemented the program?" And nobody is going to know.

Sai

I think the nutrition group has several responsibilities: (1) to help identify
the problem; (2) to point out that nutritional improvement can be one of the
indicators that planners can use in evaluating success of other improvement
programs; (3) to be able to develop nutrition indices which can be used as
sensitive markers for measuring improvement.

Ultimately, a major role for a nutritionist or a nutrition group in a country
is to help identify nutrition measures that can be used for showing the country whether they are going backward or forward in their improvement programs for the people.

Antrobus

There's just one problem in our countries: everything is urgent; everything
has to be now. You cannot have controls and leave out housing and water
supply here and leave out education there and see how it all works out. I
don't know how you will sort it out.

Montgomery

I think that you can develop ways of dealing with this.

Solimano

Just to complete the thinking: there is the question of the role of the different agencies. Of course, the government has to run the programs, but what
should or could the universities be doing at the same time to complement this
type of plan? In our countries, we don't use all the resources we have available because we don't commit other institutions to participate. Universities
are very important in research as a backup for this type of activity. Governments sometimes don't have the ability or the time to do it, but we can look
to other resources.

Latham

It seems to me, in addition, that nearly all of the Caribbean islands have a
completely different weapon to fight nutrition problems than most of the
other countries. Tanzania, for instance, can stop importing certain luxury
foods, but, on the whole, 95% of what is eaten in Tanzania is produced in
Tanzania, whereas the Caribbean countries rely so heavily on imports of food
that they have a different mechanism to play with.

You mentioned that the government now controls some of the expensive
items that are imported. It seems that a central part of nutrition and economic policy for any Caribbean island would be looking at the imports and at
what are good nutritional buys on the world market. If, this year, one can get
a thousand calories of wheat cheaper than rice, then increase wheat and reduce rice imports, and so on. This is something that *you* can use that very few
other countries can use.

Antrobus

In fact, 95% of the cereals are imported in Jamaica, and this is why these targets were set in numerical terms, reducing by 20% the food imports by a certain date. The government felt that there was some value in setting a specific numerical target, whether it was attainable or not.

Levinson

Is this a government policy? Or is this something written by the NAC?

Antrobus

This has been accepted by the cabinet as a government policy.

Latham

A central body dealing with this could save the country a huge amount of money and also have an important nutritional impact.

Antrobus

Part of the research towards this is being done by CFNI in monitoring the costs of some 60 carefully selected food items in about 10 of the territories and publishing a quarterly list of the nutrient costs in terms of calories and protein. This has been handed to the governments, and they have received it very well—as have consumer groups. Now there is some basis for a price control or food import policy if the governments choose.

Schlossberg

While the import situation may be different in terms of the amounts of foods that are imported in the Caribbean countries, the idea of relating import policy to nutrition is applicable to any country. Just as an example, the United States has a tax on imported foods, and that tax has been used to maintain a fund that traditionally was used to support American commodity producers. If there were a surplus of oranges or a surplus of potatoes, that fund would be used to buy up the surplus.

In more recent years, the fund was invaded for use in nutrition programs: to support a pilot supplementary feeding program for low income infants and children or for any other nutrition program that needed extra funds to carry it through a year. There might be an example here for taxing luxury food items that are imported and then using those proceeds for nutrition projects.

Latham

The larger the percentage of imports, the stronger is that weapon, and the more you can use it.

Levinson

It's certainly easier to affect import policies than land use policies!

Antrobus

The Institute, in its role as a catalyst in nutrition matters, has, in fact, gone a stage further and assisted the very small island of St. Lucia in developing a food and nutrition policy. This was done by exactly the same mechanism as in Jamaica. The people of the country, using the data that we helped to get together, prepared their own papers and worked out their own strategies. That policy is undergoing a certain amount of refinement now. There are at least three other countries in the pipeline interested in this type of exercise.

Montgomery
I hope you are going to do it the way you did it in Jamaica, with the technicians from the CFNI.

Antrobus
Yes, but, of course, the difficulty is a bit greater, the smaller the country.

8 SUPPLEMENTARY FEEDING INTERVENTION: A PROGRAM TO PROTECT POPULATION GROUPS AT HIGH NUTRITIONAL RISK IN THE REPUBLIC OF PANAMA

Julio C. Sandoval A.

Julio C. Sandoval A. has been closely associated with the Government of Panama's attempts to deal with nutrition problems in innovative ways, and has helped to develop and implement the supplementary feeding intervention described in his paper. At present, he is Executive Director of the National Water and Sewage Institute. Prior to his current position, he held the post of Vice-Minister of Health, Republic of Panama. Dr. Sandoval received his MD from the University of Madrid, Spain, and his Master of Public Health degree from the Johns Hopkins School of Hygiene and Public Health. He is a fellow of the American Academy of Pediatrics and Professor of Epidemiology and Demography, Department of Social and Preventive Medicine, University of Panama.

INTRODUCTION

The world demographic explosion has outlined with alarming clarity the
nutritional deficits of a great portion of humanity. It appears that a great
nutritional crisis is on its way for the world as a whole, within a relatively
short period.

Panama, like other third world countries, has nutritional problems resulting from interrelating geographic, economic, cultural, and political factors
which determine the availability, consumption, and utilization of food.

It is recognized that nutrition conditions a population's biological and social development. The search for appropriate solutions to decrease hunger and
malnutrition should be a goal of every responsible government.

For several years, the international organizations concerned with health and
nutrition have offered schemes to help with this difficult task. One of these
approaches has been to promote, within each country, closer coordination
among the public and private agencies concerned with food and nutrition
problems.

The discussion of national food and nutrition policies has appeared as a
constant subject in practically every international meeting on nutrition in the
last thirty years. Unfortunately, implementation of such policies has been
very difficult in the majority of countries. We hope that, at this meeting, a
critical analysis of specific experiences in this field will be undertaken. This
analysis and future discussion will be of benefit to all who believe that national food and nutrition policies are an integral part of the general development
policies of the various countries and the only logical and efficient means of
facing the nutritional problems that affect all our peoples.

GENERAL CHARACTERISTICS OF PANAMA

Geopolitical Characteristics

The Isthmus of Panama constitutes the narrowest and lowest part of the
Central American Isthmus, occupying its extreme southeast and serving as a
link between the continents of North America and South America.

The Republic of Panama has an area of 77,082 km^2, including 1,432 km^2
of Panamanian sovereign territory, the Panama Canal Zone, under special
jurisdiction of the United States of America, for the specific purpose of maintenance, operation, sanitation, and protection of the oceanic canal. Panama is
situated in the intertropical zone, which determines its special climatic characteristics and tropical vegetation: a moderate temperature, varying little
throughout the year, abundant rainfall, high humidity, thick rain forest and
tropical grassland. The Republic of Panama borders on the Caribbean Sea to
the north, the Pacific Ocean to the south, Colombia to the east, and Costa
Rica to the west.

The coasts of the Isthmus of Panama form a parallel double curve, providing an extensive shoreline of close to 2,900 km. To the north, there is a narrow strip of coast field, broken by the valleys of large rivers, and exposed to the direct influence of the northeast wind, laden with moisture. The area is thus extremely wet, with a rainfall average between 250 and 350 cm annually. The narrow coastal field, as well as the mountain area, is covered by thick vegetation and humid tropical forest. The lowlands are widest in the Pacific coast, where they form the Panamanian fields. These grasslands extend in an east-west direction, approximately from the central Isthmus to the border with Costa Rica. This coast, protected by a chain of mountains from the humid wind, has a dry tropical climate. The average rainfall is between 100 and 150 cm annually with 4 to 5 months of drought. Grassland and dry tropical forest are the dominant types of vegetation.

Panama's road system, as of June 1974, was 7,121 km long with 8.9% concrete, 22.4% asphalt, 25.9% revetted, and 42.8% earthen road. The Pan-American Highway will soon reach Palo Alto de Las Letras at the frontier with Colombia.

The last constitution of Panama (October 1972) divides the country administratively into 9 provinces, 65 districts or municipalities, an Indian territory, and 505 *corregimientos* (the smallest political divisions) which form the political base of the State. In each corregimiento a Local Committee operates under the coordination of a Community Board. The board is chaired by the corregimiento representative who, at the same time, is a representative in the National Assembly and in the municipal council of his respective district. The most important provincial political organ is the Provincial Coordination Board, formed by corregimiento representatives, the governor, the military chief of the province, and the provincial chiefs of all the ministries and state agencies.

Demographic and Economic Characteristics

As of July 1974 Panama had an estimated population of 1,670,000, a density of 22 inhabitants per km^2. Along with most Latin American countries, Panama has a high rate of natural growth, that, if sustained, could double the population in a short period, in our case, 26 years. During recent years, however, a slight decline has been observed in the birth rate. Along with rapid demographic expansion, there is geographical redistribution, with increasing concentration in urban areas. Natural growth during the last decade would imply an urban population increase at an annual rate of 3%, but the actual increase in the cities is 4% annually, close to double the speed with which the population of the rural sector increases (2.2%). The difference observed between natural growth and the population's actual growth in both areas is explained by rural-to-urban migration. One quarter of the total increment in urban population is due to movement of people from rural areas. At present, the urban sector represents approximately half of the total population, of which 60% resides around the Canal Strip and terminal cities: Panama City on the Pacific and Colon on the Atlantic.

However, there is also an important problem of demographic dispersion in Panama. In 1970 about 97% of inhabited localities had less than 500 inhabitants, representing almost 40% of the total population. This brings about two sets of problems—on the one hand, it becomes almost impossible to improve living standards for the dispersed population, and on the other hand, concentration of the population in a few urban localities makes expensive the provision of services necessary to a high standard of living: access to schools and jobs, adequate housing, potable water, electricity, sewage system, transportation, and so forth.

The Panamanian population structure, by age, shows a predominance of youth. Close to 43% of the population is under 15 years of age; 53% between 15 and 64 years, and only 4% over 65 years of age. The high index of dependency means that a great part of available resources must be directed toward the basic needs of an essentially consumer population.

The Panamanian economy has experienced a vigorous and sustained expansion recently. During the '60s, the gross national product increased at an average rate of 8% annually in real terms; and the product per person, close to 5%, was one of the highest registered in Latin America during that period.

Nevertheless, during the last 4 years, the country has grown at a slightly slower pace, due in part to adverse economic phenomena, such as rapid inflation and shortages of goods for both production and consumption. Economic activity is generated for the most part in the metropolitan area, containing less than half of the total population.

Thus, the manufacturing industry, banks and other financial establishments, construction and commerce, which are mostly located in this area, have experienced the fastest expansion. On the other hand, agricultural activity, predominant in the rest of the country, grew less rapidly, with lower relative contribution to the total product. In fact, the backwardness of a large part of the agricultural sector, where a large population remains at subsistence conditions, is eloquent proof that many groups have not participated in or have benefited only poorly from the gains obtained in national income.

As an effect of the long years of marginal existence of the peasant population and certain urban population strata, important deficiencies are observed in nutritional, sanitary, educational, and housing conditions. In spite of the tremendous effort that the government is making to correct the situation, it is still far from achieving adequate levels.

The illiteracy rate has been reduced considerably during the past years, down, in 1970, to a level of 18% in the population 10 years of age and older. But in the rural areas, the index is as high as 31%—five times higher than in the urban areas.

One of the major economic difficulties is the lack of productive employ-

ment for a growing labor force. In spite of rapid economic expansion during
the past decade, generating employment at an average rate of 3.7% annually,
the growth of the labor force at almost the same level (3.5%) prevented a
significant reduction of unemployment. The absolute number of unemployed
is practically unchanged over this period. In the metropolitan area, the rate of
growth of employment has been more than double that in the rest of the
country and has accounted for more than two-thirds of the employment
generated in the last decade.

The livestock and agriculture sectors contributed only 6% of the new job
positions in the same period. This great disparity in the creation of new job
opportunities, and in the income derived from them, between the metropolitan area and the rest of the country accentuated income maldistribution.

According to a recent study (1970), the top 10% income group received
43% of the total income, averaging US$6,719 per year. This is 4 times greater
than the national average ($1,561), and *54* times higher than the average
income of the individuals in the lowest 20% of income levels. This lowest 20%
received slightly more than 1.6% of the total income, with an average income
of $123 annually, equivalent to one-twelfth of the national average.*

Health Indicators

Population growth at 3% annually has increased the demand on social and
economic services. The fertility rate began to decrease in 1962; and from
1967 on the rate of decline increased. For the decade 1962-72, rates declined
a total of 14%. Birth rates decreased from 40.2 per thousand in 1962 to 36.0
per thousand in 1972, with a decline of 10% in registered births in the urban
area from 37.8 to 35.0 per thousand. In the rural areas, the decline was from
43.7 to 37.0 per thousand in the same period. Fertility rates in 1962 were
13.5% higher in rural areas than in urban areas, but only 5.4% higher in 1972.
These figures suggest a change of attitude in families, probably due to increasing educational level and better access to effective family planning methods.
It is logical to think that through the modernization of our society we will
show a faster decrease in rates, thus modifying the structure of the Panamanian population in the next 20 years. Apparently, Panama has entered the tran-
sitional demographic cycle, with more orderly growth, compatible with the
available national resources.

The implementation of new medical techniques in Panama has effected a
visible decrease in mortality, a trend even older than the reduction in birth
rates (table 1). The positive correlation between changes in these rates has
been explained by some as due to a process in which parents, realizing that
more children survive, begin to understand the advantages in having smaller

*This data is a result of a Special Study in Income Distribution in the Republic of Pana-
ma. The income figures refer to the average income of employed persons in the capital
city and should not be interpreted as the national per capita income which is approximately US$847 for fiscal year 1974.

Table 1
Health Indicators, Panama, 1966-74

Year	Birth Rate	Mortality Rate			Population Growth
		General	Infant	Maternal	
1966	38.9	7.2	45.0	1.5	31.7
1968	38.9	7.1	39.6	1.4	31.8
1970	37.1	7.1	40.5	1.5	30.0
1972	36.0	6.0	33.6	1.1	30.0
1974	31.2	5.3	31.0	0.8	25.9

Source: Ministry of Health, Republic of Panama

families.

The tendency toward urbanization and the extension of health service coverage has improved the life expectancy of the younger Panamanians. Infant mortality has declined from 42.6 per thousand in 1962 to 33.7 per thousand in 1972, with a net gain of 21% for the decade. Although there is an overall tendency for infant mortality rates to decline, this had not been of the same proportion in the urban and rural areas: changes of 28% and 14% respectively have been recorded. The urban area has been able to double rural gains in the fight against sickness in early infancy, thus amplifying the difference in infant mortality rates between the two zones from 9.5 percentage points in 1962 to 24.9 percentage points in 1972. The distribution of resources and services gives ample advantage to the urban areas over the rural population most exposed to the risk of sickness and death. Factors that have been responsible for gains in survival include:

a   Expansion of coverage of the prenatal attention program, which in 1972 reached 68.4%.

b   Professional attention at delivery, with a gain of 23% from 1962 (55.3%) to 1972 (68.2%).

c   Water supply programs covered an additional 27% of the population in the 1964-73 period and now serve 76% of the population. Despite this, only 53% of the rural population has potable water. 386,800 inhabitants, or 24% of the population of the country, does not have potable water.

d   Sewage systems are available for 84% of the population. This represents an increment of 30% from 1964. In the rural areas only 71% of the population has these services.

e   Reduction of incidence in parasitic and infectious diseases is a product of the improvement of the environment, the application of new medical technology, and the development of health programs in the communities.

The overall maternal mortality rate has declined by 39% from 1962. It is clear that service received by the mother in her pregnancy avoids abnormalities of the newborn and safeguards life immediately after birth. The maternal mortality rate in the rural area is 2.2 per 1,000 live births. In the urban areas, however, it is 5 times lower (0.4 per thousand live births), down 67% from 1962. Professionally attended deliveries include 97% of all the births. This suggests the necessity to redouble efforts in the areas least well served—the rural areas, with a delivery assistance rate of 42%.

Vaccination programs are directed to protect the population susceptible to certain diseases and there is clearly an important decrease of morbidity and mortality. Panama has achieved 74% protection for children under 5 years old with DPT vaccine, 82% with polio, and 62% with measles, from 1970-74. The reduction in mortality from measles from 13.5 to 6.5 deaths for each 100 cases during the period 1964-73 and of diphtheria from 19.6 in 1964 to 0.0 in 1973 confirms a steady pace of development in preventive health. The main causes of death and disease in the past have been infectious, but these have now been replaced by degenerative diseases and accidents, as seen in more developed societies. Nevertheless we must bear in mind that average figures hide the reality of our rural inhabitant, shadowed by social and economic marginality and in a constant struggle for new and better opportunities.

AGRICULTURAL SECTOR

Panama's development is closely related in an interdependent fashion to countries with high industrial capacity which mold the world economy to satisfy their needs for primary resources. Panama's role has been fundamentally directed towards traffic, servicing world commerce, which utilizes the isthmus to shorten distances and save time.

In this context it has not been possible to stabilize Panama's agricultural production. Panama was a metal exporter up to the middle of the sixteenth century, and began to send tropical fruits to the international market at the beginning of the present century. Yet transit has always been the principal operation of the country.

Land Tenure Systems

It was not until the present decade that the country worried seriously about promoting agricultural production and incorporating the agricultural population, which forms 50% of the total, into the development process. At present, the form of land tenure systems and of land use varies substantially from the highly technological agroindustrial enterprise, through various levels of productive relations, down to the peasant's subsistence level.

In Panama, latifundium-minifundium relations do not characterize agricultural sector socioeconomic life, nor do they exercise significant influence in political struggles. Five forms of agricultural production can be identified, all interdependent and encompassing social relationships.

1 The Enclaved Agricultural Enterprise   60,000 acres of the top quality soil are controlled by this enterprise, mainly for the production of bananas for the international market. Roughly 15,000 workers are involved in an industry responsible for approximately ¼ of the incoming foreign currency and 60% of the total of Panamanian exports. Workers are employees with a monthly average income of US$150. Due to this relatively high income, their living standards are the best within the agricultural population. Nevertheless, environmental health standards need to be improved.

2 Internal Market Agricultural Enterprise   Several agricultural operations are organized to satisfy local demand. In Panama there are two principal types: one is privately owned, either family enterprise or corporate enterprise, and one has a collective structure under the agrarian reform (almost 200 rural settlements, or *asentamientos campesinos*). Production relations are closely related to—if not dependent on—the urban market.

3 Latifundium—Minifundium   The relations characterized by semiobligatory jobs of rural workers on private ranches have been reduced to a very few areas in Panama. This situation is still predominant in the western Indian region, however.

4 Small Rural Property Holdings   Small rural property holdings are now in a process of disintegration, ostensibly due to constant migration and relative poverty. The traditional land use system is familiar in this circumstance: owners produce to satisfy their basic needs by their own effort and take a variable part of their goods to market.

5 Subsistence Rural Man   The subsistence Panamanian agricultural worker represents 50% of the total agricultural labor force. In this category are largely landless workers. According to some studies, the annual income per person of this rural man amounts to only US$60.

Agrarian Reform and the Structure of the Agricultural Sector

Agrarian movements have not been absent from Panamanian reality. During the nineteenth century civil encounters were common; and after the separation from Colombia in 1903, a sector of the agricultural group, traditionally marginal, obtained political power. In 1940 changes in laws on family patrimony were approved.

Under the influence of the Alliance for Progress, agrarian reform was promulgated in 1963. The objective was to increase production. Regulations and price control systems were installed, import tariffs and fees were established, certain agricultural inputs were freed from taxes, a production center for improved seeds was created and a credit policy was developed.

In 1970 a new stage was initiated with more emphasis in agrarian reform settlements. At the end of 1971 there were 109; in 1974 the number increased to 195, encompassing more than 5,000 families. From 1969 to 1973 agrarian reform acquired more than 700,000 acres of land, benefiting 15,549 families.

From 1974, the Panamanian government projected a policy to incorporate the agricultural sector into the development process of the country. Special interest was directed toward agricultural production. With the La Victoria sugar mill (in Veraguas), a new program was initiated which is currently being extended to other areas of the country. The country is thus undertaking agroindustrial projects that represent important land conversions, use of machinery, and technology. In addition, with the bankruptcy of a critical enterprise involving foreign capital, the state intervened to maintain production.

Panamanian agriculture is not characterized by its dynamism. In the 1960s the economically active population in agriculture increased slowly. According to a recent report, during that decade "the agricultural growth product was unbalanced and unequally shared." Growth concentrated in bananas, rice, sugar, and beef. These products are primarily for export and are cultivated in medium or large operations, with modern production techniques or systems of extensive land use. The benefits and advances only favor a few. In the majority of cases (smaller and more numerous operations), productivity did not grow. In small operations the main problem is the impossibility of utilizing all the labor available.

During 1970, in 85% of all agriculture, labor was performed exclusively by members of the family of the producer. In another 9% the jobs were done *principally* by members of the home. In only 6% was the major part of the job done by hired manpower. The operations that exist for family subsistence "are generally small, dedicated primarily to temporary cultivation, rice, corn, or beans. The work system is primitive and is based on human energy and simple instruments. Very few imports are used to increase the production of the soil."

There is another group of operations, not very numerous, that produces for market purposes. Two subgroups can be distinguished: one, a "semimodern operation, uses technological inputs and machinery for some jobs and hires manpower at certain periods of the year. Second, a smaller number of modern operations, with the latest advances in technology, improved seeds, and chemical inputs. It has hired permanent and temporary manpower."

There is no available information as to the exact number of operations in each group and no way to measure their effects on agricultural improvement. It has been shown that the yield in the modern operation, in comparison to that of the subsistence one, was three times greater for rice and six times greater for corn. In the case of bananas the difference in output was less important, due to differences in the quality of the product. It was noted that, on the average, one day of work suffices, in the traditional system, to produce 18 kg of rice or 22 kg of corn or 600 kg of cane sugar. In the modern operation output is 218 kg of rice, 86 kg of corn, and 1,700 kg of cane sugar.

Transforming agriculture and its orientation towards the market has been, without a doubt, one of the most outstanding changes of the past years. The annual growth of 5.5% in this sector during the last decade was due to important advances in job productivity. In a decade, import of tractors, machinery, and other agricultural apparatus has been multiplied by ten, and everything suggests that since 1972 this tendency has accelerated. In the decade 1960-70 the number of totally mechanized operations grew from 1,800 to 6,800. The transformations in Panamanian agriculture have profound influence on the forms of land tenure and on the people's standard of living. In addition, rapid growth in mechanization creates a rural unemployment problem and generates movement of the population toward the urban areas.

Food Availability

According to the last Food Balance Sheet report (1973) the daily availability of nutrients per capita in Panama was 2,422 kcal, 60.2 grams of protein, and 77.8 grams of fat. These figures, evaluated in terms of the average demand of calories and proteins for the Panamanian population at the same period of time, represent 108% of the average demand for calories and 129% of the average demand for protein. In other words, national production plus the imports of food were sufficient to satisfy the population's need for calories and proteins. Obviously, these *average* figures are hiding the real situation that is observed in some areas of the country.

In table 2, data related to national availability of food for the years 1970-73 is presented. It is important to point out the decrease that is observed for the year 1972-73. This fact could serve as a warning of the food crisis that is approaching unless adequate measures are taken promptly to overcome it. In the same table, information in regard to the caloric, protein, and fat contribution from foreign sources can be observed. It is interesting to point out that where there is the lowest daily availability of calories per person, in 1973, there is an increase, in percentage terms, of the calories derived from imported food. These imports were extremely significant in cereals (wheat, flour, and corn) but reduced in oil and fats. The country is generally a net importer of basic grains. Only rice production has been sufficient to cover internal demands during the past years, with exception of 1971, when bad weather resulted in very bad crops. There is a decreasing tendency to import beans, even though national production has also declined. Consequently, so has consumption.

There has been a great effort to promote national production with the implementation of a series of measures such as minimum prices for basic products, increased taxes on some import goods, and incentives for the farmers.

Table 2
Daily per capita availability of calories, proteins and fats, Panama, 1970-73 (with percent contributed by imports)

Year	Calories (kcal)	% Contributed by Imports	Proteins Vegetable (g)	Animal (g)	Total (g)	% Contributed by Imports	Fats (g)	% Contributed by Imports
1970	3,000	23.6	38.3	27.5	65.8	26.3	81.5	39.6
1971	3,136	37.6	39.6	28.6	68.2	40.0	93.2	42.9
1972	2,774	29.3	34.3	30.9	65.2	35.9	77.5	30.6
1973	2,422	31.4	30.8	29.4	60.2	33.4	77.8	22.2

Note: Table prepared from data in refs. 1, 2

The most important export crops for the year 1973 were, in order: sugar, bananas, shrimp, coffee, and meat. The struggle initiated by Panama to obtain a just price for our bananas in the foreign market received worldwide attention during the year 1974. The economic issues raised, but most important, the moral issues, have resulted in support from other nations on these claims.

In the context of national food and nutrition policy this problem claims high priority, not only because a favorable solution would result in currency increases that could be employed in the purchasing of foods for which local production is still below country demands, but also because this money could be invested in machinery, fertilizer, seeds, and other essential inputs to improve national food resources. If there is not a rapid, acceptable answer, it will be necessary to change the utilization pattern of these lands, dedicated at present to monocultivation. Already, rice plantation experiments have been initiated in some banana areas in Bocas del Toro.

Among the measures directed to increase productivity, the Ministry of Agricultural Development has placed special emphasis on improvement of the storage systems for basic products. Storage continues to be a serious problem due to the fact that, in 1974, the capacity of the storehouses of the National Board of Marketing was only 61% of its need. The remaining 39% of the products had to be stored in hired depositories, sometimes inadequate to the task.

Some advances have been registered in marketing, particularly in the urban centers. The availability of certain basic products (principally fresh vegetables, fruits, grains, eggs, chicken) has been improved, through the "Cheap Food Program." "Sales stands" are set up at strategic points in the principal cities of the country, and food is sold directly to the public, without middlemen. This program operates under the National Board of Marketing. In the rural areas, the great population dispersion and the many out-of-the-way communities present a serious food distribution problem, especially during the rainy season.

It is thus easy to imagine the contrast in the consumption of food between the rural and urban sectors, and, within these sectors, in the different economic strata. The so-called typical diet of the country is composed of rice, beans, starchy roots and tubers (such as yucca), and some corn. In some areas plaintain is a daily dish; in others it is used only occasionally. Meat, whenever it can be obtained, is a very acceptable article in the daily food pattern. With the exception of certain Indian groups (Kunas), which consume much fish, there are no taboos in regard to consumption of this food; however, intake, especially of beef and pork, is rather limited in remote rural areas.

Table 3 presents the daily average ingestion of nutrients per person in rural and urban areas, including percent adequacy of this diet, according to Central American dietary standards. In the rural area, calcium, vitamin A, and riboflavin stand out as major deficits. In the urban sector, average adequacy data give the impression that there are no serious dietary deficiencies. Yet the deceptive quality of average figures is well known, and this must be borne in mind.

THE HEALTH SECTOR

Organization and Structure

The health sector is made up of public and private subsectors, and the population uses both, without distinction, for medical service. The *private* subsector is composed of clinics, laboratories, and private hospitals situated throughout the country, although the majority are in the metropolitan area. Each of these institutions is licensed by type of services offered. The Ministry of Health is responsible for the formulation of the laws, rules, and regulations

Table 3
Average daily intake per capita and adequacy of diet, rural and urban areas, Panama, 1967

Nutrient	Rural Area		Urban Area (City of Panama)	
	Per Capita Intake	% Adequacy	Per Capita Intake	% Adequacy
kcal	2,089	104	2,101	98
Protein (g)	60	112	71	120
Calcium (mg)	301	59	419	80
Iron (mg)	14.3	141	14.9	143
Vitamin A (mg)	0.55	49	1.1	97
Thiamine (mg)	0.92	116	0.91	107
Riboflavin (mg)	0.69	58	0.98	76
Niacin (mg)	14.3	108	14.8	105
Vitamin C (mg)	87	194	107	230

Adapted from ref. 3

governing the exercise of private practice.

On the other hand, the ministry also supervises the public subsector which is composed of different state agencies, the most important being the Ministry of Health, the Social Security Agency, and the National Water and Sewage Institute (IDAAN). Other agencies, such as municipalities, health committees, and the National Lottery Office, contribute financially to health system operations. The University of Panama meanwhile participates in scientific and technical education through several of its faculties, especially those of Medicine, Natural Science and Pharmacy, and Odontology.

The Ministry of Health and the Social Security Institute implement national health policy through the development of integrated health programs, intended not only to improve individual health, but also basic community health. During the past years, more effective coordination between the Ministry of Health and other services in the health sector has been developed, especially with the Social Security Institute. There are already four provinces where Ministry of Health-Social Security integration has taken place, and the aim is to achieve a total health service integration by the end of 1976. This integration process is a response to the existing administrative and technological imbalance and the competition between agencies that should be serving the same goal. With integration, service coverage can be expanded for the majority.

In order to implement integration, the Ministry of Health was reorganized in 1974, changing from multiprovince regions to single-province regions. Each region is under a medical director, responsible for health services in the province. Nine sanitary regions were created, one for each province, with the exception of Azuero Sanitary Region, composed of the provinces of Herrera and Los Santos; Panama Sanitary Region, made up of the province of Panama and San Blas Territory; the Metropolitan Region, encompassing the districts of Panama, Taboga, and the special district of San Miguelito. Within the regions there are 17 sanitary areas, which are subdivided into health sectors.

In Panama there are three types of hospitals: the national hospitals located in the city of Panama; the regional or provincial hospitals, located in the most populated areas of the provinces; and the local or district hospitals that are located in towns, generally capitals of districts.

Services are provided to the community at the health centers or subcenters. There are 67 health centers of which 15 have a maternal-pediatric annex, and there are 96 health subcenters where paramedic personnel render services.

Budget

It is difficult to determine the *total* health budget of the country because it includes both private and public subsectors, and there is little information on the private sector. The public subsector budget for health has increased over the past five years. There are two components to this budget: operational or expense budget, and the infrastructure or investment budget. The health expenditure budget for 1975 assigns 66.1% to the Social Security Institute, 24.7% to the Ministry of Health, and 9.2% to IDAAN. Only about ½ of the Social Security share is spent on health, however, because about ½ goes to direct financial aid programs. The investment budget for the same period gives 66.0% to the Social Security Institute, 25.6% to the IDAAN, and 8.41% to the Ministry of Health. Of the Ministry of Health's *total* current expenditures, 29.8% goes to preventive medicine and 70.2% to curative medicine. In the Social Security Institute, 90% or more is destined for curative medicine.

Human Resources

The Decennial Health Plan of the Americas, 1971-80, approved a regional goal of 8 doctors per 10,000 inhabitants, 2 dentists per 10,000 inhabitants and 4.5 nurses per 10,000 inhabitants. At present, Panama's distribution is: 8.1 doctors per 10,000 inhabitants, 2.0 dentists per 10,000 inhabitants, and 7.8 nurses per 10,000 inhabitants. In addition, Panama has surpassed the goals set for paramedical personnel.

It is important, however, to note that a high proportion of the medical and paramedical personnel is concentrated in the metropolitan region of the country, which makes difficult, at times, satisfactory delivery of health service in the rural areas.

Coverage

Health service coverage reaches 64.3% of the total population, while 78% of the population that lives in urban zones of more than 2,000 inhabitants is protected with some type of state health service. It is estimated that private practice covers about 15% of this urban population.

THE NUTRITIONAL PROBLEM IN PANAMA

In general, studies aimed to diagnose the nutritional conditions of populations are very laborious and expensive. For this reason, they are usually carried out on relatively small samples, which are not always as representative as desirable. Consequently, results should be accepted with certain reservations.

Definition of the Problem

The only nutritional survey of national scope conducted in Panama took place in 1967. Its results underlined the following as the most relevant problems:

- protein calorie malnutrition
- nutritional anemias, principally caused by a lack of iron and folic acid
- hypovitaminosis A

- low intakes of thiamine and riboflavin
- endemic goiter

The Most Affected Groups

According to anthropometric and biochemical studies, the group most affected by protein calorie malnutrition is preschool children. Applying a weight indicator, developed by INCAP for Central America, the prevalence of undernutrition in children less than five years of age was, in 1967: First degree malnutrition, 48.8%; second degree malnutrition, 10.8%; and third degree malnutrition, 1.1%.

This situation produces a retardation in the growth and development of children, starting as early as three months of age. At five years of age, the accumulated retardation, in weight, is 14 months. In height, it is significantly greater. This is confirmed by the adults, who are of smaller stature than their genetic potential would have permitted if they had not been affected by malnutrition. These adults are frequently ill and have a low working capacity.

The 1967 survey findings have been confirmed and superseded in more recent studies done in selected areas of the country. A nutrition survey conducted in January 1975 in 19 rural localities in the Province of Veraguas (a total of 191 families) revealed a more severe protein calorie malnutrition problem than the previous survey. The anemia problem also appeared impressive.

The two studies are not wholly comparable, because the first study did not include populations of remote areas while the later one studied mostly such communities. Because of this, it would be fair to conclude that the 1967 national survey figures underestimated the malnutrition problem existing in the country at that time. In table 4 findings from both studies are presented.

The studies of anemias showed a high prevalence of low and deficient levels of hemoglobin in males 12 to 44 years of age. Following, in order of severity, were women between 45 and 64 and then males 65 and over. In the urban area, frank anemia appears in a smaller proportion of the population. The higher standards of environmental sanitation in these areas may be respon-

Table 4
Prevalence of malnutrition in children less than 5 years old. Data derived from two studies

Level of Malnutrition	1967 Study[a] (National Average) (%)	1975 Study[b] (Average for Veraguas) (%)
First Degree	48.8	52.4
Second Degree	10.8	21.9
Third Degree	1.1	2.6

[a]Data from ref. 3.

[b]Preliminary data from a study conducted on five districts of the province of Veraguas by the Department of Nutrition, Ministry of Health, 1975

sible for this more favorable situation.

In spite of the fact that dietary studies point out a deficient intake of sources of vitamin A, clinical studies do not reveal severe signs of this deficiency. Biochemical studies do nevertheless show low levels in the blood serum, especially for rural children under 10 years of age.

The low intake of riboflavin, revealed through dietary studies, correlates well with the biochemical data. Clinical signs suggestive of deficiency (e.g., angular stomatitis and nasolabial seborrhea) were found, but on a much lesser scale than expected from dietary and biochemical findings.

For thiamine there are conflicting results from dietary and biochemical studies. Calculated food nutrient values, from the Food Composition Tables, do not match data derived from urinary excretion studies. This apparent discrepancy disappears when dietary values are calculated from chemical analysis of exact "replicas" of the food consumed. It seems that the preparation and cooking methods for rice traditionally employed in Panama are responsible for this situation: in effect, the repeated washing and, later, overcooking of this main staple food causes considerable loss of thiamine, exceeding 50% of the vitamin. No clinical evidence of niacin or ascorbic acid deficiency has been found, though the latter nutrient is, at times, absent from the diet of low economic status individuals in urban areas.

The high prevalence of endemic goiter (national average, 16.5%) that was revealed in the 1967 survey, must have changed considerably by this date on account of the iodized salt program promoted by the Ministry of Health and put into operation in 1970 for the whole country. In 1975 an evaluation of the program was carried out with clinical and biochemical data. Results are not yet available as the data are still being tabulated.

Calcium, of which the intakes are very low in relation to recommended levels, presents no nutritional problem since organic and functional evidence of deficiency has not been documented by surveys.

Conditioning Factors

The multicausal origin of nutritional diseases is clear, but the role of the effective demand for food, that is, the purchasing power of the population, must be emphasized. Table 5 represents the 1971 and 1975 purchasing power of laborers in Panama City, in the lowest classified job activity, in regard to 7 food items usually consumed by urban Panamanians. Purchasing power is expressed in terms of working time needed (in minutes) to buy each of the articles on the basis of the official minimum salary for this group. The slight increase in salary in 1975 does not compensate for the price increment of the food articles listed. Specifically for beans, one of the basic foods in the Panamanian diet, the working time required, according to the chart, is, in 1975, twice as much as that in 1971.

In December 1969, calculations revealed a daily cost of US$2.10 for the

Table 5
A laborer's purchasing power, based on minimum salary, City of Panama, 1971[a] and 1975[b]

Item	Amount	November 1971[a] Average Cost (US$)	Working Time Required to Purchase Food (minutes)	March 1975[b] Average Cost (US$)	Working Time Required to Purchase Food (minutes)
Beef Loin ("Falda")	1 lb	0.45	54	0.70	76
Cow's Milk (fresh)	1 lt	0.25	30	0.30	33
Powdered Milk	4 oz	0.24	29	0.32	35
Evaporated Milk	14½ oz can	0.23	28	0.34	37
Rice (med. quality)	1 lb	0.12	14	0.21	23
Beans (average of different kinds)	1 lb	0.19	23	0.42	46
Bread	1 lb	0.19	23	0.32	36

[a]Standing salary for the lowest classified job activity for the City of Panama 1971 (US$0.50/hour).

[b]Standing salary for the lowest classified job activity for the City of Panama 1975 (US$0.55/hour)

"minimum cost adequate diet" for a family of five, in Panama City; in 1971 it was $2.32 and in March 1975 it rose to $3.62, which represents a 72% increase in six years' time. A special study on income distribution in 1970 revealed a per household average income in Panama City of $3,666 per year. Applying the "minimum cost adequate diet" for December 1969, we find that to feed a family of five cost $766.50 per year, or 21% of the *average* household annual income reported for the area. On the other hand, if we relate the cost of the diet with the average household income of the families in the lowest 30% bracket ($358) we find that the annual cost of such diet represents *more than double* (214%) *the annual income* received by such households. The logical conclusion is that the economic factor is notably important, at least for a large part of the eighteen thousand and more households of the metropolitan area classified in the lowest 30% income range. Recently, the government reduced prices 20-24% for rice, beans, and evaporated milk. This was done because of a surplus of these commodities and will be implemented by the institute that controls consumer prices. This institute oversees the merchants and ensures that market prices do not exceed set prices. We do not know, yet, the nutritional consequences, if any, of this price adjustment.

Insufficient knowledge of basic principles of food and nutrition on the part of the housewives makes a precarious situation even more delicate. In the rural areas, this picture becomes even more complicated because of low levels of sanitation and correspondingly high prevalence of infectious diseases.

ACTIVITIES INTENDED TO SOLVE THE PROBLEMS

Background Information

Nutritional problems have been recognized for quite a long time in Panama. Forty years ago, the school lunch program began to take shape due to the interest of a group of socially minded public school teachers, alert to the nutritional condition of their pupils. The present coverage of the lunch program was notably increased with the aid of bilateral food distribution program (US PL 480, the Food for Peace Program).

Scientific consideration of nutritional problems, however, did not begin until 1951, with the establishment within the Ministry of Health (at that time, Ministry of Work, Public Welfare, and Health), of a Nutrition Section. This office came into being as a consequence of Panama's ratification of the basic agreement that created the Instituto de Nutricion de Centro America y Panama (INCAP), an institution promoted by the Pan American Health Organization, with the objective of studying and finding solutions to the nutritional problems of the six countries of the Central American isthmus.

During its first ten years of operation, the Nutrition Section, with the help of INCAP technical staff, concentrated attention mainly on basic research and the collection of information about the magnitude of the nutritional problems in Panama.

During the same period, in 1952, with the help of UNICEF, a Supplementary Feeding Program for the benefit of mothers and children (infant, preschool, and school age) was also started. This program was taken over in 1956 by CARE and, on a lesser scale, by CARITAS. Both agencies continue to operate in our country, acting as intermediaries for the distribution of the Food for Peace products. As is traditional in this kind of program, the Government of Panama covers the cost of administration, storage, and internal distribution of the products. For 1974, this represented an expenditure of approximately US$135,000,000. 84% of the beneficiaries of this program were schoolchildren.

In 1962, with UNICEF financial help and the technical cooperation of FAO and WHO, the so-called "Programa de Nutrición Aplicada" (Applied Nutrition Program), was initiated. In its general structure it was very similar to other programs started about the same time in more than a hundred countries over the world. In Panama, the program was concentrated at the primary school level. Its main objective was to educate the population in basic principles of food and nutrition. Hence there arose the idea of utilizing the extensive network of schools and teachers in this important task.

Prior to participation in the program, teachers were given special seminars in the basic philosophy of applied nutrition work. Information in specific areas such as nutrition, horticulture, and general health was very profitable for their work within the school, but other factors prevented them from carrying on the same work in the community at large. The school gardens, some of them excellent examples of applied technology, helped to reinforce the theoretical concepts about food and nutrition learned in the classroom. Also, the gardens were magnificent motivation for the acceptance by the children of a variety of previously unfamiliar vegetables, rich sources of carotene.

UNICEF aid extended from 1962 through 1968. The most outstanding contribution of the program was the coordination that was established among the Ministries of Agriculture, Education, and Health, by means of a national and several regional committees. Its main failure was the extremely weak community involvement.

In 1969, the Ministry of Health was separated from its previous administrative attachment to the Ministries of Labor and Social Welfare. At the beginning, the minister and a lot of the new officials were pediatricians, and the group was sometimes described as the "Pediatric Ministry." The medical group that is most sensitive to nutritional problems is pediatricians, so there began to be a great concern for this subject. With a new philosophy, exemplified in the motto *"Salud Igual Para Todos"* (Equal Health for Everyone), officials underscored the importance of the nutritional problem in the country, emphasizing the poor availability of foods in the rural areas as one of the main causes of undernutrition. A campaign for the promotion of communal gardens was started in which the campesinos were invited to participate, in groups, under the guidance of qualified agronomists and with the aid of modern technology, including small garden tractors. The political and technical impact of such an intervention was enormous because of its origins in a ministry of health. For the first time, the health sector recognized its responsibility in improving the availability of foods at the community level.

The entire health team, with members at all levels of the health organization, participated in the many phases of this task: preliminary health diagnosis of the communities involved in the projects; joint discussions between campesinos and health officials of the problems encountered and ways to solve them; and above all, the work of making the people conscious of their "rights and duties" in the field of health. In 95% of the communities approached, the people expressed their desire to participate in the communal food production experiment, employing modern technology. At present, the Ministry of Health is integrating this work into the rest of the programs dealing with health promotion and protection such as those related to water supply systems, general environmental sanitation, and immunizations.

While pursuing these programs, the Ministry of Health has also been conscious that the extent of malnutrition in the country could be reduced by an integrated approach, with the active participation of all the sectors of government that have some responsibility in this area. From this concern, shared equally with the Ministry of Planning and Economic Policy, came, late in 1973, the formulation of a "Program of Protection of Population Groups with High Nutritional Risk." This program, which was put into effect in 1974, represents the closest approximation to effective multisectorial coordination, an indispensable element in the definition and later execution of a national food and nutrition policy.

Thirty years after the first creation in Panama of a National Nutrition Council, replaced soon after by another equally nonfunctioning group, it is only now that we have a glimpse of some significant action in this area. The evaluation of this experience, with special attention to its problems and accomplishments, constitutes the central theme of the presentation that follows.

Supplementary Feeding Intervention: Part of a Program to Protect Population Groups at High Nutritional Risk

This section summarizes the outstanding facts related to the origin and initiation of a nutritional intervention as a component of the major *Programa de Proteccion a los Grupos de Poblacion con Mayor Riesgo de Desnutricion en el Pais.* The present government of Panama has proposed this program as an emergency solution to the nutritional problems suffered by some marginal groups. This intervention is considered as the first approximation to effective multisectorial coordination, an indispensable element in the definition and further execution of a national food and nutrition policy.

Condensing the process by which this nutritional intervention came into being, we recognize at least four important aspects:

1 Motivation at the highest political level of decisionmaking.

2 Interest by a group of very qualified government technicians—professionals in various disciplines, well acquainted with the nutritional problems of Panama, eager to capitalize on the interest shown at high levels, who designed a plan to solve the problem of malnutrition in the country by approaching it in a more rational manner and taking into account all the factors that condition the problem.

3 Execution of this intervention at the local level, with active participation at national as well as provincial levels.

4 Finally, the outstanding importance of political and economic endorsement in the solution of nutritional problems is recognized. In the absence of such powers, accomplishments in this field become very dubious and weak.

In regard to the first of these phases, it is important to point out the great changes produced by the revolution of 1968, and the elections four years later, including a marked concentration of government effort in the rural areas, trying to increase local participation in decisionmaking, in an approach we call direct democratic participation. At present, the trend in the government is progressive, very much task-oriented, with a technocratic push, dedicated to the establishment of social justice, concerned with the fate of the poor people, the children, and especially the campesinos. This political setting must be kept in mind because it explains much of what one sees in Panama.

The chief of state, in constant dialogue with the campesinos and marginal groups, promised to elevate their living standards. His closest collaborators encouraged him to undertake studies about poverty. As a result of this scheme, the Ministry of Health accelerated the gathering of information on the health status of very isolated communities as a means of promoting the community organization required to initiate aggressive, basic programs of environmental sanitation (potable water and construction of latrines) and immunization.

Ministry of Health technicians were challenged to propose a plan to solve the problem of malnutrition, recognizing that the complexity of nutritional problems are a reflection of the low standard of living of rural areas. This implied that attention had to be paid to the lack of land, low level of education, reduced income and deficient diet of the people.

The Plan   The working group in charge of formulating the plan were conscious that the National Nutrition Plan would require a "maturation period," involving innumerable meetings and conversations with all the different sectors of the government. At the same time, this group was terribly pressured from the highest levels of the political world to present concrete and rapid answers to the most urgent problems of nutrition. Because of this situation, the technical group unanimously determined to give first priority to a program oriented toward the groups most severely affected by malnutrition and/or with the highest risk of suffering from it. The program established two very well defined stages:

1 The first, or urgency stage, would consist of the distribution of food rations to the groups in most need. This is the so-called Supplementary Feeding Phase.

2 The second stage would proceed with the development of production projects (in agriculture, chicken and pig raising, craftsmanship, and so forth) with the objective of increasing family productivity by full use of the economically active population.

Both stages of this program have the family as the target point of all help. It is recognized that the undernourished child comes from an "undernourished family," in the fullest meaning of the term. The program is conceived as an integral part of the Economic and Social Development Policy of the country, and is accepted as one of the first strategies conducive to the formulation of a definite national food and nutrition policy.

The Population at Risk—How to Define It?   Undoubtedly, one of the most difficult problems facing the working group in preparing this program was the delineation of the population exposed to the "risk" of suffering malnutrition, especially at the community level. Previous nutritional studies had always evaluated the situation at a national or regional level. Thus, for this program, the population at risk was determined by means of indirect indicators: at the district level, the proportional mortality in groups 1-4 years of age (figure 1) was applied; at the village level (the smallest political divisions) the deterioration index excreta/potable water (percent of homes without latrines + percent of homes without potable water) was used. As complementary indicators, illiteracy and level of agricultural development were employed.

In this fashion, it was possible to separate, from the 65 districts and the Indian region of San Blas, those in most urgent need. Fifteen districts were chosen, distributed in seven of the nine provinces, and in those districts approximately 9,000 families with a total population of about 50,000 persons were selected for attention. This corresponds to 25% of the total population of these fifteen districts.

The supplementary feeding activities include basic health activities, as well as the distribution of food rations. The health activities are related to sanitation of the environment, which requires, in turn, intensive educational work at the village level. Logically, these actions presuppose some sort of community development. The promotion of this development constitutes one of the main goals of the program, and is carried out mainly with the help of trained auxiliary personnel.

Due to the differences in cultural patterns in the various geographic areas and due to the variations of resources within the families and communities, no minimum duration for the continuation of this food help has been assigned. There only exists a maximum period of duration, set at three years. Because of this, the second stage of the "Program to Protect Population Groups at High Nutritional Risk" does not have a definite initiation period. The ideal is to start it as soon as communities are ready for it.

The following goals have been established for the supplementary feeding intervention itself:

1 To eradicate third degree malnutrition in the group 0-5 years of age.
2 To reduce by 80% the prevalence of second degree malnutrition among the group 0-5 years of age.
3 To reduce by 80% the prevalence of anemias within the program population.
4 To reduce the prevalence of hypovitaminosis A in the same population.

Nature of the Food Rations   The type of food rations to be distributed to the beneficiaries was discussed at length in regard both to the food items and the nutritive composition. It was considered very important that the latter not be too high in order to lessen the risks of the ration becoming a substitute, rather than a supplement, for the family diet. The negative effects of such substitution are obvious. It was decided that the contribution of the ration should be between 20-30% (maximum) of the daily demand for calories and proteins of the different members of the family groups. For other nutrients, the percentage is a little higher.

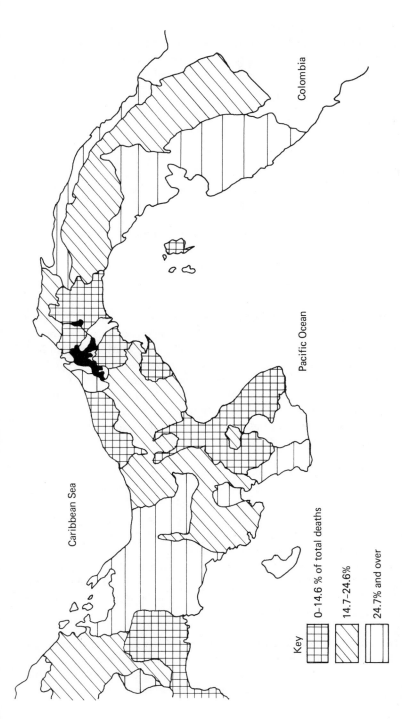

Figure 1
Deaths of one to four year olds, 1971.

On the basis of local dietary habits and facility of preparation, two different types of rations were established from the beginning: one for children 6 months to 3 years of age, and one for the rest of the family members. The "regular" ration (3 years of age and more) included the following:

Rice	75 g
Beans	25
Skim milk powder	10
Oil	15
Sugar	10

With the exception of skim milk powder (which is included because of its calcium and riboflavin contribution), all the other foods are commonly consumed in the Panamanian diet. This is a great advantage, as the danger of refusal on the part of the families is minimized.

The infant food mixture, called NUTREBIEN, is equally acceptable. Its formula includes:

Rice	60%
Whole milk powder	16
Sugar	24

and a concentrate of iron and vitamins. This mixture is industrially prepared and is distributed in 42.5 g (1.5 oz) bags. The recommended daily ration is 85 g, the equivalent of two bags per day for children 6 months through 3 years. Its nutritive contribution for this age group varies between 29-39% for calories and proteins; it is higher for iron, thiamine, riboflavin, niacin, and retinol. Our most serious problem is that we are able to store the ration adequately for only four weeks, since the milk tends to become rancid in the high humidity. All the rations for each family are put together in one "15 day" package; packages are provided twice a month.

Execution of the Plan in the Country at Large Although there is great urgency to help the 15 districts identified as of the "highest nutritional risk," action must be conditioned by the financial conditions of the country. It is important to point out that the budget of this plan is totally financed by national funds. In spite of its high priority, therefore, it cannot demand expenditures beyond national financial possibilities.

Logistic considerations suggest the initiation of a comprehensive project in a single province. By doing this, it would be possible to acquire valuable experience which, in turn, would permit easier evaluation of methods and procedures, undoubtedly beneficial for the future.

Execution of the Plan in Veraguas Although the first conversations in regard to this subprogram took place in April 1973, becoming more technical and definite starting in August of the same year, it was not until September 1974 that the actual distribution of foods was initiated in the province of Veraguas.

The organization of the administrative aspects indispensable for beginning this task was a long, tedious process given special attention by the Ministry of Health and the Provincial Coordinating Committee of Veraguas. The Ministry of Health, whose budget allocated US$0.5 million for the initial phase of this nutritional intervention, integrated the personnel required to carry out these new responsibilities into the health system of the province.

In the province of Veraguas, aside from the four districts originally selected as of "highest nutritional risk," a fifth district was added, because a recent flood had caused great damage to the crops.

By November of 1974, food rations were reaching all the communities chosen as beneficiaries of this intervention, and the last census showed that 4,244 families, distributed throughout 224 villages, were enrolled. This amounted to a total of 24,676 persons, or approximately 20% of the total population of the entire province of Veraguas. The tremendous effort necessary to buy, store, and pack rations adjusted to the ages and number of family members, and the distribution of these goods to very remote places has required constant revision of a system that is still very primitive. There is little mechanization, with the exception of trucks to transport the food rations to 30 distribution centers located at strategic points within reasonable distance of the five beneficiary districts.

Coordinating Bodies This feeding subprogram has a principal coordinating body, the National Nutrition Committee, composed of the undersecretaries (vice ministers) of Planning and Economic Policy, Education, Agricultural Development, and Health. The latter official acts as general director of the program. At the provincial level is the Interministerial Provincial Coordinating Committee, strongly reinforced by representatives of ministries and official agencies in addition to those on the national committee. These additional members include the governor of the province, the chief of the National Guard at provincial level, and the representative of the Minister of Public Works. The Provincial Health Director, by delegation of the Vice Minister of Health, acts as provincial director of this subprogram. Both the national and provincial committees are assisted by their respective technical groups.

It is extremely interesting, from the point of view of process, to note how the Provincial Coordinating Committee became linked to this nutritional intervention. The committee was not the outcome of the supplementary feeding experience. On the contrary, this subprogram made use of an already-existing coordinating structure. The first contact with this committee was made early in 1974, by the Minister of Health, who travelled to Veraguas with a draft of the Plan of Operations to "sell" the Program to Protect Population Groups at High Nutritional Risk. It was widely discussed and the committee, a political body, saw the political implications clearly, and unanimously gave approval. Immediately, the members pledged to involve their respective offices in the execution of the tasks necessary to the initiation of the supplementary feeding stage in the province.

The *representantes de corregimientos* (political officials of the five target districts of the program) offered collaboration in the selection of the villages, in accordance with the criteria established in the Plan of Operations. Although the application of the selection criteria was not strictly observed in all the cases, the involvement of the representantes in this task represented great political backing, very badly needed at this initial stage.

Community Development In the majority of the selected villages, the community organization is very weak. Organization, essential for the adequate development of the supplementary feeding stage, becomes still more important for the second stage of the program, the phase of development of production projects. The hope is to synchronize this second phase with the level of community development that each of these villages attains.

Execution will demand vigorous coordination with the Ministry of Agricultural Development and other official and private agencies. The program has been somewhat slow in Veraguas in the preliminary studies of feasibility of specific community projects. The only research studies done so far are the nutritional evaluations of the target population and some sociological explorations on the acceptability of the program. Both studies have been carried out by technical personnel of the Ministry of Health. There remains an urgent need for integration with technicians from other official agencies in the work on these tasks.

Real integration of different disciplines and agencies at this stage is the only way to prevent this tremendous effort from ending as merely a glorified supplementary feeding intervention, unable to carry out the next step: communal social and economic development.

The Scope of the Education Task Educational work with the communities is one of the very important components of the program. Thirty positions of "health assistant" have been created whose principal functions are the *administration* of the 30 family ration distributing centers and the *educational* activities at the community level in basic aspects of health, with special emphasis on food and nutrition. Each assistant is responsible for 10 to 15 communities, depending on their accessibility. The assistants travel, giving lectures and making sure that the people receive the foods. No doubt, the success of the supplementary feeding subprogram will depend substantially on proper understanding of the objectives of the program by the beneficiaries themselves.

The creation of consciousness of the real meaning of food assistance and the pledge to work on agriculture or other projects aimed to raise living standards constitutes a very special task, requiring very special personnel with a high degree of social sensitivity and great dedication. Although the minimum academic requirement for health assistants is the completion of the first secondary (9th grade), graduate teachers are preferred. A positive attitude toward communal work in rural areas is considered a basic and indispensable qualification for the work.

Considerations on Future Expansion of the Program   The future expansion of the program, beginning with the supplementary feeding stage, will be the responsibility of the National Interministerial Committee, duly assisted by the technical groups. Logically, economic aspects will count heavily in any expansion decision. At present, the average annual cost per capita is about US$40.00. This represents an appreciable sum of money. During 1975, the $1 million assigned to the execution of the supplementary feeding stage in Veraguas will barely cover the expenses, for two reasons: (1) the increase in beneficiaries over the maximum assigned figure, and (2) the rise in the price of foodstuffs. In addition, the NUTREBIEN packages are relatively expensive, just under 14¢ each, mainly due to the paper wrapping. We are working with the producer to find another kind of paper, which can serve the same purpose more cheaply.

This represents a real challenge to the planners, who must work out alternatives so decision makers can choose the best course of action for the future evolution of this program.

Outstanding Problems Encountered in the Development of the Supplementary Feeding Subprogram in Veraguas

It does not take great effort to imagine the series of problems that the initiation of such a complex activity can generate. Many of them have been solved already or are in the process of solution. Their recognition, nevertheless, constitutes a major advance. Among the most relevant, the following must be mentioned:

1 Difficulty with intersectorial coordination at all levels. We try to interest other people in nutrition, but often it appears that nobody cares: it's nobody's problem. So we have to pick up the problem in the health sector in terms of sickness.
2 Rudimentary food packing system.
3 Delay in the training of health assistants, who must have education themselves before they can function effectively.
4 Difficult access to some isolated communities, especially during the rainy season, which interferes with the travel of beneficiaries to the distribution centers.

Positive Aspects of this Nutritional Intervention

It is impossible to think in terms of accomplishments of the supplementary feeding stage, scarcely 10 months after its initiation. Periodic evaluations of the administrative and technical aspects, nevertheless, do point to some positive effects:

1 This program has stimulated the execution of health promotion and protection activities in very remote communities, which had never before received any health services, except possibly malaria control. This change is a result of the fact that the program is dependent on the *local* provincial health officer who thinks about whether the food recipients are vaccinated, and so forth.

2 The inclusion of adults in the food distribution program represents a new concept: the recognition of a nutritional problem among the economically active group and its importance in their future work performance. On the other hand, it also represents a protection of the children's food ration, which in former programs had only a "theoretical" value.

3 The distributional impact of the program is of great significance. The economic contribution of the food rations represents more than 50% of the average annual income received by families in the lowest 30% of income levels in the rural area. Many of the families benefiting from this program fall within that category.

4 Although intersectorial coordination still remains a problem, some observed advances bode well for the future. There is no doubt that the health group has had a major role in promoting such a propitious and indispensable situation.

Finally, any program geared to improve the nutritional conditions of any country can only be successful if it receives the proper political and economic backing. In the absence of these powers very little can be achieved. In Panama, the political endorsement of this program is presently very ample. Economic support is also generous, in accordance with our abilities. We firmly believe that this important backing will progressively increase and that interagency coordination will consolidate, giving rise to the structure of a real and definitive national food and nutrition policy.

DISCUSSION (PANAMA)

Sandoval

I know everybody wants to know how this all began: that's why we are here.
As I mentioned, the government's one important objective was to improve
the living condition of the campesinos, the poor people, and the children.
Someone in the government decided that we had to increase production in
order to overcome inflation and other economic problems. Then it was mentioned that some people in Panama were so poor that they have nothing to
eat, and, if they can't eat, they can't work.

So the government challenged the health sector to come up with a program
for that population. Funds were allocated *before* the program was designed.
This is very important: they trusted us to come up with some kind of effective program. The first six months were a learning experience. When we started this program, we tried to obtain the new tractors and we tried to hire
technicians. It caused all kinds of problems because we were told we should
be in the hospitals taking care of patients or out vaccinating people. We had
all kinds of opposition within the country—even some of the recipients of the
program, at the beginning, were distrustful and afraid. They asked questions
such as, "Must I go to the army if I receive a package?" It was an innovation,
and, as with all innovations, there are problems.

Now, however, the political impact of this program is very, very impressive.
This program, with its concern for the living conditions of the people, is generating very positive feedback. In the health sector, we suddenly found ourselves with money which we were trying to obtain for years and years. We
thought that we would get results by way of a national coordination committee, but we got it directly, at a top political decisionmaking level. This may
not be the best way for *every* country, but it is one sure way!

Mellor

You say the feedback is important, but to whom is it apparent?

Sandoval

Within each corregimiento there is a national representative who is a spokes-
man for his community. Some of these representatives come from communities so remote that most people don't know if they are in Panama or in Costa
Rica—practically no one has ever *heard* of them! Such a person comes and
says his people are receiving food. The political implication is that the government is doing something to solve problems rather than promising such things
as a highway or bridge. This is something the people can grasp within their
small context, and, as I said before, we have thousands of small communities.

Wray

How do you choose which areas receive supplementary feeding?

Sandoval

Within each district, there are a number of corregimientos, the smallest political division of the country. They have to present hard data showing that they
really need the program. Then, within the corregimiento, we serve several
communities. We have to know the number of the families and number of
children under three years of age so we can prepare the packages of
NUTREBIEN and the proper ration. We are currently covering roughly
25,000 people, half the population at risk.

Maletnlema

Who is responsible for collecting the data within each corregimiento? Do you
go out, or is the district responsible? We had a similar program, with food
distribution to needy children, and the district had to convince us of its need.
Eventually we realized that some of the districts which were very needy did
not have the people who could collect the data to convince us while the better-off districts had very good people. They were able to do the convincing,
and get the money!

Sandoval

In Panama, data is all collected at a district level, so it is easy to know immediately what district has what mortality. Of course, there are some overesti-
mates and underestimates, but the picture is clear, over all, at the district
level. Within the district, we went to the corregimientos and did surveys.

We had an idea, beforehand, of where the problem was, but we had to have
objective evidence in order to tell those who don't get the food: "We are
sorry, but we have to give it to someone else." Everybody wants this program. It's a political issue, so we need hard facts to say, "You just don't qualify." When a community with poor indices is bigger than 500 inhabitants, we
decide family by family, but if the community is smaller than 500, all the
people receive food. This is so nobody trades and nobody steals. Since it is
local food, nobody sells it. Where would you sell it? To whom? Local shops
have the same product and are perhaps selling it cheaply already to those who
have some money.

Montgomery

How is the ration distributed? Could you tell us more about the actual process?

Sandoval

All the food is bought locally with national funds, then the entire packing
operation is done in a packing center by hand in a very primitive way. We
have just ordered two machines to do this job, but when we began the project, we packed by hand. When I took over, there had been discussions for six
months about what type of uniforms to use! I just went ahead and started it,
even without packing machinery.

Each ration package varies according to family composition and is made up individually. Packages are then loaded onto trucks which take them from the packing center to a distribution center or depot. We use any place we can find as a distribution center: sometimes we use a jail, sometimes we use part of a school, and sometimes we have to pay rent.

Each family has a card with its ration figures, and the packages are double-checked before they are handed over. Recipients are double-checked, too! One problem is that, for large families, the sacks of food are so heavy, it presents a problem to transport them home!

Wray
Julio, by using local food, were you able to avoid the need for education in food preparation?

Sandoval
We tried to use local foods for that reason, and we were generally successful. To our surprise, however, some of these people were not used to cooking with oil, and, after they boiled the rice, they poured the oil *over* it! So we needed some educational component, but not too much.

López
You emphasize that this is a supplement, not the total consumption. How did you choose the 20-30% of requirements as the level of supplementation?

Sandoval
According to the nutrition survey of 1967, it was calculated that the nutritional deficit was around 25%. So, what we are trying to cover with the program is that 25% deficit. We are not trying to replace all the food that a family needs.

Soekirman
For how long will the family get the supplement?

Sandoval
That is the big question. The program was designed for three years. We want to incorporate these people into some kind of productive work before it ends, but it's not very easy to do. How long the government will continue this plan depends on a lot of factors: the national budget situation, what the government feels about the program, the kind of feedback they get, and so on.

The only way the people will progress is by working together. This program needs to be attached to the whole program of rural development that Panama is pushing. The Ministry of Economic Planning is providing the funds on the understanding that the program will be put into the main rural development plan.

Winikoff
Can you tell us a little about the community development projects and your successes and failures?

Sandoval

We have a nutritional technician who works as part of an educational group
and we work with the people to set up communal gardens. One problem is
that these projects have to be way, way out in the mountains because that is
where one can find unoccupied land. The gardens are from six to ten hectares
each and are worked with a mechanical plow. The plows are two-and-a-half
horsepower, Japanese-made, and run on diesel. They are very easily driven,
and can be managed by children! They can also serve as a water pump. They
also do not cost too much. First, we got local donations for purchase; then
we persuaded UNICEF not to send isolettes and incubators but more tractors.
They bought a hundred. Then we persuaded AID to put some money into
some of these tractors. We also have some animal projects, such as communal
chicken projects.

Montgomery

In the same community as the gardens?

Sandoval

No, we cannot afford to have several interventions in one community. We try
to spread them out.

Wray

How large a population would be served by one communal unit?

Sandoval

It depends on money!

Mellor

Will you be able to calculate the dollar effectiveness of these three different
local interventions?

Sandoval

There is no way we can evaluate this in absolute terms. We can only evaluate
the changes. Not all communities are making good use of what we try to do
with them. Sometimes we work with a community and donate the small
tractor and fertilizer, plus give technical assistance, but, either for lack of
trust or laziness or some other reason, it fails to work. In that case, we remove the tractor and take it to another community because we have over
8,000 communities, and I don't think we're *ever* going to get 8,000 tractors.

Now, we are trying to transfer at least some of the communities from the
supplementary food program into one of the production programs. The idea
is not to keep this supplement going forever but to see if we can't shift it to
other communities that are equally in need.

Another significant feature which must be taken into account is that, in
Panama, we have started with the most backward and rural and isolated population, which is not the usual approach. Most supplementary feeding programs start giving food to the people that are much nearer, and more acces-

sible, but those people are the ones that probably have less needs in many respects.

Levinson
It strikes me that there are some very positive things about this program:

1 It was developed in a way that would integrate it into a broader program of rural development.
2 The areas were chosen sensibly, quickly, on the basis of some simple, but reasonable, indicators.
3 It didn't require years of planning.
4 It didn't require the 15 or 20 different factors that certain planning experts call for.
5 The basic premise was learning by doing.
6 It is a program which does transfer real income.
7 It is a program which seems to have utilized foreign aid sensibly.

It seems, from what you've said, that all of this happened and funds were allocated because there was a generally receptive government, and then *you,* Julio, came along. You had a fair amount of political clout, and you made it happen.

Sandoval
When I arrived, they had everything written down, but they hadn't done anything. They were waiting for the next meeting. I took the planning paper, and I read it. I had no experience, and I am not a nutrition expert, but it sounded good. So, I took an administrator, and I sent him to the province with money and orders to buy the trucks, to rent space, and to begin to pack the food. I don't know what happened next, but for the rest of the year, we never had time for another meeting!

Schlossberg
I think that the idea of using a food package as an incentive to a health program is a very good idea. We do it sometimes in the United States.

Antrobus
The whole topic of supplementary feeding merits some further discussion. There are certain implicit philosophical questions, and we must explore how it ranks as an intervention alongside education, medical service, transport, and so on.

9 NUTRITION AND GOVERNMENT POLICY IN THE PHILIPPINES   Florentino S. Solon

Florentino S. Solon is the internationally known manager of what is perhaps the most comprehensive nationwide nutrition program to date. Solon was trained as a medical doctor and did most of his initial work in Cebu City, the Philippines. There, in association with the Cebu Institute of Medicine, he developed skills as a program initiator and coordinator, as well as a reputation for clinical nutrition research. At present, Solon serves concurrently as Executive Director, Nutrition Center of the Philippines, and Executive Director, National Nutrition Council of the Philippines. He works closely with multilateral, bilateral, and Philippine government agencies and also with the First Lady of the Philippines, Mrs. Imelda Marcos, in helping to translate her personal interest in the nutrition of children into a functioning national program.

INTRODUCTION

July 2, 1974 was a milestone in the history of nutrition in the Philippines. On this day two events awakened national consciousness of the problem that plagues two-thirds of the entire world: malnutrition.

First, was the pronouncement into law by His Excellency, President Ferdinand E. Marcos, that thenceforth nutrition would become a priority of government action, to be implemented by all agencies in an integrated fashion.[1] In pursuit of this policy, the president created the National Nutrition Council (NNC), charged with the formulation and coordination of the Philippine Nutrition Program (PNP).

The second event, no less auspicious, was the commitment of the First Lady of the Land, Mrs. Imelda Romualdes-Marcos, to lead the private effort in the nationwide nutrition campaign. To institutionalize this commitment, Mrs. Marcos founded the Nutrition Center of the Philippines (NCP), a private foundation dedicated to gather the resources of the private sector in support of the Philippine Nutrition Program.

These two bodies, the NNC and the NCP, represent the merger of government and the private sector in the massive effort against malnutrition. This partnership is deemed to be a crucial feature for the success of the program.

It should be recalled that the beginning of the Development Decade found the Philippines in a period of severe economic dislocation: an economic slump with political disturbances, especially in the country's rural areas, increased unemployment in the cities, and worsening criminality. It was a period of intellectual ferment and of introspection, a period of social upheaval.

In an effort to bring order out of chaos, President Marcos declared a state of emergency on September 21, 1972 and embarked on a planned program of development, instituting sweeping economic and political reform directed at improving the quality of life of Filipinos rather than merely at registering impressive gains in economic statistics.

Inevitably, a reassessment of the government's public welfare projects was in order, and one area which needed major realignment was nutrition. In contrast to previous administrations, the present government viewed malnutrition not as an isolated phenomenon, but as attributable to a wide variety of social parameters. Any solution definitely had to encompass more than mere feeding programs or increased food supply. To combat malnutrition, effective national leadership had to campaign simultaneously against the related social ills of unemployment, ignorance, uncontrolled population growth, and the generally low purchasing power of the people. Thus, the nutrition program entered into the stream of national developmental planning.

It was within this perspective that the NNC and the NCP were established as organizational expressions of the bond of partnership between the public and private sectors in the common effort against the menace of malnutrition. Together, the NNC and the NCP have formulated the Philippine Nutrition

Program which approaches the problem from a development perspective.[2] An integrated program involving a broad cross section of the country's government and business sectors, the PNP, in little more than a year, has already made its influence felt in awakening the nutritional consciousness of the population.

HISTORY OF NUTRITION IN THE PHILIPPINES

This does not mean, however, that nutrition activities in the Philippines started only two years ago. Indeed, over the past five decades the Philippine government, with private sector support, has strived to formulate a comprehensive nutrition program that would adequately respond to the needs of a growing population. During the embryonic stages of its development, however, the concept of nutrition as an input to national growth was largely confined to scientific circles and did not become a matter of government policy until 1947. Consequently, interest in nutrition during the period 1928-39 was more evident in sporadic activity than in any consistent long term program. Nonetheless, the prewar years contributed significantly to defining nutrition as a "mission" of government rather than merely another welfare activity.

Institute of Nutrition

It was not, however, until after the Second World War that central nutrition planning was institutionalized. In 1947, President Manuel Roxas established the Institute of Nutrition[3] under the leadership of Dr. Juan Salcedo, Jr. Charged with the responsibility of unifying, centralizing, and coordinating all nutrition activities, the institute began the continuing process of investigating the people's nutritional status with a view of developing appropriate methods suitable to local conditions.

To supplement the Institute's planning activities, President Roxas appointed a Nutrition Board made up of experts from the fields of health, labor, agriculture, finance, and social welfare. It was hoped that by drawing together a group of people from various spheres of expertise, nutrition planning could have a broader perspective. Creation of the board had a dual significance:

a   The national leadership had come to realize that any integrated nutrition campaign demanded an interdisciplinary and intersectorial approach.
b   The leadership had also realized that food and nutrition policies must be based on studies of food consumption habits and the nutritional status of the population.

Among the first activities undertaken by the Institute of Nutrition was the Rice Enrichment Project, better known as the Bataan Rice Experiment. The project, undertaken by Salcedo and others, experimented with rice enrichment as a public health measure for the prevention of beriberi.[4] This project reaped worldwide acclaim and boosted international research on the efficiency of rice enrichment in predominantly rice-producing regions.

The Bataan Rice Experiment's success in virtually eliminating a disease traditionally classified as endemic, gave impetus to the enactment of a Rice Enrichment Law in 1955.[5] Political developments, however, stood in the way of effective enforcement of the law. The Huk rebellion in Central and Southern Luzon and the Visayas threatened to envelop the country in a national conflagration barely a decade after the Second World War. Again the campaign against malnutrition had to assume secondary importance. Furthermore, the Rice Enrichment Law was found administratively impractical because rice milling was generally a private enterprise without sufficient fiscal control by the government. Rice millers simply refused to enrich the rice since the quantity of milling could be judged from the amount of enrichment—and their tax adjusted accordingly!

Food and Nutrition Research Center

Until the year 1958, government programs were still attempting to strike a working balance between research and application. Although research work continued, the results were hardly sufficient to warrant large scale action. To deal with this deficiency, the Institute of Nutrition was reorganized. It was transferred from the Department of Health and placed under the National Science Development Board (NSDB), the central science agency of government. The Institute of Nutrition was renamed the Food and Nutrition Research Center (FNRC) and was given the principal function of being a clearinghouse for nutritional data and information, as well as conducting systematic research on locally available food sources and actual nutritional needs.

Through regional nutrition surveys from 1958 to 1969, the FNRC was able to pinpoint protein calorie, vitamin A, iron, and iodine deficiencies as the most common forms of malnutrition in the country.[6] Through intensive laboratory and field studies, the center has established calorie and nutrient allowances for Filipinos, defined standards of height and weight, compiled information on nutritive value of Philippine foods, conducted metabolic, clinical nutrition, and diet therapy studies, published and distributed nutrition education materials.[7] It has developed nutritious food formulations for use in feeding operations after extensive animal assays and acceptability tests.

Nutrition Foundation of the Philippines

Within the private sector, public health programs were dependent on individual initiative. Understandably, instances of this type of initiative were few and far between. The organization of the Nutrition Foundation of the Philippines (NFP) in 1959, initially supported by the Williams-Waterman Fund, can be described as the proverbial ripple which eventually swelled into a tide of private sector enthusiasm for the program. Pioneering in community-oriented activities, the NFP led the way in grassroots information campaigns and leadership training as the foundation for any public welfare program.

National Coordinating Committee on Food and Nutrition

To enhance the coordinative role of government in nutrition work, the Food
and Nutrition Research Center, led by its director, Dr. Conrado R. Pascual,
worked hard for the formation of the National Coordinating Committee
(later changed to Council) on Food and Nutrition.[8] This was organized in
July 1960, drawing its members from both the public and private sectors. The
NCCFN can be considered the forerunner of the present NNC, except that
the former was not vested with the powers of law, and the members were
representatives (not heads) of ministries concerned with nutrition. Through
the data-gathering campaigns and the postsurvey conferences from 1960-67,
the NCCFN was instrumental in formulating a common language among participating institutions and a common definition of problem areas. In addition,
the NCCFN was able to forge a harmonious working relationship among the
various disciplines involved in the solution of community problems. By the
mid-1960s, therefore, the NCCFN served as the rallying point for community
nutrition programs.

One of the offshoots of the NCCFN's postnutrition survey conferences was
the establishment of a pilot project on Applied Nutrition in Bayambang, a
town in Northern Philippines, in 1964. The project was led by the Department of Education with assistance from the Department of Health, Department of Agriculture, Food and Nutrition Research Center, Presidential Assistance on Community Development, as well as from UNICEF, FAO, and
WHO. The project included school and community food production, supplementary feeding of school children, and nutrition education in schools and
communities. The project, later known as the Philippine Applied Nutrition
Program, was expanded to some 600 schools with a thousand more on a self-
help basis.

The Bureau of Agricultural Extension also started integrating nutrition into
the activities of their technicians. An important component of their campaign
was the supplementary feeding of preschoolers through the Targeted Maternal
and Child Health Program (TMCH) assisted by US AID. Home Management
Technicians organized Rural Improvement Clubs and Homemakers Courses to
teach mothers in the community about proper nutrition practices.

National Nutrition Program

It should be emphasized that, at this point, although the nutrition effort was
attracting an increasingly broad cross section of public and private institutions, and although significant headway was being made on the research end,
there still existed no comprehensive program that could eventually embrace
the entire country. Furthermore, the question of who should be the recipients of nutritional aid had not been sufficiently narrowed down so that the

limited resources could be used optimally.

Conscious of these facts, the Department of Health, with the assistance of US AID, launched the first government program on public health nutrition in 1967. The National Nutrition Program synthesized the research and coordination work undertaken by the government and the community-oriented methodology introduced by the private sector. It also added a novel approach, however, that of educating mothers towards acquiring a basic appreciation of proper food values.[9]

Proceeding from the premise that mothers assumed the principal responsibility for the family's dietary needs, mothercraft teams were fielded in targeted areas. Model centers were put up specifically to train mothers in ways to rehabilitate malnourished children.

As mothercraft activities were invariably undertaken in the field, most of the published knowledge from this period was acquired through actual experience. For instance, mothercraft teams had to devise practical methods of pinpointing malnourished cases. The consequent standardization of weighing procedures added immensely to the growing fund of expertise on nutrition and public health techniques.

In the field of research, the National Nutrition Program put a premium on the development of locally available, highly nutritive, yet low cost food combinations, suitable to the average family budget.

At the leadership level, the NNP conducted short term courses and seminars in a campaign to, at minimum, familiarize public health administrators, as well as regional- through municipal-level government officials, with the fundamentals of nutrition work.

The First Malnutrition Ward (Malward)

In 1967, the first Malward was established by Solon and others in Southern Island Hospital, a government hospital in Cebu City. The primary purpose was to give intensive rehabilitation to the malnourished children referred and admitted to the hospital; another purpose was to give thorough nutrition and health education to the mothers. It has served as a teaching ward for doctors, nurses, medical students, and applied nutrition workers. This Malward became the model for 150 Malwards later established all over the country. The first 20 wards were established with the assistance of UNICEF.

Cebu Institute of Medicine

While a national nutrition program was still in the embryonic stages, private initiative was shaping what would, in the future, prove to be handy, practical models for nutrition and health services delivery. This initiative was demonstrated most vividly by the example set in Cebu City, south of Manila, by a partnership between a medical institution, private hospitals, civic and business

groups, and the population of several communities. Here, a succession of
experiments in the Cebu Institute of Medicine (CIM), a medical college in
Cebu City, set up a malnutrition ward and a community training program
for medical interns in order to expose the interns to health and nutrition
problems at the village level within their total ecologic background.

Over the five years since the program was established, the CIM has demonstrated a comprehensive health care delivery system based on a unique organizational scheme in which public services are delivered to the people through
organized community effort.[10] A special feature of the approach is the development of local leaders, each one to head a small cooperative unit. The strategy is to render total health care, centered mostly on nutrition of the preschool child, family planning, and disease prevention with a systematic expenditure of the efforts of each worker and maximum utilization of time made
possible by the help of a network of barrio health aides. The system entails
spot mapping activities to pinpoint each family according to classifications
such as level of nutrition, family size, morbidity and mortality incidence, and
so on.

Philippine Food and Nutrition Program

From the wide range of experience accumulated by groups working in nutrition during the '60s, it became increasingly evident that nutrition intervention and food production were inseparable and had to be pursued with equal
stress. In 1971, the National Food and Agricultural Council (NFAC) created
by Executive Order No. 285, not by law, was assigned to coordinate and
supervise all activities pertinent to the twin areas of nutrition and food production.[11] The council was headed by the Department of Agriculture, and, as
we usually see with councils, there were interministerial jealousies which
weakened the whole operation.

Out of this development, however, evolved the four-year Philippine Food
and Nutrition Program which gave emphasis to this dual approach in program
planning and implementation.[12] The program solicited multiagency participa-
tion, involving both the government and the private sector: Department of
Health (DOH), Department of Agriculture and Natural Resources (DANR),
Department of Education and Culture (DEC), Department of Social Welfare
(DWS), Department of Local Government and Community Development
(DLGCD), National Science Development Board (NSDB), Philippine National
Red Cross (PNRC), Nutrition Foundation of the Philippines (NFP), Philip-
pine Business for Social Progress (PBSP), Catholic Relief Services-National
Secretariat for Social Action (CRS-NASSA), National Council of Churches in
the Philippines, Peace Corps/Philippines, National Media Production Center
(NMPC), Kilusan ng Wastong Pagkain, CARE, US AID, UNICEF, WHO and
FAO.

The four-year Philippine Food and Nutrition Program (PFNP) was based on the concept that efficient attainment of improved nutrition hinged on simultaneous and synchronized efforts to provide adequate food supply, promote wise selection and utilization of the food produced, enhance family life and social environment, develop manpower resources for food and nutrition, and promote relevant family-income-generating activities. It also established priority groups who would be the direct beneficiaries of the program. These were the vulnerable groups: infants, preschoolers and schoolchildren, as well as pregnant and lactating mothers.

A Management Committee for Nutrition was organized at the national level to formulate implementing guidelines for program personnel. An Inter-Agency Action (INTACT) Group served as the link between the Management Committee and the field by rendering technical assistance and making periodic field visits. At the local level, provincial, municipal, and barrio nutrition committees were established. A provincial staff was organized in each program province to supervise the barrio (village) team of workers in their role as initiators of barrio projects in nutrition. The PFNP included five different projects: nutrition training, nutrition education, supplementary feeding, food production, and nutrition rehabilitation wards, each under the supervision of a project officer at the provincial level. In addition, support activities, including food and nutrition research, nutrition communications, and income-generating activities were undertaken.

Because of limited resources, however, the PFNP had to be confined initially to only 11 (of more than 70) provinces. In the first few months of program implementation in a province, five "pilot" barrios in five "pilot" municipalities were selected as targets, after which the program was allowed to expand to other barrios and municipalities according to available resources. The program called for expansion at the rate of 10 to 20 provinces per year, so that by the end of June 1974, 42 provinces scattered throughout the entire country were covered.

At the same time, business groups started to muster their resources to help the government's nutrition program. One such group is the union of 150 private firms that forms Philippine Business for Social Progress (PBSP). This group was formally established on December 16, 1970. It sought to organize financial assistance in supporting social development through an integrated approach based on total involvement of the community.

The Applied Nutrition Program (ANP) is a big component of PBSP-assisted projects.[13] Its objective is to test and validate a scheme for delivering nutrition services to low income communities through development of working models, both urban and rural.

National Nutrition Council and Nutrition Center of the Philippines

Until 1974, however, there existed no clearly defined policy on nutrition supported from the highest levels of national leadership. Although initial efforts had been made to coordinate nutrition activities, there still remained the task of organizing a system to oversee program implementation from the national to the barrio levels.

The simultaneous establishment of the National Nutrition Council and the Nutrition Center of the Philippines expressed in concrete terms the government's concern for an integrated nutrition program to marshal effectively the technical expertise and financial resources of the public and private sectors.

With the coordinating activities of the NNC and the private sector support represented by the NCP, the nutrition campaign entered a new stage. In this stage, the struggle against malnutrition began to be viewed within the developmental framework, not merely in terms of stopgap feeding schemes but as long term policies designed to prevent rather than merely cure this age-old problem.

THE MALNUTRITION PROBLEM IN THE PHILIPPINES

The Philippines is an archipelagic nation of more than 7,100 islands occupying a land area of 300,000 km^2. Slightly more than a third of the total land surface is cultivated. One-half of the land is retained in forests while another large area is uncultivatable grasslands, swamps, and marshes. The climate is tropical, with distinct dry and rainy seasons.

The Philippines is distinguished by an intermingling of people from many cultures and has been accordingly influenced by each. Filipinos are mainly of Malayan stock with a mixture of Chinese, Spanish, and Indian stock. According to the 1970 census, there were 36,684,484 Filipinos, making the Philippines the seventh largest nation in Asia and the sixteenth most populous nation in the world. The population is a young one, with 43% below 15 years old. Moreover, the population is growing at a rate of 3.0% per year, faster than any other nation in Asia, so that by the end of 1975, it is estimated that there will be 43 million Filipinos. Roman Catholicism is the predominant religion, encompassing 90% of the total population. There are 8 major dialects and 50 or more mutually unintelligible dialects in the Philippines. However, 44% of the population can speak the national language, which is Pilipino or Tagalog, and almost 40% can speak English, the major second language. 83% of the population over 10 years old can read and write.

The country is reasonably endowed with the natural resources necessary for economic development except, for the moment at least, petroleum. The Philippines has ample forests, mineral deposits, extensive marine and inland fishing resources, as well as fertile agricultural lands. The country's main industries include agriculture, fisheries and forestry, mining and quarrying, construction, and manufacturing. Principal agricultural products are rice, corn, coconut, sugarcane, tobacco, and rubber.

Rice, the main staple food, traditionally has been imported, except in 1973 when the rice production campaign of the government was totally implemented. In that year, rice production equalled 4.4 million metric tons of palay (rough rice), while corn production was 1.8 million metric tons (table 1).[14] Aside from rice and corn, the main food crops are bananas, sweet potatoes, fruits, and vegetables. Wheat is imported up to a maximum of 1.4 million metric tons annually. Fresh cow's milk is virtually nonexistent, and the milk industry consists of mixing skim milk powder with vegetable oils such as corn and coconut oil. Fish is the principal source of animal protein, and, in 1973, production amounted to 1.2 million metric tons. Livestock production consists of hogs, carabao, cattle, and poultry. In spite of the production of copra, only 174,000 metric tons of fats and oils were produced in 1973 (table 2).[15]

From these data alone one can discern the average diet of the Filipino: rice (corn in certain areas) plus fish and succulent vegetables or bananas. This has been repeatedly confirmed by the FNRC regional nutrition surveys which were conducted from 1958 to 1969.[16] These surveys, covering 9 out of 10 regions of the Philippines, revealed prevalent dietary inadequacies giving rise to the following major problems: protein calorie malnutrition, vitamin A and iron deficiencies, and endemic goiter. Of lesser importance are riboflavin and thiamine deficiencies.

Dietary Inadequacies

The FNRC surveys showed that the average Filipino diet was adequate only in cereals—meaning rice, corn, and wheat products (table 3). The only other food group that satisfied the recommendation was "other fruits and vegetables," consisting of such foods as legumes, eggplants, bananas, etc. All the rest of the food groups fell far short of allowances. Thus, sources of vitamins and minerals such as leafy and yellow vegetables and vitamin-C-rich foods were grossly inadequate. So were the protein-rich foods: meat, poultry, eggs, milk and milk products, and dried beans and nuts. Fats and oils were also grossly deficient. In short, the total food intake was very much below recommendation.

Table 1
Crop production, Philippines, 1973

Selected Major Crops	Production (Metric Tons)	Value (₱)
Palay (rough rice)	4,414,630.0	2,650,048,400
Corn	1,831,130.7	828,209,700
Fruits and nuts	1,803,431.2	1,445,661,700
Banana	1,012,604.3	814,672,600
Rootcrops	1,220,496.5	490,518,300
Vegetables (except onion and Irish potato)	271,797.6	280,616,000

Table 2
Gross available food supply, Philippines, 1972 and 1973

Food	Supply 1972	1973	Percent Increase
Vegetable Origin			
Cereals	5,069	5,581	10.1
Rice (milled)	3,149	3,479	10.4
Corn (shelled)	1,920	2,102	9.4
Starchy roots, tubers	1,290	1,406	9.0
Sugar, syrups	769	770	0.1
Dry beans, nuts (excl. coconuts)	56	55	−1.8
Vegetables	1,159	1,283	10.7
Fruits	2,057	2,271	10.4
Fats, oils	139	174	25.2
Coconut for food	157	120	−23.6
Miscellaneous	902	1,053	16.7
Total of vegetable origin	11,598	12,713	9.6
Animal Origin			
Meat, poultry	615	682	10.9
Fish, other marine products	1,517	1,614	6.3
Fish	1,298	1,406	8.3
Crustaceans	82	137	67.1
Mollusks	137	68	−50.4
Milk (whole)	27	29	7.4
Eggs	147	151	2.7
Total of animal origin	2,307	2,476	7.3
Total	13,905	15,189	9.2

Note: Supply is given in thousands of metric tons a.p. (as purchased)

Translating this food intake into calories and nutrients, we find that the calorie intake was only 83% of allowance (table 4). At first glance it seems surprising that the calorie intake was deficient, considering the adequate intake of cereals. The deficiency was, in fact, due to inadequate intake of calorie-rich foods such as fats and oils, as well as animal foods.

The protein content of the average Filipino diet was also found to be somewhat low. This was due to inadequate intake of meats and poultry, dried beans and nuts, milk and milk products, and eggs. This protein lack was aggravated by the deficiency in calories. Moreover, the largest part of protein intake (60%) came from rice; a much smaller portion came from animal foods.

Table 3
Average daily per capita food intake compared to recommended allowances, 9 regions of the Philippines, 1958-69

	Actual Intake (g)	Recommended Allowance (g)	% Adequacy
Cereal	345	325	106
Roots, tubers	65	73	89
Sugars, syrups	18	28	64
Beans, nuts	7	16	44
Leafy vegetables	28	85	33
Vitamin-C-rich foods	30	72	42
Other fruits and vegetables	138	135	102
Meat, poultry, fish	119	139	86
Eggs	5	15	33
Milk, milk products	21	90	23
Fats, oils	8	30	27
Total	784	1,008	78

Source: Nutrition Profile of the Philippines. Unpublished data, FNRC, NSDB, 1975

Table 4
Average daily per capita nutrient intakes compared to recommended allowances, 9 regions of the Philippines, 1958-69

	Actual Intake	Recommended Allowance	% Adequacy
Energy (kcal)	1,671	2,003	83
Protein (g)	46.2	49.2	94
Calcium (g)	0.34	0.57	60
Iron (mg)	9.0	10.0	90
Vitamin A (IU)	1,812.0	4,066.0	44.5
Thiamine (mg)	0.73	1.02	72
Riboflavin (mg)	0.47	1.02	46
Niacin (mg)	14.0	13.0	108
Ascorbic acid (mg)	67.0	69.0	97

Source: Nutrition Profile of the Philippines. Unpublished data. FNRC, NSDB, 1975

Another important dietary deficiency that was found in the surveys was a shortage of vitamin A. The deficiency in this nutrient was brought about by low intake of green leafy and yellow vegetables, as well as animal foods, especially milk. No doubt the deficiency in fat intake aggravated the vitamin A deficiency.

The intake of iron seems to be high, but it must be pointed out that most of this iron intake came from rice, vegetables, and other plant sources where the iron is not readily available to the body. This is borne out by high prevalence of anemia among the population (see below).

The intake of riboflavin was also far below recommended allowances. The deficiency, of course, is a reflection of the general inadequacies in food intake. The calcium deficiency was due to the low intake of leafy vegetables, milk, and eggs.

In general, the average diet found in the dietary survey contained 79% of the calories as carbohydrates, 10% as protein, and 11% as fat. The diet in metropolitan Manila differed from the rest of the country in this regard: carbohydrate contributed 66%, protein 11%, and fat 23% of calories.

Types and Extent of Malnutrition

The extent of protein calorie malnutrition may be gleaned roughly from the results of weighing surveys. In the FNRC regional surveys cited earlier,[17] as many as 69% of 1-4 year-old children were underweight by more than 10% of the standard. In fact, about 29% of the children of this age group were classified as suffering from second or third degree undernutrition according to the Gomez Classification, using a Philippine standard (FNRC).

In the weighing operation ("Operation Timbang") of preschool children below 6 under the Philippine Nutrition Program, in which we have weighed over 1 million children, 20.6% were classified as normal by weight, 47.7% as first degree malnutrition, 24.7% second degree, 5.9% third degree, and 1.1% overweight. A total of 1,012,166 preschool children have already been weighed in this program.[18]

Xerophthalmia is another serious condition that has been identified in nutrition surveys. In the FNRC surveys, serum vitamin A and carotene levels were in the "deficient" and "low" categories in the majority of subjects examined. The problem is most acute in the 1-6 year age group where 82% of those examined had deficient or low serum vitamin A levels (table 5). Schoolchildren and pregnant and nursing mothers were not spared.

Clinical surveys have also shown that a sizeable percentage of the population show physical signs of vitamin A deficiency. Taking only one such sign, dryness of the conjunctiva, the FNRC surveys found 11% of the 1-6 year age group showing symptoms, as did 26% of the 7-12 year age group, and 30% of pregnant and nursing mothers.

In an intensive study of vitamin A deficiency in Cebu province by Solon,[19] involving 1,700 children aged 1-15 years from different ecological zones, 58% of the children were found to have deficient or low serum vitamin A levels using ICNND standards. Seventy percent of the children displayed clinical symptoms of xerophthalmia (table 6). Defining xerophthalmia as only those cases with concomitant presence of clinical signs *and* low or deficient serum A levels, the incidence of xerophthalmia was 40%. Children of both sexes in the 4-9 year-old category were the most severely affected. At the same time, the largest age-specific incidence of blindness directly associated with xerophthalmia appeared in children below 6 years old. It was estimated that 15.14 out of 10,000 children aged 1-6 are blinded from xerophthalmia.

The biochemical phase of the FNRC nutrition surveys revealed the presence of another important nutritional problem: anemia. As a whole, almost 50% of all the subjects examined had either deficient or low hemoglobin levels using the WHO standard of 11 grams hemoglobin (table 6). A closer examination

Table 5
Biochemical findings, 9 regions of the Philippines, 1958-69

	Percent of Population Suffering from:				
Group	Anemia[a]	Vitamin A Deficiency[a]	Protein Deficiency[a]	Thiamine Deficiency	Riboflavin Deficiency
Children					
1 - 6 years	71	82	10	b	b
7 - 12 years	52	76	5	b	b
13 - 20 years	41	47	2	81	82
21 and over	41	27	3	83	82
Other Groups					
Pregnant women	78	30	36	76	84
Nursing women	52	41	1	80	83
Total population	49	50	5	80	83

[a]Includes those with deficient/low levels of hemoglobin, serum vitamin A, and serum albumin.
[b]Not examined.
Source: Food and Nutrition Research Center, NSDB

Table 6
Prevalence of xerophthalmia (percent)

Zone	Clinical Symptoms	Biochemical Deficient or Low/ICNND	Both
Urban			
Squatter	72	54	40
Barrio	50	59	29
Rural			
Coastal	83	62	41
Hinterland	83	56	48
Total	70	58	40

Number of cases: 1,715. All 3 factors have significant F-test at the .01 level.
Source: F. S. Solon, Cost and Effectiveness of Alternate Means of Controlling Vitamin A Deficiency (Xerophthalmia), 1974

revealed that 71% of 1-6 year olds had low to deficient hemoglobin levels, and 78% of pregnant women and 52% of nursing mothers were anemic. In another study by Tantengco et al.[20] the prevalence of anemia among school-children 6-14 years ranged from 15-23%.

Ariboflavinosis also seems to be very common. In the FNRC surveys, angu-lar scars were found on the lips of 16% of the 1-6 year age group, 36% of the 7-12 year age group, and at least 44% of pregnant and nursing mothers. The majority of the population 13 years and above also showed deficient or low levels of urinary thiamine and riboflavin. These findings were not surprising in view of the dietary inadequacies. On the other hand, pellagra, another B vita-min (niacin) deficiency disease, has never been found to be a problem.

It has long been recognized that goiter is endemic in many areas in the Philippines. The FNRC surveys showed about 12% of pregnant mothers with goiter, and, in fact, this condition was present in 4% of the total population. The Goiter Control Project of the Department of Health,[21] launched in 1967, has resulted in much greater awareness of the goiter problem than heretofore. The disease was found to be most prevalent in mountainous areas of the country, although it was also found even in coastal areas. In certain regions, almost everyone was found to have goiter. Adolescent girls and preg-nant women were most prone to the disease.

Another factor that contributes to the generally low nutritional health of the population is the high incidence of intestinal parasitism. Even old people were found, on examination, to have intestinal parasites. Ascaris was the most common, and hookworm, which no doubt contributed to the anemia prob-lem, was found in more than 16% of the surveyed population.

In summary, then, the Filipino diet is deficient both in quantity and quality. This has resulted in high incidence of protein calorie malnutrition, especially among preschool children. Vitamin A deficiency remains a major cause of preventable blindness. Iron deficiency anemia is widespread. The high incidence of riboflavin deficiency is an indication of the generally poor quality of diet, and endemic goiter is more prevalent than was generally be-lieved. Intestinal parasitic infestation continues to be a population-wide phenomenon.

FACTORS CONTRIBUTING TO MALNUTRITION

Some Filipino economists contend that low purchasing power and unequal distribution of income are the primary causes of malnutrition, signifying that malnutrition is not merely a physical disease but, perhaps chiefly, a social and economic disease. Other people, including those associated with movements for proper feeding, point out that ignorance brings about malnutrition. Such disagreement inevitably has raised the issue of whether singling out the cause of malnutrition can be achieved at all, but the conflict itself is an indication that malnutrition has generated a healthy interest among policymakers and development planners.

Basically, what governs current programs on nutrition in the Philippines is the setting down, albeit roughly and broadly, of the interrelationships between the various causes of malnutrition. Somehow, the low purchasing power of the population, inadequate food supply, ignorance and lack of education, limited health services, and high population growth all appear interrelated. Identification of the social, economic, and environmental causes of malnutrition helps planners to appraise the malnutrition problem in the Philippines, and will, in the long run, allow the stripping of the problem to its barest, primary indicators. This, in turn, will guide the policymakers in formulating a broad program to combat the condition.

Low Purchasing Power of the Population

The per capita income of the Filipinos has grown at a moderate pace from ₱311 in 1961 to ₱647 (roughly US$108) in 1971.[22] This per capita income does not, however, reflect the purchasing power of the average Filipino, due to unequal distribution of income. Table 7 depicts income distribution in 1971.[23] It can be seen that the lowest 20% of families receive less than 5% of total income and that the lowest 50% of families receive approximately 18%

Table 7
Percent distribution of family income, Philippines, 1971

Income Class (in ₱)	Families	Income (₱)
Total	6,347,000	23,714,284,000
Percent	100	100
Under 500	5.2	0.5
500 - 999	12.1	2.4
1,000 - 1,499	12.2	4.1
1,500 - 1,999	11.8	5.5
2,000 - 2,999	9.6	5.8
2,500 - 2,999	8.1	6.0
3,000 - 3,999	12.5	11.5
4,000 - 4,999	7.5	8.9
5,000 - 5,999	5.0	7.3
6,000 - 7,000	6.4	11.7
8,000 - 9,999	3.6	8.5
10,000 - 14,999	3.7	11.8
15,000 - 19,999	1.1	5.1
20,000 and over	1.3	10.8

₱7.50 = US$1.
Source: Table A, p. xxxii, BCSSH Bulletin Series No. 22; Table 3, p. 2, BCSSH Bulletin Series No. 34

of total income.

Based on a minimum food basket for a reference family of 6, a food poverty line of ₱8.85 per family per day or ₱3,230 per year for 1973 has been derived.[23] Since about 60% of total income is spent for food, the total poverty line is ₱5,283 for Manila for the same year. Adjusted to 1971 prices, it can be shown that more than half of the families are below this poverty line (table 8). Hardest hit are manual workers, where the incidence of poverty was 83%; farmers, 68%; and skilled workers, 51-59% (table 9).

It is estimated that it would take 135% of the total 1971 national income to eliminate poverty altogether.[23] Transfer of income from the top 20% of families, who receive more than 50% of income, could totally eliminate food poverty, however. Thus, unequal distribution of income works against poor families and has grave repercussions, most particularly on nutritional status. Previous administrations geared development programs towards increasing and redistributing income. Among the most significant of these were land reform programs which attained real support during President Diosdado Macapagal's term (to 1965), but legislative rigmarole obstructed final approval despite strong public demand, notably from peasants' unions and students.

Agrarian reform aimed at solving land tenancy problems and giving property to the landless to boost their incomes received impetus when, two days after declaring martial law on September 21, 1972, President Marcos announced the emancipation of tenants from their bondage to the soil and directed the start of land distribution.[24] Although operating at a slow pace, agrarian reform is expected to cover the entire country.

Policies have been set by the National Economic Development Authority to stimulate regional dispersal of production, as well as labor-intensive and export industries. To keep prices within the reach of low income families, low tariff rates are maintained on live animals for breeding and for food. Price control is imposed on basic commodities and consumer items.

Price control, however, has not yielded the desired results. The country's

Table 8
Incidence of poverty and percent of total poor population by age of head of household, Philippines, 1971

Age of Head of Household (Years)	Incidence of Poverty	Percent of Total Poor Population
25 or less	81.19	6.17
25 - 34	71.03	26.65
35 - 44	69.65	28.34
45 - 54	57.24	18.20
55 - 64	57.67	12.63
65 and over	67.88	8.01

Source: Family Income and Expenditure, 1971, Series No. 34, BCS Survey of Households Bulletin, May 1966, table 8, p. 19

Table 9
Incidence of poverty and percent of total poor population by occupation, Philippines, 1971

Occupation	Incidence of Poverty	Percent of Total Poor Population
Professional, technical, related	14.91	0.93
Administrative, executive, managerial	13.60	0.47
Clerical	36.83	2.03
Sales	45.84	5.89
Farmers, farm laborers, fishermen, hunters, loggers, related	64.60	55.91
Miners, quarrymen, related	53.33	0.22
Transport, communications	51.11	5.04
Craftsmen, production-process workers, related	59.36	12.24
Manual workers, laborers	83.12	3.50
Occupation not reported	—	—
Unemployed w/o work experience and not in the labor force	61.68	9.83
Service, sports, related	49.15	3.94
Total		100.00
Employed Wage and salary workers	49.57	27.91
Self-employed workers	79.78	72.09
Total		100.00

Source: Family Income and Expenditures, 1971, Series No. 34, BCS Survey of Households Bulletin, May 1966

inflationary trends, arising from the increased price of oil products and the instability of the American dollar, brought about spiraling prices. This made it hard for Filipinos to meet their food budgets. Since 1961, average income across regions has worsened. Income growth is much slower, and wages increase at a snail's pace. On the whole, inputs aimed at generating higher incomes and distributing revenues equally have not raised the buying power of the average Filipino family even to a manageable level.

Inadequate Food Supply

In a country that has abundant natural and mineral resources and has been involved in international trade for hundreds of years, it is hard to understand why the population cannot be fed adequately. Ideally, other factors remaining constant, if food production is maintained at a rate adequate to supply the country's growing aggregate consumption needs, food intake should inevitably be sufficient. This is not true, however.

In 1973, total food crop production was 9,900 metric tons lower than 1971's 13,958,000 metric tons. Rice production went down by 13.4% or 0.7 million metric tons. Comparatively speaking, food crop production in 1971 was 82,000 metric tons, (0.6%) lower than the 1970 level of 14,040,000 metric tons.[14] The net available for human consumption in 1971 was 13,378,000 metric tons, 0.6% (or 87,000 metric tons) lower than the 1970 level. The decrease in crop production was due, in part, to drought in some critical areas. Lack of fertilizer and lack of irrigation compounded the problem.

On a per capita basis, 950.2 g of food from all sources was available per day in 1972 and 995.0 g in 1973, reflecting an increase of 45.2 g (or 4.7%). The 1973 supply almost fulfilled the FNRC's recommended allowance of 1,006 g* (table 10). Indeed, if one compares the Food Balance Sheet with food intake figures from nutrition surveys, one will note a marked parallel between sufficiency of intake and sufficiency of supply (table 11). Closer examination, however, reveals that in a number of food groups, food supply was significantly higher than intake. The gap was particularly large in the case of sugar, fats and oils, milk, and eggs. While this may be partly due to intakes "hidden" from dietary surveys such as the use of these items for commercial purposes in the production of soft drinks, cakes, bread, etc., the gap could very well be the target for nutrition education, such as in the case of leafy greens, milk, and eggs. Undoubtedly, unequal and inefficient food distribution has led to the unequal distribution of food intake.

The government has taken steps to bridge the gap between inadequate supply and food consumption requirements. Crop growers are given assistance ranging from credits on fertilizers and insecticides to agricultural equipment. Extensive research is being conducted on increasing the rice yield at minimum cost to the farmer. Nutrition campaigns have been launched calling on parents to join the Green Revolution by raising vegetable and fruit crops in the backyard. Programs such as *Palayan ng Bayan* and *Masagana 99* have been designed to increase agricultural yields and utilize idle lands. There has been a recent move to mill and eat second class (undermilled) rice rather than white rice both to increase nutritional value and also to raise the yield of the milling.

*While the demand for food grows annually by 3.0% to 3.9%, there has been a marked slowdown in the rate of growth of agricultural output—from 4.5% per year in the 1950s to 3.8% per year in the 1960s. The imbalance has been felt more strongly within the food crop sector than within the commercial crop sector.

Table 10
Daily per capita food allowance and daily per capita food supply, Philippines, 1973

Food	Recommended Allowance Per Capita Per Day[a] (a.p., g)	Food Supply Available for Consumption Per Capita Per Day (a.p., g)	Percent of Sufficient Food Supply
Vegetable Origin			
Cereals	325	368.2	113.3
Rice (milled)	—	250.7	—
Corn (shelled)	—	86.0	—
Wheat flour	—	31.5	—
Roots, tubers	74	83.7	113.1
Sugars, syrups	28	50.3	179.6
Dry beans, nuts (excl. coconuts)	16	3.6	22.5
Fruits, vegetables	290	192.7	66.4
Leafy and yellow vegetables	85	29.9	35.2
Vitamin-C-rich foods	71	21.8	30.7
Other fruits, vegetables	134	141.0	105.4
Fats, oils (incl. fats from coconuts)	30	12.9[b]	43.0
Coconuts for food (excl. fats)	—	7.1	—
Miscellaneous	—	72.0	—
Total of Vegetable Origin	763	790.5	103.6
Animal origin			
Meat, poultry	140	156.2	105.9
Milk, milk products	87	38.2	43.9
Eggs	16	10.1	63.1
Total of Animal Origin	243	204.5	77.2
Total	1,006	995.0	98.9

[a]Recommended allowance based on e.p. (edible portion) converted to a.p. (as purchased). Data obtained from an unpublished mimeographed report by the Food and Nutrition Research Center, NSDB.
[b]Containing about 99 g pure fat/100 g a.p., i.e., equivalent to 12.8 g pure fat.
Source: Food Balance Sheet, 1972/73

Ignorance and Lack of Education

Ignorance of proper nutrition practices, as well as persistence of erroneous food habits and beliefs, undoubtedly plays a major role in the problem of malnutrition. This, however, has been difficult to quantify. Sporadic and

Table 11
Daily per capita food intake end supply, Philippines, 1973

Food	Intake Per Capita Per Day (a.p., g)[a]	Available Supply Per Capita Per Day (a.p., g)[b]	Available Supply as Percent at Intake
Rice, Other Energy Sources			
Cereals, cereal products			
Rice	253	250.7	99.1
Corn	73	86.0	117.8
Wheat flour	19	31.5	165.8
Subtotal for Cereals, etc.	345	368.2	106.7
Roots, tubers	65	83.7	128.8
Sugar, syrups	18	50.3	279.4
Total for Rice, etc.	428	502.2	117.3
Fruits, Vegetables			
Leafy and yellow vegetables	28	29.9	106.8
Vitamin-C-rich	29	21.8	75.2
Other	138	141.0	102.5
Total for Fruits, etc.	195	192.7	99.0
Fat-Rich (Fats, Oils)	8	12.9	161.2
Protein-Rich			
Meat, poultry, fish, other marine products	119	156.2	131.3
Milk, milk products	22	38.2	173.6
Eggs, pulses, nuts (except coconut)	5 7	10.1 3.6	202.0 51.4
Total for Protein-Rich	153	208.1	136.0

[a]Intake of e.p. (edible portion) converted to a.p. (as purchased) obtained from the table of average daily per capita food consumption, Food and Nutrition Research Center, May 10, 1974.
[b]Obtained from the 1973 Food Balance Sheet.
Source: Food Balance Sheet, 1973. NEDA, Manila

localized studies have indicated extensive lack of information and misinformation, particularly on infant feeding and weaning practices and nutrition during pregnancy.

Whether formal education has any influence on nutrition in the general population is still being debated. A prevailing concept is that as the number of years of schooling increases, the average diet rating improves (table 12).[16]

Table 12
Average diet rating and average years of schooling

Household Average Years of Schooling	Number of Households Surveyed	Average Diet Rating, Percent
Below 5 years	1589	61.8
5 - 10 years	1140	67.9
Over 10 years	84	77.8

Source: Nutrition Profile of the Philippines. Unpublished data, FNRC, NSDB, 1975

Of course, this is only true within limits, as other variables come in at the extremes to influence nutritional intake. In fact, more than one-fourth of the total population attends school,* but because of the dropout rate,[25] only a few attain optimum education. Many children have only limited access to formal education at the high school level. 29,500 of the total of 41,000 barrios are still without public secondary schools.

Inadequate Health Services

1972 vital statistics data reveal that of the total deaths, 23% were of children less than 1 and 39.7% were less than 5 years of age (table 13).[26] Infant mortality for the same year was 68 per 1,000 live births. Among the leading causes of death in the postneonatal period were pneumonia, gastroenteritis, bronchitis, and nutritional deficiency states.

A cursory look at the country's health services reveals serious problems which have been disturbing the health authorities for years. In her survey of maternal and infant nutrition in four Tagalog communities, Guthrie[27] found that 42% of the babies had never been seen by a doctor. She also estimated that only 15% of the births in the communities had been attended by a physician.

Medical manpower and services fall short of medical requirements of both infants and adults. There were, in 1974, 52,783 available health personnel for a population of 40 million.[28] Of these, 13,107 were physicians (1:3,000 population), 8,283 were nurses (1:5,000), and 320 were nutritionists (1:22,400). The total number of hospital beds was 52,136, or 1 bed per 797 people. At the municipal level, where 70% of the population resides, there were in 1973 only 1,967 health centers (1:21,136), unequally distributed, and mostly concentrated in urban areas. There are 46 existing Malwards, many of them located in Manila and other urban centers.

The immunization campaign in 1974, aimed at 34,106,047 people, reached only 12,225,571—35.94% of the total.[29] Aside from the shortage of health

---

*In 1968, 65% of the 5-14 year age group and 35% of the 15-19 year age group were in school. In 1971, there were 7 million in the primary, 2 million in the secondary, and 800,000 in the college level.

Table 13
Distribution of population and deaths by age group

Age Group	Total Population[a] (1970)	% of Total Population (1970)	Number of Deaths[b] (1972)	% of Deaths (1972)
All ages	36,684,486	100.0	285,761	100.0
0 - 4	5,836,618	15.9	114,602	40.1
5 - 9	5,894,618	16.1	12,494	4.4
10 - 14	5,025,876	13.7	5,492	1.9
15 - 19	4,079,731	11.1	6,196	2.1
20 - 24	3,150,634	8.6	7,686	2.7
25 - 29	2,460,222	6.7	6,929	2.4
30 - 34	2,071,530	5.6	7,804	2.7
35 - 39	1,898,645	5.2	8,765	3.0
40 - 44	1,484,876	4.0	8,159	2.8
45 - 49	1,282,192	3.5	8,832	3.1
50 - 54	1,015,600	2.8	9,835	3.4
55 - 59	807,601	2.2	10,077	3.5
60 - 64	613,621	1.7	12,360	4.3
65 - 69	388,179	1.0	11,024	3.8
70 - 74	292,265	0.8	14,253	5.0
75 - 79	130,573	0.4	7,905	2.8
80 and over	221,848	0.6	32,139	11.2
Not stated	29,658	0.1	2,209	0.8

[a]Source: Age and Sex Population Projections for the Philippines by Province.
1970-2000 UNFPA-NCSO Population Research Project. NEDA, NCSO, MANILA
[b]Source: BCS Special Release, Series of 1974

and immunization services, the frightening costs of hospitalization to the patient discourages sufferers from seeking immediate medical treatment.

To compound the problem, environmental sanitation is below standard. In 1970, 20,840 wells, 2,081 springs, and 1,377 water supply systems of all sizes, served a total of between 15 and 18 million people in urban and rural areas (38-45% of the total population). The rest did not have access to potable water.

In the fiscal year 1973/74, 3.4% of the total Philippine government budget was spent for health. Although total expenditure has increased in the last decade (₱112 million in 1963 to ₱477 million in 1974), the proportion of the national budget spent for health has declined from 6.0% in 1963 to 2.4% in 1975.[28] The per capita expenditure on health in pesos, at constant prices, increased slightly, from ₱4.76 to ₱5.43. In terms of international currency, however, this has actually declined from US$1.22 in 1963 to US$0.81 in 1974, at constant prices.

The National Health Plan that is now being formulated calls for the strengthening of health services, especially in the rural areas. To this end, the Department of Health has adopted the strategy of training and using medical auxiliaries to be assigned to the villages.[28] These subprofessional workers, mainly midwives, will be expanded in number and retrained to treat simple and common ailments. They will man the first level of health care in the villages known as Barangay Health Centers. A system of referrals to higher levels (public health nurse and sanitary health inspector for second level, and rural health physician at the third level) will be established for more difficult cases. In addition, rural practice programs for medical and nursing graduates as well as volunteer service programs will be undertaken.

Rapid Population Growth

The meteoric rise of population has been viewed with alarmed concern in the Philippines. In view of the handicap the increased members present to improvement of the per capita food supply, population control has received priority in development programs.

The population increases by over a million persons annually. During the 70-year period from 1903 to 1970, population increased by 380% (table 14).[30] Accelerating at a faster pace than many other nations in Asia, Africa, and Latin America, Philippine population growth showed an increase in annual average from 1.9% in the 1940s to 3.1% in the 1950s. With the present growth rate of 3.0%, population will double in a little over 23 years.

The rapid population growth has been brought about by the spectacular decline in mortality while births remain at a high level. The death rate has dropped from 58 per 1,000 in 1903 to about 12 per 1,000 during the 5-year period 1965-70. This reduction has increased the life expectancy at birth, from less than 20 years in 1900 to 56.3 years in 1960.[30] While the fertility rate has gone down slightly, from 6.46 in 1958-62 to 5.89 in 1968-72, it remains at a high level. Even with a continuing drop in fertility rate during the coming years, population will continue to grow at a high rate because of the increasing proportion of women entering the childbearing ages. The Population Commission estimates that by the year 2000, the population will have increased to somewhere between 78.6 and 95.2 million.

As recently as a decade ago, it was unthinkable to start a population program in this predominantly Catholic country. With increasing realization of the dire consequences of runaway population growth, however, the government in 1971 formalized its policy on population matters through the Population Act. A presidential decree further strengthened this law in 1973, creating the Commission on Population and declaring that "for the purpose of furthering the national development . . . a national program of family planning involving both public and private sectors, which respects the religious beliefs and values of the individual, shall be undertaken." Thus a nationwide

Table 14
Population, the Philippines, 1903-1970

Year	Population	Annual Rate of Increase (%)
1903	7,635,426	
1918	10,314,310	1.9
1938	16,000,303	2.2
1948	19,234,182	1.9
1960	27,086,685	3.1
1970	36,684,486	3.0

Source: Bureau of Census and Statistics, Population Census of the Philippines. Census Year data

population program is now being pursued by both the government, through the Population Commission, and the private sector, through the Population Center Foundation.

THE PHILIPPINE NUTRITION PROGRAM

Organization

The New Society, announced by Proclamation 1081 declaring martial law on September 21, 1972, stressed the urgent need to bring about social, economic, and political reforms in the country.

Recognizing the gravity and extent of malnutrition in the country, and the important role that proper nutrition plays in socioeconomic development, the president and the first lady gave nutrition priority status in the national development program. The president signed Presidential Decree 491 in July 1974, creating the National Nutrition Council, and at the same time, the first lady founded the Nutrition Center of the Philippines as the lead agency for the private sector. There is no doubt that without this recognition by leadership at the highest level, nutrition would not arouse the present high levels of interest in the nation, from department heads to national planners, technocrats, local leaders, community workers, and the people at large.

The setting up of an active organizational structure at all levels of operation is of utmost importance. At the national level, the National Nutrition Council (NNC) is the nerve center for planning and coordination, and the Nutrition Center of the Philippines (NCP) harnesses the private support for the program (figure 1). The unique feature of this arrangement is that the Executive Director of NCP is concurrently the Executive Director of NNC in order to afford the closest coordination possible between these two agencies in the implementation of the PNP.

As the top-level coordinating body, the NNC is composed of the highest

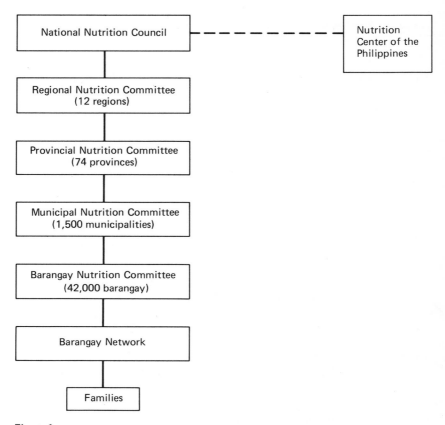

Figure 1
Organizational structure of the Philippine Nutrition Program.

officials of various sectors of the government: the secretaries of the ministries of Agriculture (chairman), Health (vice-chairman), Education, Social Welfare, Local Government and Community Development, and the chairman of the National Science Development Board. The private sector is represented by the heads of the Nutrition Center of the Philippines, Nutrition Foundation of the Philippines, and the Philippine Medical Association. To date, there are 25 cooperating agencies from government, private, and international institutions who are committed to an implementation of the Philippine Nutrition Program in an integrated fashion.

The executive director implements the policies, programs, projects, and decisions of the council, and heads a secretariat which facilitates and monitors NNC activities and operations. The chairman of the secretariat is the Secretary of Agriculture. At the same time, he is the chairman of the National Food and Agricultural Council. The chairman of the Council for Nutrition and the Chairman of the Council for Food is the same person, so the secretariat further ensures coordination.

There is a planning division and an operations division, as well as a management committee. This committee is crucial because the full council only decides major policy and meets with the cabinet members only four times a year. The management committee, however, meets every month and provides continuity. It is comprised of the nutrition heads of every ministry. If there is anything needed immediately, the management committee can deal with it. There is also wide freedom in operations because the council is under the Office of the President. The Nutrition Center is under the Office of the First Lady.

At the local level, provincial, municipal, and barangay nutrition committees are composed of government and civic leaders. These committees are headed by the highest government official at each level: the governor at the provincial level, the mayor in the municipality, the barangay chairman in the barrio (figures 2-4). The responsibility for implementation of the nutrition program rests primarily on the local government leaders.

The municipality is the focal point of implementation of the program. The Municipal Nutrition Committee creates a planning staff and invites representatives of different agencies in the community to discuss problems of malnutrition, share experiences, and give information on their own ongoing programs (figure 4). When fully organized there will be a total of 1,500 municipal nutrition committees all over the country.

Under the city/municipal nutrition committee is the Barangay (village) Nutrition Committee (figure 5). The committee assumes the responsibility for implementing and coordinating the nutrition program at the barangay level. It organizes the Barangay Network which is composed of three types of personnel. First, there is a teacher-coordinator. Since we have 265,000 teachers (an average of 5 to 7 in every village), we are making use of them as coordinators. Second, there are *purok* (zone) leaders. Every village is divided into zones, with a leader for each. Third, in the villages, we have what we call a unit leader for every 20 families. This is the final link between nutrition agencies and the program's target: the family. To coordinate this group, one must have surveillance, monitoring, and delivery of information. These workers are really like teachers, but outside of a classroom. At present, some 1,573 villages have organized Barangay Networks which serve as a two-way system for delivery of nutrition services, educational materials, and the conduct of other nutrition-related activities.

For the first year, 1974-75, ₽3.4 million of NFAC (National Food and Agriculture Council) funds have been stipulated for the nutrition program. The sum of ₽10 million is also appropriated from national government moneys as operating funds for the National Nutrition Council starting in fiscal year 1975/76. These amounts are hardly enough to cover the expenditures necessary to bring nutrition to the people effectively, and this is understood by the program administrators. However, this is not an absolute obsta-

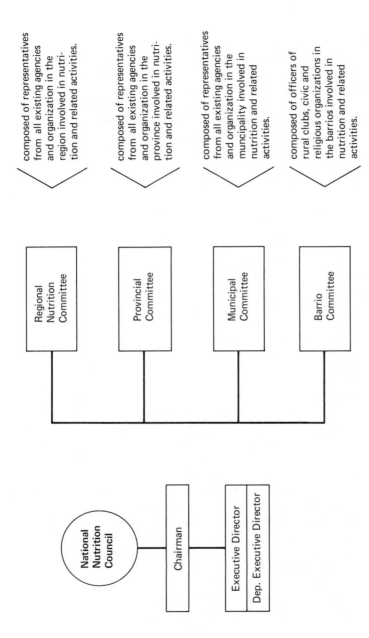

Figure 2
Composition of Nutrition Committees at the field level.

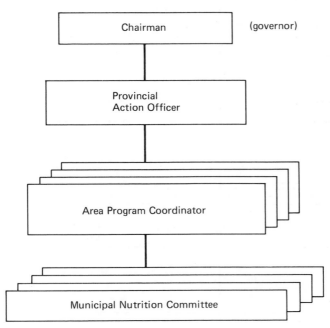

Figure 3
Provincial program staff.

cle to successful implementation since the program's components are practical, effective, and inexpensive strategies which are of double value: (1) The
program hinges largely on local organization down to the village and family
levels. This assures effective distribution as well as effective monitoring and
delivery of services, goods, and information. The Philippine Nutrition Program may be seen as the sum of municipal nutrition programs organized,
formulated, and implemented by locally manned multisectorial committees.
(2) The package of interventions intended to eradicate malnutrition and raise
the general nutritional level will be delivered mostly by local branches of
national agencies and through local funds. Because of the employment of
local leaders, developed through intensive training in various aspects of nutrition, implementation will create less strain on the program's budget and on
personnel from cooperating agencies.

   The PNP represents individual and collective efforts, planned and organized
to solve the malnutrition problem of the Philippines.[2] It forms an integral part
of the government's development program. A broad and comprehensive national nutrition program is being formulated at present. Meanwhile, an interim
program is being implemented.

Objectives

The general objective of the Philippine Nutrition Program is to improve the

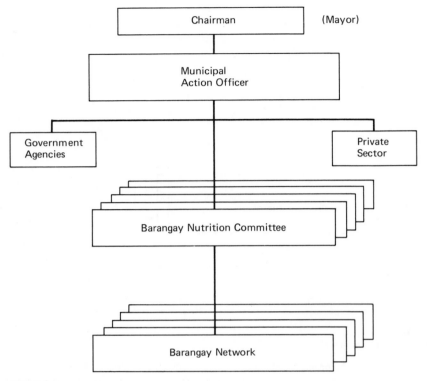

Figure 4
Municipal nutrition committee.

nutritional status of the population, paying particular attention to the vulnerable groups: infants, preschoolers, and pregnant and nursing mothers.

Specifically, the PNP aims to:

1   reduce the incidence of third degree malnutrition among infants and preschoolers by at least 25% and lower mortality rates by at least 25%
2   decrease the prevalence of second degree malnutrition among infants and preschoolers by at least 10%
3   motivate 50% of the pregnant and nursing mothers to adopt desired nutrition, health, and family planning practices as well as the proper food production techniques
4   improve nutritional status of at least 40% of the school children suffering from malnutrition
5   identify and treat cases of vitamin A deficiency and anemia
6   promote nutrition among all families such that no more than 50% of infants and preschool children will have weights below 90% of normal

Policy Directions

General policies give directions to the program, as follows:

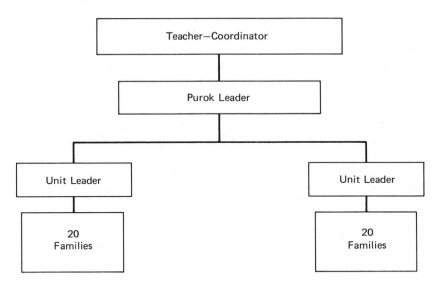

Figure 5
Barangay network.

1 Priority is given to improving nutrition status of the vulnerable groups.
2 Services will be provided to protect, cure, and rehabilitate the malnourished.
3 Information and education programs to stimulate the demand for local
foods and encourage their maximum use will be designed.
4 Increased production of low cost foods will be encouraged. Those engaged
in family planning will be encouraged to cooperate.
5 Applied and basic research in nutrition and related fields will be promoted.

Strategies

The strategies established are aimed at maximizing the implementation of the
Philippine Nutrition Program at all levels of operation:

1 establishing organizational structures at regional, provincial, municipal,
and barangay levels to coordinate and facilitate program implementation and
monitoring of activities
2 conducting nutrition training activities for various categories of personnel
at different levels
3 locating the malnourished in the community
4 formulating and implementing appropriate nutrition interventions aimed
to cure and prevent malnutrition of vulnerable groups
5 identifying agencies involved and their responsibilities, the inputs required,
and resources

Operation Timbang

To pursue its objectives of reducing the incidence of malnutrition in the country and improving nutritional status, the PNP has a very simple strategy: locate and cure the malnourished and prevent malnutrition among the vulnerable groups. As a means of locating and pinpointing the exact location of the malnourished (and at the same time arousing awareness in the community about nutrition), a nationwide body-weight survey dubbed "Operation Timbang" (OPT) has been started. The aim of this project is to weigh all children under 6 years of age and classify them by level of nutrition. This will enable the local nutrition committee to identify and locate families with malnourished children so that they can be given emergency food and medical assistance.

Since Operating Timbang is being carried out on a mass scale, so is the training of teachers and village leaders who conduct the weighing in each village. Training of these field workers has been tied in with the nutrition training program involving training officers and other personnel affiliated with the nutrition movement.

There have been obstacles to OPT, however. The most difficult is that the recommended clinical scale is rarely available in the villages. Even when it is available, it is so costly (about US$68) that the mayor cannot afford to buy it with his limited budget. To keep the operation going, the NCP has devised a good substitute, a renovated bar scale popularly known as an *espada*. Costing P70 (about US$10) on the retail market, the bar scale is being mass-produced for distribution to the villages.

Intervention Programs

While OPT paves the way for the thrust of the program, five different intervention schemes form the substance of the PNP. These are: food assistance, food production, nutrition education and information, health protection, and family planning (figure 6). It is in these programs that the real contributions of government and private agencies can be measured.

Food Assistance   Food assistance seeks to give the severely malnourished preschool child supplementary protein- and calorie-rich food to rehabilitate his nutritional status and prevent him from dying. This objective can be achieved in several ways. One approach is for a municipality, or several municipalities together, to produce, using local funds and resources, a package of food supplements for third degree malnourished children within their jurisdiction, as identified in the OPT. For this scheme, the NCP has formulated what is known as "Nutri-Pak." Distributed free or given at token cost, each pack contains ground rice, protein-rich food (such as mini-shrimp, dried *dilis* (anchovies), or mung bean powder), skimmed milk powder, and cooking oil. The package is cooked by the mother herself and given to the child until he or she

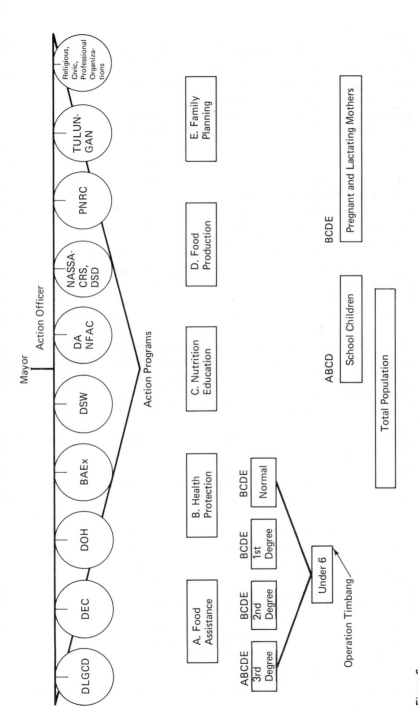

Figure 6
Municipal nutrition program.

is out of danger, as a supplement to the usual diet. It is estimated that a municipality with 150 third degree cases will spend less than US$1,000 per year for raw materials for a six-week feeding program conducted twice a year. Only simple local equipment is needed to put the pack together.

A second approach is through existing feeding programs, using donated food commodities. Feeding programs of such groups as the National Secretariat for Social Action-Catholic Relief Services (NASSA-CRS) and the Ministry of Social Welfare will be fully coordinated under the PNP in order to retarget their commodities to the children who most need them.

Finally, in the absence of a municipal Nutri-Pak system or donated food commodities, mothers of severely malnourished children may be given individualized instruction by a village worker. The mother will be given specific instructions on how to prepare a Nutri-Pak herself using family resources. Or, she may be told what food from the family pot to give her child, including details of preparation and feeding. This way, emergency feeding would have a distinct educational component, thus ensuring long term success.

Health Protection   While food assistance will relieve the malnourished child of his nutritional deprivation, health protection will prevent and treat the illnesses associated with malnutrition. Health services are primarily of two types: (1) medical treatment either through the provincial Malwards, Medicare Clinics, Rural Health Units, or home care services; and (2) institution of appropriate measures to increase resistance to illnesses, such as immunization, and diet and hygiene advice. In other words, nutrition will simply be integrated into each of the basic health services provided by the government's health team: medical and nursing care, communicable disease control, maternal and child health, health education, environmental sanitation, and epidemiology and vital statistics.

Malwards will be established in more government hospitals so that more cases of severe malnutrition, especially those with complications, may be treated. Malwards not only serve as intensive care units but as a place for educating the mother on how and what to feed her child, teaching her about nutrition for her family, as well as motivating her on family planning, home food production, and income-generating activities. She returns to her neighborhood as a nutrition communicator with her rehabilitated child as evidence. In the absence of hospitals, more limited wards—called Nutreunits—run by rural health personnel have been installed.

Rural Health Units, each manned by a municipal health officer, a public health nurse, a sanitary inspector, and several midwives, are also part of the program. Retrained midwives will handle routine and simple cases; more difficult cases will be referred to the main health center.*

The Philippine Medical Association, a private group, has committed its

---

*Of the total demand in rural health units and barrio clinics, nearly 64% has been found to be manageable at the first level. Around 55% of cases dealt with by the municipal

voluntary services to the program. Each private physician is enjoined to "adopt" severely malnourished cases for treatment free of charge. Malwards are being established in private hospitals through the intercession of the Philippine Medical Association and the Nutrition Center of the Philippines.

Information and Education   Another intervention scheme, nutrition information and education, aims to create mass awareness and consciousness of proper nutrition. Intended to change current attitudes and to promote adoption of desirable nutrition practices, this campaign utilizes three approaches: (1) mass media, (2) schools, and (3) nutrition classes.

A large scale information campaign is being mapped out under the leadership of the Nutrition Center of the Philippines. Radio is being given emphasis, although print, film, and television are also being utilized. A few simple and very specific nutrition messages are the subject of the information campaign.

The integration of nutrition into school curricula is being managed by the Ministry of Education and Culture. Other agencies responsible for conducting nutrition classes are: the Bureau of Agricultural Extension; the Ministry of Health, which maintains the Mothercraft Centers; the Philippine National Red Cross; Nutrition Foundation of the Philippines; and Philippine Business for Social Progress.

Food Production   This intervention enables families to have sufficient quantities of nutritious foods to supplement daily food intake and augment family income. There are two aspects of the implementation of the food production intervention: (1) the establishment of at least one food shop in each municipality for the production of nutritious food supplements, and (2) the production of selected crops in the homes, schools, and community. The crops are those which the agriculturists call "plant and harvest" varieties. The Green Revolution Movement, initiated by the first lady, has added momentum to food production efforts in both the home and in the schools. Livestock, poultry, and fish production is also encouraged.

One of the most pressing problems of food production is a source of good and viable planting materials. At present, the Bureau of Plant Industry is assigned the task of procuring, producing, and distributing vegetable seeds, and so on. The Green Revolution Command Center also receives donations, and procures and distributes seeds. A novel scheme in which a bank distributes free seeds to its depositors is gaining momentum.

Family Planning   As family size directly affects the nutritional status of family members, the PNP recognizes the importance of family planning as a complementary program. The priority targets of family planning are mothers of malnourished children and mothers of closely spaced children.

---

health officer could be tackled by the public health midwife and 16% of conditions seen by the midwife would have to be referred to a physician.

Information on family planning will be integrated into relevant educational activities for homemakers and into information materials to be developed cooperatively by the Population Commission and the National Nutrition Council.

At the municipal level, the nutrition workers' role is to assist in locating family planning acceptors through established barangay systems and to facilitate referrals to family planning clinics.

Role of the Private Sector

When the first lady founded the Nutrition Center of the Philippines, the Philippine Nutrition Program was assured of sustained, organized support from the private sector in a manner that was never before available to nutrition efforts in the country. The NCP, first of its kind in Asia, not only gathers the resources contributed by the international and private sectors, but also enlists and leads these sectors to active participation in sponsoring projects supplementary and complementary to the government program.

The organizational setup of the center reflects three areas of activity in which it lends support to the Philippine Nutrition Program, namely, project development, finance, and information and education. In order to maximize contributions to the program, the NCP identifies specific inputs needed under each intervention scheme or activity of the PNP. Thus, since its founding about two years ago, the center has begun its task by supporting activities such as Operation Timbang, Food Assistance, Nutrition Education, Health Protection, Food Production, and Family Planning, as well as Training and Research. It has illustrated how private involvement can be harnessed through encouragement of individual and organizational initiative and the utilization of existing resources or structures.

The NCP is the agency under the PNP responsible for the conduct of a massive nutrition information campaign intended to reach down to the grass roots. The center identifies specific and simple nutrition messages designed to correct important prevailing misconceptions about nutrition. It also conducts a nationwide awareness campaign about aspects of the program such as Operation Timbang, Nutri-Pak, and so on.

The center is at present the lead agency for the training needs of the PNP. It organizes training programs and orientation courses for administrators, trainers, and program implementors. It puts out training materials and manuals and contributes staff for these programs. Thus a well-organized training scheme is now being implemented, starting from the regional level, which eventually will reach the workers in the village.

The center also endeavors to support meritorious research projects in applied nutrition, especially those of immediate application. It continues to explore innovative approaches for the intervention schemes of the PNP, such as the formulation of Nutri-Pak for the food assistance program, the design for a simple village processing plant for Nutri-Paks, the design of a locally manufactured, cheap, and portable weighing scale for use in OPT. The NCP has been able to make this scale available to local governments at minimum cost. It has provided thousands of Nutritional Level Calculators, especially designed for the OPT, to enable workers to assess quickly and accurately, the age, standard weight, and nutritional level of preschool children. It has taken the lead in designing a system of reporting the results of OPT by providing special workbooks for the purpose, and collating the results using a computer. The NCP is also starting a data bank where nutrition-related data from the field are organized for easy retrieval and analysis. Finally, the center renders technical assistance to communities in starting nutrition programs. For this purpose, a Community Nutrition Task Force (CONTAF) has been created under the auspices of the Nutrition Foundation of the Philippines and the NCP.

To support all these activities, in addition to maintaining an office, library, and training complex, the center maps out fundraising activities and manages an investment portfolio and trust fund.

Aside from the NCP, there are many private groups involved in the program, although in more circumscribed ways. Mention has already been made of the Nutrition Foundation of the Philippines (NFP), the PBSP, and NASSA-CRS.

The NFP continues to render technical assistance, upon request, to communities as well as to civic, religious, and professional organizations desiring to undertake nutrition programs. NFP nutritionists assist in planning programs, training of personnel and field workers, conducting baseline surveys, and even initial implementation. The NFP has also participated in Operation Timbang and in the training program under the PNP.[31]

The PBSP is at present involved in developing prototypes of community development schemes under both urban and rural settings. Three communities—one in a relocation area for squatters, one in an urban area, and another in a small town in Southern Luzon—serve as working models for the applied nutrition program of PBSP. The program being tested has six components: nutrition education, nutrition rehabilitation, food production, food preservation, income-generating projects, and evaluation.

NASSA-CRS is a religious group that has done much in providing food commodities for feeding programs. While the scheme is parish-based and directed through the dioceses, coordination with the PNP is now being developed in order to ensure that recipients are those most in need: the third degree malnourished preschoolers.

Other groups include Tulungan Foundation and the Green Revolution Project, both projects of the first lady. The former is concerned with mothercraft centers in communities not reached by the government. The Green Revolution Project emphasizes backyard and community gardening as well as livestock raising to augment income and improve family nutrition. It works closely with the nutrition program, since the latter also includes home and community food production as an important component.

A novel approach has recently been devised in answer to the problem of rice shortages, which too often plague the country. General Order 47, promulgated by the president in 1974, has made it mandatory for all corporations operating for profit and with 500 employees or more to "provide rice and corn requirements of their employees and the latter's immediate family." Such corporations have a choice of importing or engaging in the production of rice and/or corn. The program will not only activate idle private agricultural land but harness private technology, managerial expertise, and managerial capability in the field of agricultural production. Already, some 225 firms with a combined payroll of 287,632 workers are either in the early stages of production or are ready to implement the scheme.[32]

International Agencies

A discussion of the PNP would not be complete without mention of the role international assistance agencies have played in the history of its development and in its present implementation.

It can be said that the nutrition rehabilitation component of the present PNP evolved from the mothercraft and feeding programs first introduced here by such agencies as US AID, CARE, and CRS. Some examples of these programs are nutri-bun distribution for elementary school children, the introduction of the high-protein supplementary feeding for preschool children in several provincial areas, and, even back in the '50s, the distribution of rolled oats, bulgur wheat, skimmed milk, and fortified margarine throughout the country. It is only lately, however, that the food supplementation programs of these agencies have been woven into a total approach involving not only nutrition education for mothers and schoolchildren, but also health protection, family planning, and home food production.

US AID committed US$403,000 for fiscal year 1975/76. This supports supplementary feeding programs through the Bureau of Agricultural Extension, TMCH (Targeted Maternal and Child Health) program, the Department of Social Welfare's Day Care Centers, and the Department of Education and Culture's Philippine School Nutrition Program. In addition, a number of pilot research and development projects will continue to be supported such as the Barangay Health Aid Project, cost/benefit analysis of nutritional health delivery systems, pilot manufacture of coconut skim milk, community canneries, and others.

UNICEF has also been contributing generously to the program. For 1975, the support program calls for $398,000 in the form of supplies, equipment, and transport, as well as stipends for training at the national, provincial, and village levels.

There are other international agencies which contribute in one way or an-

other to the program. CARE and CRS are actively involved by providing food
commodities for food assistance programs. The International Development
Research Center of Canada (IDRC) and Virginia Polytechnic Institute and
State University are assisting specific research projects under the program.

NUTRITION IN THE DEVELOPMENTAL STRATEGY

Although past administrations consistently announced priority for provision
of adequate food for Filipinos, close scrutiny of past development efforts
reveals a lack of definite policies or programs which would support the claim
that improvement of nutritional levels was a major objective of national development. The impression gathered from state-of-the-nation reports and past
programs is that food adequacy was pursued largely for political ends.

On the other hand, malnutrition and related concerns were, until lately,
treated apart from the total development effort. Even when programs were
introduced, they were short-term measures that addressed only certain aspects of the problem and were usually considered to involve only the health,
civic, or welfare sectors. Most indicative of this attitude is the fact that it was
the private sector which led the way in promoting nutrition and agitating for
nutrition programs in the country.

Economists can point out several underlying reasons for the usual approach
to the food adequacy issue by national leadership in past periods, and why
emphasis was placed on self-sufficiency per se as the answer to a country's
food problem.[33] Motivations included maintenance of political stability,
avoidance of leverage by foreign states, elimination of inflation, and improvement of incomes of rural families.

At one time or another, the Philippine government has tried many different
policies in support of the food adequacy objective, but aside from investment
in irrigation, there has not really been much continuity from one administration to the next. It is ironic that while the main goal of these policies is intensified food production, provisions for implementation have been wanting or
weak. A case in point is the unsuccessful setting of floor prices for rice and
corn which depended on government purchases of the crops from farmers.
Because there were insufficient government funds available for the program,[33] however, the floor price followed the market price. Only in the last
few years has the problem been solved and the prices of rice and corn been
stabilized.

Food adequacy can be interpreted as the attainment of a balance between
available food supply and consumption requirements of the total population.
Food balance sheets from 1953 up to the present represent the preoccupation
of all administrations in achieving such a balance. It should be noted, however, that food balance statistics are only *average* figures, i.e., the total food
supply divided by the total population. Hence, they do not take into account
access to food, distribution, and levels of adequacy. A review of the country's

statistics on income distribution would reveal how many families are, in fact, able to buy the FNRC recommended food basket. This would underscore the grossly unequal distribution of food adequacy, so that while a small percentage enjoys an oversupply of food, the large majority of the population are only able to buy food far below the standard requirements.

Moreover, it should be noted that FNRC standards are relatively low compared to FAO standards; hence one is fairly sure that the number of persons not consuming enough food will be underestimated.[33] It strikes an alarming note, then, when one sees that in 1971 the food supply available for Filipinos was only 80% adequate based on "conservatively low" FNRC requirements.[34] Even judging from the 1973 food balance sheet,[15] which shows 99% adequacy in total food, one can assume a sizeable percentage of the population are still inadequately fed.

It is clear then, that food adequacy alone, as pursued by past government administrations and as reflected by food balance sheets, does not indicate, or even less, assure that Filipinos will be well-nourished and healthy participants in efforts for national progress. A more accurate manner of measuring how much of the available food supply has contributed to overall well-being (through lessened mortality and morbidity) and eventually to productivity is clearly in order. Such a measurement would, in fact, reflect how much a government has done for its people, who are, in the final analysis, the recipients of the benefits of development. There is a cycle in which social development contributes to national development and progress which are, in turn, aimed at the social good.

For this reason, health and nutrition occupy a prominent place in the system of social indicators recently devised by the Development Academy of the Philippines (DAP), and adopted by the present New Society administration.[35] The social indicators system will measure national well-being by quantifying targets and achievements of development programs, and measuring them over time. It is hoped that the system will depict changes objectively, whether positive or negative, in order to guide national leaders and planners in setting priorities.

The system recommends an output orientation for national development programs so that at the end of each year, for example, one can see how much the total program and each of its components have contributed to national well-being. Illustrative of this output orientation is the DAP indicator of Net Beneficial Product (NBP), a consumption concept for social goods and services. In addition to this and present indicators (mostly economic), the DAP recommended supplementation of basic data by annual surveys of family income and expenditures, ownership of wealth, housing, and utilities, and disability due to illness. The DAP also recommends indicators on the level of educational capital, the number of families below the poverty line, and polls of citizens' attitudes and perceptions, among others.

The DAP indicators identify two of man's major concerns in health: length
of life, and quality of health in those years of life. Two aspects of health are
the most socially important: freedom from morbidity and good nourishment.
Thus, the DAP lists the following indicators of Filipino health:

1 *Infant mortality rate.* This is considered the single, most telling indicator of
health status of the population.
2 *Life expectancy.*
3 *Disability due to illness.* This is difficult to estimate because of different
degrees of disability caused by different illnesses. It has been shown, however,
that it is possible to estimate the number of full disability equivalent days lost
due to illness.
4 *Average daily supply of calories and protein.* Because of relative importance of calorie and protein vis-à-vis other nutrients and the prevalence of
protein calorie malnutrition in the Philippines, the DAP indicators focused on
the available supply of these nutrients. Besides, protein and calorie intakes are
positively correlated with intake of other nutrients.
5 *State of malnutrition.* Aside from usual indices of levels of malnutrition,
the DAP recommended serial weighing of preschool children, such as Operation Timbang, as monitor for the health status of the population.

Actually, information flowing PNP operations in the field will constitute
basic indicators not only of the population's nutritional level, but also of its
general well-being. Through a systematic spot-mapping surveillance of every
family in each community by local leaders, basic data—on morbidity/mortali-
ty, pregnancy, family planning practice, and malnutrition—can be gathered
with an accuracy that has never been possible in the past. The PNP, in fact,
has set up a potential mechanism for gathering social indicators and monitoring the flow of other government goods, services, and information.

At present, the National Economic Development Authority is in the process
of revising the 4-year National Development Plan (1974-77), to adjust to the
rapid pace of reforms under the New Society. Substantial changes are being
made in the social programs area particularly in nutrition, because of the
introduction of a strengthened PNP in mid-1974 through presidential decree.
Since implementation of the PNP is to be carried out by many sectors of
government, it is expected that the revisions will incorporate nutrition functions in new areas. For example, since the PNP is to be carried out by nutrition committees from the national to the village level, new provisions have to
be made in the section on local government and community development.

In effect, the revisions being made in the development plan of the country
represent a total reorientation because of the emphasis on social development
and the importance of the PNP. In the words of President Marcos, the 1974-
77 plan is a social plan, with specific, defined objectives aimed at eliminating
malnutrition in the country and raising the nutritional status of the people.
For its first year of implementation the PNP has set numerical goals against

which achievements can be measured at year's end.

A healthy, well-nourished population is a prerequisite to the attainment of national goals. This is a key to the promotion and maintenance of health and economic productivity, the attainment of which intersects with government objectives in family planning, education, job opportunities, food and agricultural progress, and a wide range of efforts to enhance socioeconomic progress. The Philippine Nutrition Program is a means to achieve these goals within the context of other socioeconomic development programs.[2]

The 1974-77 National Development Plan

In addition to the general goal of improving the standard of living of the greater mass of the population, the plan sets forth the following objectives:

1 promotion of employment
2 maximum feasible economic growth
3 more equitable income distribution
4 regional development and industrialization
5 promotion of social development
6 maintenance of acceptable levels of price, and balance of payments stability

Specific programs and activities have accordingly been mapped out in the development plan to cover the various sectors of the economy during 1974/75.[36] Most of these will affect nutrition directly and indirectly.

Expansion of food production to attain self-sufficiency, nutrition education, and the provision of basic health services are among the primary concerns of the plan, as embodied in both its economic and social development provisions. Agrarian reform, accelerated food production, and cooperative development programs have been developed in order to raise agricultural productivity, attain self-sufficiency in food, and raise the level of rural income.

The development of export-oriented industries and medium- to small-scale industries is a top priority in the industrial development program. This will promote employment opportunities, diversify and expand manufactured exports, and increase efforts at regional development and industrialization. To sustain the overall development effort, the infrastructure program provides for the setting up of an efficient system of roads, posts, railways, and airports, as well as of power-generating, telecommunications, and water resources facilities.

In view of the glaring growth imbalance among regions, more emphasis will be given to regional development and industrialization. Thus, in addition to the correction of policies which artificially favor a few selected areas, the integrated approach to regional development is being utilized. This approach calls for the integration of physical development with the economic, social, administrative, and financial aspects of development into a common plan for a given area. Under the New Society, the New Plan, released in October 1974, emphasizes the magnified role of nutrition and health in the country's total development effort.

CONCLUSIONS

Nutrition in the Philippines has bright prospects, indeed. After years of struggling and elbowing for due recognition of the gravity and urgency of the problem, it has finally attracted the attention of the top echelons of government. This has triggered the national consciousness to a dedication of efforts towards the eradication of malnutrition in the country. The expressed commitment by our national leaders, the president and first lady, to the cause of nutrition is the most important single factor reinvigorating nutrition activities in the country.

Until the 1974 4-year development plan, the government was somewhat vague in its commitment to the priority of nutrition. It is indeed heartening that this time there is a concrete commitment from the highest level to bring about improved nutrition. This commitment has led to the formulation and enforcement of a comprehensive program that combines the goals of adequate nutrition and total human development through family and community level efforts. This is the program's biggest asset and the largest difference from previous nutrition drives: it is not only grassroots-oriented, but grassroots-originated as well. The PNP is the sum total of individual local nutrition programs developed as close to the people as possible, organized by local leaders, and based on local needs and capabilities. The Barangay Network is the expression of the grassroots orientation and a most significant approach to the problem of dissemination of services and information as well as assurance of sustained and immediate identification of the target population. Because Barangay Nutrition Programs are planned and carried out by and among people in the village, it is certain that these programs will be responsive to village needs and problems. Local leadership also provides inexpensive outlets for effective delivery of program goods, services, and information materials.

Another factor that augurs well for the program is the concerted commitment by the private sector to the program. The vital contributions that the private sector can make, such as generation of interest and awareness, material and technical support, and innovative insights and approaches to the nutrition problem have been amply demonstrated from the earliest days of nutrition in the country. The PNP recognizes the boost that the private sector can give the program, and, in fact, private efforts make up a large part of the PNP history and present activities. Private cooperation, effectively harnessed by the Nutrition Center of the Philippines, fills the gaps in the government program, and lends credibility to the government's sincerity in the undertaking.

Finally, the trend of success registered this early by the government's socio-economic development programs, particularly land reform, agricultural development programs, and infrastructure, gives added optimism for nutrition in the country. Already we see evidence of increasing prosperity through land reform, the beginning effects of redistributing wealth through taxes and other measures, bumper harvests through the advent of modern technology and farm credit, and increased mobility arising from intensified infrastructure projects.

In short, we have evidence that the average Filipino is at last starting to liberate himself from the shackles of poverty. It is hoped that with continuing support from the leaders of the country, the dedication of men and women from all walks of life to the goal of the nutrition program, and the contributions of the private sector—all in the background of peace and economic development—nutrition in the Philippines will finally come of age.

DISCUSSION (THE PHILIPPINES)

Solon

Let me start the discussion by thanking the Foundation for allowing me to discuss the one-year history and the future of the nutrition program of the Philippines.

Winikoff

Could you tell us a little more about the unique administrative organization: two independent bodies with one director?

Solon

As Executive Director of both the Nutrition Center of the Philippines, a private body, and the National Nutrition Council, the government coordinating body, I represent both the government and private sectors. There is no conflict of interest. The council formulates, implements, and coordinates nutrition policies and programs in the country, while the center plays a supportive role by mobilizing the resources of the private sector in support of the Philippine Nutrition Program.

We have defined our targets as the under-six-year-old group, the pregnant and lactating mothers, and the schoolchildren. We decided that health protection would be part of the whole program. The economic status of the families would be improved through the cooperative work of pertinent agencies. It is obvious, for instance, that we cannot raise the economic status of the families through our own effort but only with the cooperation of the Economic Development Authority. We also designed an information and education program geared towards increased production of low-cost nutritious foods and promotion of family planning.

The general objective, as in any other country is to improve the nutritional status of the population. Specifically, we want to recognize, locate, and cure the malnourished. We were informed that out of 9 million children, 3.5 million are malnourished; but where are they? We want to locate them and help them. So we have launched a systematic nationwide weighing program. It is ambitious, but I think we are developing a model by which it can be done.

One thing that I would like to emphasize is organization. Unless we have organized the community effort, I do not think we can really run any kind of program for the people. If the people, themselves, are not organized to receive the program, it will not work. It will collapse when the nutrition workers leave.

Another very important ingredient of the program is systematic assignment of responsibility. One must formulate nutrition interventions that identify the agencies involved and their responsibilities, covered by a memorandum of agreement stating that each agency agrees that their personnel have certain duties in nutrition at the national level, the regional level, the provincial level, the municipal level, and the village level. On this basis, it is now easy to evaluate who is not doing what and where. It also avoids redundancy. In the past, agencies crowded into one geographic area, rendering similar services, while other places lacked attention.

Montgomery
This memorandum of agreement defines functions?

Solon
Yes, at different levels. The agencies found at the municipal level usually include the local government, education, health, extension work, social welfare, and agriculture. The functions of each of these workers are spelled out in the memorandum. The target population is also very clear: children under six years first, pregnant and lactating mothers, then schoolchildren.

Montgomery
It doesn't mandate how much money each agency is going to put in?

Solon
The amount of money each has to allocate to nutrition is in each agency budget. Thus, I don't have to beg for money: each member agency must appropriate money even for transportation, material, personnel, and other inputs in nutrition within the agency budget.

In addition to agency participation at the national level, there is participation in regional and local organizations all the way down to the village committees.

Sandoval
Do those nutritional committees just work on nutrition and nothing else?

Solon
No. Since there were no committees at those levels previously, the nutrition committees are now composed of representatives from the different related agencies such as health, welfare, and agriculture, all of which offer nutrition services. I would even propose to change the name of these committees to something like "Family Development Committees."

I have seen applied nutrition where the national agencies try to lead the way, but I think this approach is obsolete. It will never succeed unless the *local* government takes the lead. Governors and mayors are the managers and executives. They are the administrators of the community, and giving them the authority and responsibility is crucial.

The day the first lady appointed me, I asked if I could meet the cabinet members and orient them on nutrition. She arranged it, and she was there for one hour, listening to the nutrition lecture. That was the turning point. The members of the cabinet saw the reality of the problem of malnutrition and the whole program got off the ground. Now, it extends through every level of government.

Schlossberg
What happens if a local official isn't enthusiastic?

Solon

That's a very good question. You know, we don't have local elections yet. The president appoints the governors and mayors. Before the president reappoints the officials, there is a performance audit. So, all the local governments are now being audited under the Secretary of Local Government, and we take advantage of this. Local officials earn merit points for nutrition inputs in their communities. Once I invited all seventy-six governors to Manila and asked each of them to bring two of their best mayors so they could implement nutrition programs as an example to the rest. We gave a nutrition lecture to them. Many representatives from international agencies told me, "I've never seen a group of governors and mayors taking notes on nutrition before!"

As Mr. Thomson said, there *is* such a thing as administration of nutrition, and that is what we are teaching these leaders. One mayor has been helping me for a year. He gives lectures to other mayors, board members, and governors on the administration of nutrition. I do not use community nutrition workers to lecture on this topic, because mayors are the best persons to teach other mayors how it can be done.

The governor and mayors are, thus, the chairmen of local nutrition committees at their respective levels. One action officer and a program area coordinator are appointed per 4 or 5 municipalities. On the municipal level, the local nutrition committee, composed of an action officer and representatives of government and private agencies, is the focal point of our program right now. When we delegate authority to the local governments we give them a nutrition manual for administrators, describing the planning, organizing, and implementing of nutrition programs. We remind governors and mayors that, no matter how many roads and bridges they build, if their population is malnourished, there is no development.

When mayors and governors asked, "Why didn't you start this ten years ago?" I told them, "You were politicians ten years ago." Today they are more interested in social development and are no longer preoccupied with the preparations for elections. The governor is audited on the number of municipal nutrition programs begun, and the mayors themselves are audited on how many village nutrition committees have been organized to implement the programs. Where there is no village program, there is no national program.

How do we set it in motion? After organizing the committee, and after organizing the village, we start training for the "Operation Timbang," or mass weighing. The weighing scale, incidentally, held us back somewhat. We have only 2,000 currently, and they are heavy and made in New York and cost US$70, illustrating Michael's point that technology transfer is not always appropriate. Finally, we designed our own bar scale, accurate to 0.1 kg and with a capacity of up to 20 kg. Now we are the sole manufacturer and distributor.

We also invented a "nutritional level calculator" which did not require a pen and paper for calculating the weight for age. If you know the child's birthday, you can get the child's standard weight and, then, on the other side you will be able to get the nutritional status immediately. A private firm covered the cost of this calculator, another example of how we involve the private sector.

The Nutrition Center also puts out an official Timbang workbook, where all the weights are entered at the unit level. In this workbook, you can see the "critical list," so, if you go to a village you can easily identify "critical families." Again, this item has been sponsored by a private company, illustrating the role of the Nutrition Center: to look for contributors of items not included in the government budget.

Montgomery
The children in Timbang are all in school?

Solon
No, they are under six years old.

Montgomery
How do you get to them?

Solon
We target the population by dividing the entire municipality into villages for weighing. Then, we divide the responsibility in the village among teacher coordinators and unit leaders or village leaders. We require a spot map of each village, and results are registered on the map. The compiled data are submitted to the Rural Health Unit at municipal level.

After weighing, the target area can be reduced to the priority villages, those with a high incidence of third degree cases: a village with more than 5% third degree cases will be designated a high risk area. Within these priority villages, one can target high risk families: first, those with third degree children, then those with second degree cases. Within the family, you reduce intervention to the under-six-year-olds and pregnant and lactating mothers. After weighing and identifying the cases, we give food assistance, "Nutri-pak."

Nutri-pak is a high calorie and protein ready-to-cook food supplement (50% of child's Recommended Daily Allowance) distributed to third degree cases from six months to six years. Each polyethylene pack contains packets of ground rice, a high quality protein food (rice/mini-shrimp powder, anchovy powder, or mung grits), and cooking oil. The rice and protein is ground so that the food is specifically for the young child, and adults are discouraged from sharing it.

Nutri-pak is given, usually for a period of six weeks, one pack a day, to assure rapid recovery. It has two purposes: rehabilitation and education. The mother can see clearly that the contents—fish, bean, rice, and oil—are traditional food items with high nutritional value. The rehabilitation that follows intake of the food makes the nutritive value apparent.

The production of Nutri-pak involves the simple process of cooking, drying, grinding, and packaging. A simple hand grinder is used in the villages by rural workers and villagers. Some municipalities have their own processing plants, especially in areas where fish and shrimp abound. Currently, we are trying to conserve our supply of shrimp since there is the possibility of this food being exported and its price becoming prohibitive. In addition to the fish, legumes are planted in vacant lots for use in the Nutri-pak.

If there is no municipal subsidized Nutri-pak system, you can teach the mother to make homemade Nutri-pak. We have 70,000 variety stores in the 42,000 villages, and there is always dried fish. The fish is sold salted to preserve it, so we teach the mother to desalt it in water, then dry and grind it and mix it into the rice porridge. Mothers can also use mung bean powder, instead of fish, for added protein in the rice mixture. After adding the high protein food, mothers add oil to the rice porridge to increase caloric density and then mix chopped vegetable leaves in the rice porridge. Finally they have "Nutri-pak" for children: high in calories and rich in proteins and vitamins.

Sandoval
Nutri-pak is just for children?

Solon
Yes. Preschool children.

Solimano
How can you be sure it is going to be used only by children?

Solon
This is always a problem with donated commodities, but mothers are told that the pack is only for the young child, that her child is sick, and Nutri-pak, although food, is also medicine.

Wray
Florentino, what did you do about acceptability, palatability, and so on?

Solon
That is no problem here because the food is exactly what the people already eat every day. Sometimes, however, there is not enough of it and none at all is given to the child. For this reason, I am not in favor of a technology that removes the odor and the taste of fish because this is what the people look for in their food!

Health protection is another important intervention, and here the health units can really be of great help. Under our new procedures, after isolation of third-degree malnutrition in a municipality by Operation Timbang, all the cases identified are given medical assessment by rural health personnel and the affected children are placed under surveillance.

Wray
What do you use as a standard for the classification of "normal" weight, from

which you derive your first, second and third degree categories?

Solon
We are using a Philippine Standard. It is Filipino 90th percentile. It is a little lower than the Harvard Standard.

Mellor
Is there general agreement that the second and third degree, whichever way they are calculated, and which in your graph make up about 30% of the population studied, were, to use a layman's expression, "unhealthy"? Do they all have a problem that really should be rectified? Can we say flatly that about 30% of the population was pretty unhealthy, simply from a caloric point of view?

Wray
Those children might be walking around, in fact one might see them on the streets and not think them sick. However, they're much more susceptible to infections, and they've got problems.

Solon
I would say the third degree child is sick. As for the second degree, I would say that potential for sickness is so great that something ought to be done for them.

Mellor
And the first degree, one would debate whether there is a problem or not?

Wray
That's right.

Solon
In two municipalities, for almost a year now, using the isolation and treatment procedure, we have reduced by 50% deaths of those under 6 years old in comparison with the same period last year, probably because the mayors provided medicine for third-degree children. Now there is real need that the mayors continue to provide medicine to the identified third degree cases. A mayor is made aware of his responsibility for every child that dies every month in his community without medical attendance. Appropriations for medicine are increasing because the mayors realize how many of the severely malnourished children will die without their help.

The approximately 1,600 Rural Health Units (RHUs) are responsible for protecting the third degree cases identified through community weighing. We estimate an average of 200 third degree cases in every municipality of 24,000 population based on the nationwide Operation Timbang results. The Rural Health Unit will have to give curative and protective care and place families with third-degree cases under surveillance.

Severe cases with complications that need hospitalization are brought to Malnutrition Wards (Malwards) or to Pediatric Wards where Malwards are not available. In the ward, mothers are given nutrition, education, and training. The rural ward has a native kitchen and a backyard garden.

Wray
Do you have any special approaches to education?

Solon
The principal technique in nutrition education is to establish and deliver priority messages, the most pertinent messages for the mothers. The information, education, and communication committee of the National Nutrition Council has listed 17 priority messages, and all agencies with nutrition activities are given guidance in the dissemination of these priority messages. We have built up our capability to produce slides and scripts, all municipalities are provided with flipcharts, and there is one training manual. All this leads to uniformity in content and methods of teaching nutrition. For the first time in the country, industrial and commercial firms spent sizeable amounts for advertisements on food value and proper diet. These are tremendous boosts to the nutrition program of the country.

Winikoff
Have you made any attempts at policies to change the nature of the national food supply?

Solon
Many people asked about rice enrichment, but we felt this would only increase the price. Besides, there would be all the 10,000 millers to supervise. Instead, our national grain authorities enforced a regulation of second class milling of all rice, except that which will be sold in hotels and restaurants.

Schlossberg
Is this as acceptable to the people?

Solon
Yes, it is. However, we are also formally promoting it through broadcasting and print media.

We also have a price control system which regulates both rice and oil. In our nutrition survey findings only about 7%, instead of 25%, of total calories were found to come from oil. Oil is expensive and does not generally reach poor people, but now we are teaching the mothers to put it in rice porridge for children. The only way we can lower the price of oil is by changing its packaging from cans to bottles. We discovered that the container was more expensive than the contents, so now, there is cheap cooking oil available in bottles, and the poor may increase their use of it. The tin can manufacturers, of course, are complaining, but we must have social conscience: we lack calories, and now we hope oil will reach the low income groups.

Schlossberg

Florentino, what about actual numbers? How many people have you identified who need the assistance of Nutri-pak and the education and the changes
in marketing? And what percentage are you reaching and at what cost?

Solon

In one year of "Operation Timbang" we have weighed one million preschool
(0-6) children. We hope to increase the rate with the availability of the bar
scale which we are producing. With the present number of weighed children
we projected 400,000 third degree cases from 0-6 years old who will need
food assistance. The cost is about 10 centavos a pack. The suggested duration
of feeding is six weeks, so the cost would be about US$0.60 for adequate
rehabilitation of one third degree malnourished child.

The Nutri-pak production is run either at the municipal or the provincial
government level. The governor can provide Nutri-pak by establishing his own
plant. More frequently, it is done at the municipal level by the mayor. Almost
all areas can afford it because the grinder and siever are the only important
equipment needed in this process. The sun can take care of drying.

Antrobus

What is the total cost of this, and what percentage of the health budget does
this represent?

Solon

It is not from the health budget. It is from the local government's budget.
That is why every municipal mayor must submit his program, and we give
guidelines on how to spend the budget for nutrition. The Bureau of Internal
Revenue is giving some money, 20% of which goes to social development. Out
of that, a slice goes to nutrition. So it is not through the health fund, but
through the mayor's municipal fund that Nutri-pak is supported. It will cost
the mayor something like US$1,000 in outlays per year to feed 300 third
degree cases six weeks twice a year.

Previously, the financial input from the municipal and provincial levels was
zero for nutrition. Now, nutrition and health are considered top priority as
indicators of community development. The Secretary of Local Government
has allowed the mayors to use some money from the social development fund
for nutrition after submission of a plan and program. For example, mayors
are now allowed to purchase weighing scales and Nutri-pak equipment from
social development funds.

Of course, some support comes from the national level in order to motivate
the local people—something like: "If you buy 10 weighing scales, I'll give you
3 free." There must be this national input in order to show national concern,
but the program must be planned at the local level. It must emanate from the
local people so that the program will be their own responsibility. We give only
guidelines on what to spend and for how long.

I wish to emphasize here that the authority and responsibility of administration of the nutrition program rest on the local government in contrast to other national programs where local officials do not enjoy full autonomy. The beauty of this approach is that the local government becomes responsible even for funding for evaluation.

Barnes
What is the source of municipal funds? Is there a municipal tax, or does the state send the money down to the municipality?

Solon
There are two sources of funds. One from local income and the other from their national share. This is why local authority is the best level: it has legislative power, taxation power, police power, and it's the nearest you can get to the people. In only one year, happily, we were able to generate funds from the local government and dependence on national funding decreased.

Thomson
I would be very glad to have some idea of the criteria for evaluation that will be used in the Philippine program. I think this would be of use to others.

Solon
Evaluation will be very simple and very specific, based on how much third degree malnutrition is reduced and how much second degree how many mothers reached with nutrition information, and how many of the specific deficiencies controlled. This is an interim program for one year, and we will use parameters which we can quantify. Our goal is to reduce third degree by about 25%, and reduce the death rate in third degree cases to about 10%; reduce second-degree about 50%; and to reach 80% of the pregnant and lactating mothers.

Winikoff
In reviewing nutrition activities we often see that projects did not have a nationwide impact for a variety of reasons. Often, the role of international aid has been viewed critically by its recipients. How have your projects meshed with the international efforts in the Philippines?

Solon
The Applied Nutrition Project (ANP), led by the Department of Education, began about 1962 but had, after ten years, covered only about 600 schools. International agencies, like US AID, came in and gave support to the Department of Health, which then became more independent in its program and seemingly moved away from the ANP. The Bureau of the Agricultural Extension likewise was supported by AID in targeted maternal and child health. Again, it became independent from the ANP. International aid to agencies in ANP somehow affected the coordination of nutrition projects. The concept of applied nutrition was actually eviscerated when it was supposed to be reinforced.

When I took over the responsibility of coordination, the first thing I did with international agencies was to meet with them. I informed them that we have a *Philippine Nutrition Program* (PNP), not an AID program, not a UNICEF program, but within the PNP there is lots of room for assistance.

We spread the whole program before the aid agencies and asked them to realign their assistance according to our priorities. What happened was that UNICEF and US AID and CARE realigned all their inputs to the program relevant to our needs. Our requests were directed to strengthening our capabilities for training and education. As the old Chinese proverb says, "If you give a man a fish, you feed him for one day only, but if you teach him how to fish, you feed him for many days."

Wray

It seems to me that it is helpful to think of these program inputs from abroad, or from the top, or from the local level as being multiplicative rather than additive. The difference between the two models is, with A plus B, if A is zero, you still have B. Right? With A times B, as A approaches zero, your product approaches zero.

Think about the effectiveness of a nutrition assistance program, let's say AID, UNICEF, and so on. This effectiveness, then, is a function of the foreign inputs times the national inputs. Now I think that, in the past, the foreign inputs have dominated, and very often national inputs have approached zero, and thus the results, finally, approached zero.

The same thing applies, I think, in the relationship between central and community levels. There, the effectiveness is a function of inputs from the central level times inputs at the local level. In terms of long-term program effectiveness, you can make a great splash with a lot of central input, but it finally depends on the local input, and, if that's zero, your long-term effectiveness is also going to be zero. From the early '50s to the late '60s or early '70s, national inputs were often limited, but that has changed because people like Florentino and Julio and others have come along. The same thing is happening now at the local level.

It seems to me that the most important thing to keep in mind is the basic intelligence of the people at the national and local levels. They have had a lot of things dumped on them in the name of community development or health or nutrition for many, many years, and they are now skeptical. In fact, they are almost hostile. The secret of getting the kind of local input which you need is in getting their trust by offering something that is obviously for their benefit. I do not think that we can get the kind of community support we need just by preaching at people. They are too intelligent to believe what we tell them without seeing for themselves.

Latham

The only thing I don't like about your mathematics, Joe, is that you more or less say that *foreign* input is essential.

Sai
What the formula means to say is, if the project is truly a function of *two* inputs, then if either input approaches zero, the effectiveness approaches zero. This is stating it in theoretical terms.

Antrobus
Is it desirable that the foreign part of the function should approach zero?

Wray
In the long run, yes.

Mellor
I would like to take issue a little with the objective of dropping the foreign input to zero. I think that it is extremely important to national programs that there be an international interchange of ideas, and getting the foreign input up may, in fact, raise the productivity of the local inputs very substantially.

On first thought, I agreed with dropping to zero, also, because of the self-consciousness typical of Americans in the aid business. We are used to thinking of foreign assistance and interchange as being done in a patronizing context, and a lot of us are uncomfortable with that. But that doesn't mean foreign assistance is a bad idea in a different context. It follows, for example, that the United States could benefit greatly, in looking at these kinds of problems, in having some inputs from other people's programs. We are in no way psychologically ready for that, but one would hope that some day we would be.

Winikoff
We have talked a lot about the importance of strong political will from the top, as well as the necessity for community participation from below. How do you see these two inputs in relation to each other? Are they always multiplicative, as in Joe's model? Can they conflict? Are they mutually reinforcing? Can they be independent variables?

Solon
In our case, we use both mechanisms. The first lady put up the Nutrition Center of the Philippines, which reinforces the government agencies working in nutrition by harnessing private resources. When she appointed me as Executive Director of the center, she told me, "You are not working for me; you are working for the people." Up to now, she has fully entrusted the work to us, and she just wants us to call on her when there is a need for support. We need the central commitment, but the people of the community are still the backbone of our program.

Solimano
We thought in the early '70s that one of the big questions was how to convince governments to undertake nutrition activities. It seems that, in four

years, we have advanced quite a lot, because now there are first ladies and
first ministers trying to do something. That's good, but I think what we are
missing is some information from the other end. What happens when the
process is initiated by the people and not at the level of the "First"? That, I
think, is something that has to concern us in the future because some of these
presidents and ministers and first ladies leave office. In some countries, they
don't change very often. But at some time they have to change in any case,
and I think we are lacking information related to the inputs from the people.

I think it might be very important to have a comparison, not of what is
presently going on, but of the long run: how stable will the different types of
programs be? In our countries, when the government changes, there are often
new priorities. Currently, nutrition, of course, is one of the top priorities
because it has appeal, because it has money, because there is a sort of international awareness. But I think we have to be careful to look out for the
future and to see how much of these things is going to last as definitive progress.

Latham

We should note, however, that Florentino has been very modest in what he
has said. When he first began in the Cebu Institute of Medicine, everybody
was struck by his ability to generate from the community a desire for something to be done about their problems. And it was he who, at the stage when
the Philippines *wasn't* under martial law, was able to get 10-unit and 20-
family groups organized and looking at their own problems. It is very interesting that, under the martial law government, they are getting this same local
organization of a sort that is not unlike that in China. Yet, the two countries
have very different political philosophies. This is working to Florentino's
advantage, as far as nutrition is concerned, in that he can get the organization
of local interest so that much of the work is being done right now at the local
level.

The same comments that John made about Indonesia apply here: there is
an attempt at land reform in the Philippines, but there are major problems
with overall production of food. Also, the relationship of this to Florentino's
grass roots programs is uncertain. I think there *is* now support from the top
that didn't exist three or four years ago, but also there is enthusiasm coming
from the bottom. This is largely a program down at the local level, though,
again, it is within a system where, if the local mayor doesn't improve the
nutrition of the people, he is no longer going to be the local mayor. That is a
little nearer to China than it is to some other countries. It will be interesting
to see what happens in Tanzania, where an African socialist system is also
developing its organization down at the village, grass roots level.

Solimano

What we are really thinking about is the problem of community participation
and what participation means. From experience, we realize that you can

encourage participation, but it's not real participation if you are too paternalistic. Requiring *real* participation means, often, you may not be able to work
in some areas. Real participation means that the people have to be committed
to a political will. It's very interesting that in both the Panamanian and the
Philippine cases, the responsibilities at the different levels are given to the
political leaders in the communities: the governor, the mayor, and so on.
That is something that also needs to be studied because, just recently, we
thought that the responsible individual had to be a nutritionist or a person
well trained in nutrition. Probably that was false.

Levinson
Michael said yesterday that it would be interesting to hear some dialogue between Florentino and Joe about the applicability of the China model to this
problem. I think it is particularly important, in light of this discussion, to talk
specifically about the efforts to mobilize local decision making. I think,
Giorgio, that the two are not so different: in China this didn't all just suddenly emerge at the bottom; the initiative was taken at the top. As Joe points out
very eloquently in a paper he wrote on China, Chairman Mao's attitude was,
when the people are ready and the local decision makers are ready, they will
pick it up. If they are not ready right now, we will wait until they are.

This may have some relationship to John Mellor's comment that the Indian
community development program, in pure development terms, may not have
accomplished very much but that it had some important political development multipliers simply by getting national and provincial attention paid to
those villages.

Montgomery
As Giorgio mentioned, we have often heard that it takes a strong, central,
authoritarian direction to make these things work. Yet I have conviction,
based on studies in several policy areas, that it *is* possible, in a democratic
state, to bring about effective interventions.

It looks to me, moreover, as though there is a possible sequence demonstrated here which points to the future. It is that you get concern, starting
first at the bureaucratic-technocratic level, which later begins to become
politically interesting. Then comes the political opportunity—which may or
may not require the context of an authoritarian state. Then a program gets
started. The politician says: "Why didn't we do this five years ago or ten
years ago?" You say to him, "Because that wasn't the way politics was five or
ten years ago."

Now, the question is, what happens when it's no longer a martial rule situation? The answer, I think, is already suggested here. What you have been
doing is to build a strong, viable political base. You have identified a target:
two or three or four hundred thousand malnourished children, one to three
years old, or one to five years old, with new children entering the "at risk

group" each year. You are not going to get rid of that problem in five years of martial rule. It is going to last for a generation. You have a viable, visible, long-term target, which no politician, once this has been called to his attention, can ignore. You have developed an institutional infrastructure to perpetuate his concern, not because he is going to lose two points and might get fired by *this* president but because, in the future, sometime, he is going to win votes or lose votes in accordance with his performance.

In other words, the process raises the consciousness of people and builds political infrastructure to support it. I want to emphasize this in contrast to John's negative view of the possibility of doing *anything* unless you have just exactly the right amount of total agriculture productivity *and* a strong national leadership. There are lots of ways you can start, and there are lots of ways you can perpetuate interest. I think this is the pattern that one will see during the periods of transition.

Mellor

First, my "background scenario" is not *"exactly* the right amount of production" but simply enough calories to provide adequate calories for the poor. I see caloric requirements as basic to all else. Second, I want to make it clear that I, in no way, favor the laissez-faire approach to helping nutrition problems. I am inclined to say that we will not have much success unless we have the right kind of basic background, though I have a somewhat open mind on that question. But once you get the right kind of background, I think that there is a great deal to be said for trying to change consumption patterns in the world. I think that a laissez-faire approach, even with the right context, will lead to consumption patterns (using "consumption patterns" in a very broad way) very much like those in the United States. It is not an accident that we in the United States have ended up where we are. Yet, I'm not sure that this is best for human welfare. It seems to me that you could look at what you are trying to do as trying to change national, community, and family consumption patterns. This needs a lot of study.

Also, I would like to see, sometime, a bit of discussion between Florentino and Giorgio as to how far one can go with the Philippines' sort of program, but in the historical Chilean context. It may not be the context that you actually have in the Philippines, but it may not be so different either. In any case, there are a lot of countries that have a context such as that of Chile. I'm curious whether Giorgio thinks Chile made a substantial effort within that context to reach the poor or not and whether he thinks the types of things being done in the Philippines will really catch the lower third, second, and first deciles of income distribution. I think this is an important question.

10 TANZANIA: NUTRITION AND GOVERNMENT POLICY—SOCIALISM AS A SOLUTION

T. N. Maletnlema

T. N. Maletnlema was born in Tanzania and educated at Tabora Secondary School there. He graduated as a medical doctor from Makerere University College, Uganda (1963), and served as a medical officer in Dar es Salaam. Later he was District Medical Officer in Nzega District. Maletnlema joined the Nutrition Unit of the Ministry of Health of Tanzania in 1965 where he served as a Medical Officer, Nutrition. He then studied nutrition in Nigeria and England and, in 1973, obtained a Ph.D. in Nutrition in Pregnancy from London University. In 1974, Tanzania created an institute to plan and coordinate all food and nutrition activities (the Tanzania Food and Nutrition Center) and Maletnlema was appointed the Managing Director. His writings reflect his broad nutritional interests and include publications in both English and Swahili. Maletnlema's paper reflects the thinking not of a political official but of one who is involved on a professional level with nutrition policy in Tanzania, a society whose goals and methods are often poorly understood outside that country.

INTRODUCTION

Malnutrition is a multifaceted, global problem seen in both developing and developed nations of the world. In the developed world, the lowest income groups may suffer from protein and energy deficiencies while *all* income groups may suffer from excessive protein and energy intake.* In short, both high and low income groups may suffer from malnutrition.

Tanzania, as the rest of the developing world, faces similar problems of malnutrition, although the balance is somewhat different. In our circumstances, too many people have too little to eat. The message of Tanzania's socialism is very simple: we should share the food available and avoid excess or deficiency malnutrition. On the international level, this should not be accomplished by transfer of food from, say, America to Tanzania, but by the conduct of trade in a more equitable manner. The implementation of this principle is not easy, but Tanzania is determined to put it to the test.

The ruling party, TANU, and the government of Tanzania share the aim of making all Tanzanians understand that:

• all human beings have the same rights
• all Tanzania citizens should receive all the basic essentials of life (adequate food, water, clothing, shelter, health services, education, and freedom of speech, worship, and work)
• all Tanzanians will recognize their rights and fight for them, given proper enlightenment

BACKGROUND INFORMATION

Political Organization

The political organization of the country is extremely important because it institutionalizes the principle of local initiative and grassroots participation. Tanzania is divided politically into 20 regions; each region is further subdivided into two to four districts. The regions vary greatly in size, but none is larger than 10% or less than 1.5% of the total area of the country. Population density in these regions also varies greatly: from 61 persons per km^2 in Mwanza region to 5 persons per km^2 in Tabora. Under the new decentralization system, each region is an administrative entity with a political head (Regional TANU Secretary) and a functional head (Regional Development Director). These two regional heads have counterparts at the district level. Districts are further subdivided into divisions, subdivisions, and villages. Since TANU

---

*The problem in the United States, for example, is that obesity—a measurement of excess consumption—is *more* prevalent in low income groups than high income groups, although it is quite prevalent in high income groups as well. The relatively infrequent indicators of *inadequate* intake are predominantly confined to low income groups. Thus, low income groups suffer from both *too much* and *too little,* whereas high income groups just suffer from *too much.* —BW

policy is to reach each citizen individually, a further breakdown of the community was instituted in 1968. In this system, households are organized into
groups of ten; these cells are known as TANU Roots. Each cell has a head
elected by all the adults in the ten households. This political structure ensures
a quick and efficient way of contacting groups or even individuals in any
Tanzanian village, town, or city, including Dar es Salaam. We believe that any
effective program must start by getting down to the heads of these small
units. One must meet with them, explain the program to them, and get their
support—otherwise the project will fail.

Demography

Projections from the 1967 census indicate that the total population now
stands at 15 million people in a land area of 919,580 km^2. The population
has exactly doubled in the past 27 years. On the average, national population
density is 15 persons per km^2; but the range is fantastically wide, from a low
of 1 (Nachingwea) to a high of 220 per km^2 (Marangu).[1] The population
pyramid is still very much that of a developing agricultural country with
about half the population under 16 years of age (table 1).
    Due to the difficulty of collecting birth and death rates, it is impossible to
compute these figures accurately. Population growth rates have been worked
out for two different plausible assumptions: one is that the birth rate will fall
steadily and the other is that it will rise gradually. Both scenarios envision a
falling death rate (table 2). From these figures it may be computed that the
rate of natural population increase lies between 2.3% and 3.2% (probably
near 2.7%).

Table 1
Age group distribution, Tanzania, 1957, 1967

Age Group (Years)	1957		1967	
0 - 4	16.7		17.8	
5 - 9	13.0	41.0	14.0	43.7
10 - 14	11.3		11.9	
15 - 19	10.4		10.2	
20 - 24	9.5		8.8	
25 - 29	8.5		7.4	
30 - 34	7.3	50.6	6.3	46.0
35 - 39	6.1		5.3	
40 - 44	5.0		4.4	
45 - 49	3.7		3.6	
50 - 69	8.4		10.3	

Table 2
Crude birth and death rates, Tanzania,
1965-80

Year	Rising Birth Rate		Falling Birth Rate	
	CBR	CDR	CBR	CDR
1965-70	48	22	48	23
1971-75	49	20	44	20
1976-80	50	18	40	17

Life expectancy is about 40 years, but with the extensive immunization
system introduced recently this is likely to rise rapidly. A future decrease is
expected in infant mortality, which now stands at an average of 155 per thousand (but varies greatly by locale from a high of 203 to a low of 93).

Similarly, child mortality averaging 261 per thousand ranges from 151 to
312. In a healthy environment children display the lowest of all age-specific
mortality rates, but in Tanzania child mortality is still very high because of
malnutrition, malaria, respiratory infections, and intestinal parasites. Partly as
a response to this high mortality, total fertility is also high: averaging 6.6
(range 4.3-8.4).

THE NUTRITION PROBLEM IN TANZANIA

There are three main pillars of Tanzania's malnutrition problem. The most
obvious is *poor production* of foods and other commodities including all
agricultural, educational, and medical products. Soil erosion is so severe in
some areas, for instance, that production of food is almost impossible. Food
is often very poorly handled and almost a third gets destroyed by vermin,
insects, and molds. In addition, families in rural areas often have access to
only the one crop that is most frequently grown in their region. For example,
the home may be totally surrounded by banana or cassava plants.

The second factor is *ignorance*. The food which is not spoiled or destroyed
is often inadequately prepared and distributed among family members with
the youngest child at a disadvantage in the shared family pot. Another common detrimental practice is the habit of taking only one or two meals per
day. In addition, in some communities sick persons are treated by the withholding of certain foods, usually the most nutritionally necessary. For example, a baby suffering from diarrhea may be taken off the breast until the
diarrhea has ceased. The result is often marasmus. For years, the ignorance of
parents has been said to be the root cause of malnutrition, but we must reexamine our reasoning. Is the poor mother's ignorance a main factor? What
about the ignorance of the leaders and the elite? Think of the commerciogenic factors leading to malnutrition; think of the example elites hold up for

rural mothers and think of the small amount of government revenue spent on nutrition programs. These, I believe, are the effective "ignorances." In Tanzania, I am glad to say, the ignorance of the leaders is slowly disappearing.

The last important factor in the picture of malnutrition is *disease*, especially measles, tuberculosis, and gastroenteritis.

Poor stamina and resultant poor work output, impaired intrauterine and early childhood growth, impaired mental capacity and frequent illness, are all consequences of the three factors mentioned above.

The Nutritionally Vulnerable Groups

Countrywide nutrition or dietary surveys have not been conducted in Tanzania, mainly because the government could neither afford it financially nor supply adequate staff. This is not a regrettable situation, for large surveys are rarely as useful as they are expensive! Regional surveys conducted in 7 regions of the country indicate various problems of malnutrition (figure 1).

The most outstanding and economically suppressive form of malnutrition is protein energy deficiency (table 3). In the first year, and especially the first

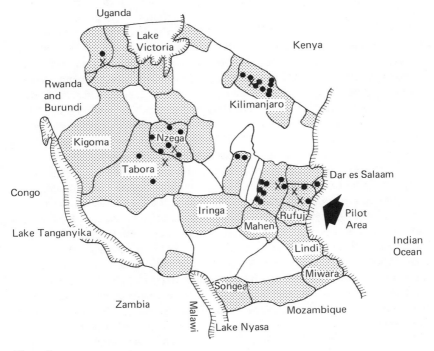

Figure 1
Tanzania map, showing areas studied, 1965-75. x, villages where dietary and nutritional status surveys have been conducted; •, villages where only nutritional status surveys have been conducted. Dotted areas have less than five years' service and staff (nutrition).

Table 3
Childhood malnutrition in Tanzania

Age (Months)	Percent with Protein Energy Deficiency			
	Kisarawe (Coast Region)	Tabora	Hombolo (Dodoma Region)	Karagwe (West Lake Region)
0 - 5	4	0	3.0	5.0
6 - 11	14	10.0	17.0	4.5
12 - 17	41	23.1	56.0	26.3
18 - 23	50	26.2	56.0	25.0
24 - 29	39	9.1	18.0	15.1
30 - 35	46	9.8	10.0	16.0
36 - 47	29	3.5	14.0	9.8
48 - 59	18	0	8.0	5.2

Note: Any child with two low anthropometric measurements (i.e., below 80% of standard for weight/age, height/age, weight/height, arm circumference, or skinfold or head/chest ratio over 1.0 after 6 months of age) plus one clinical sign (i.e., wasting, hair changes, edema, depigmentation, stunting) was taken as malnourished.

six months of life, Tanzanian children grow quite well, on the average. Between six months and one year, however, they often start to grow poorly. Indications are that the problem is mainly that of energy deficiency rather than protein deficiency. Hospitals in the country admit many cases of marasmic kwashiorkor and marasmus, but very few cases of pure kwashiorkor (sugar baby type). Such cases are seen only in banana and cassava staple areas, where, because children are fed only a starchy gruel, there is a very high incidence of severe cases (below 60% of Harvard Standard). Seven percent of the children in one area fell into this third degree classification. I estimate that if one increased intake by about 10% of the present diet, the protein gap would be covered. The energy gap, however, would require a 20-30% increase.

Economically this situation is a great drawback. The colonial rulers' misapprehension that local people were "lazy" was based on this nutritional problem, although they did not realize it. Three energy expenditure studies indicate an increase of work output with increased energy intake and a decreased output with decreased intake. Communities reputed to be lazy were found, in most cases, to be consuming much less than 8.0 MJ per capita per day (approx. 2,000 kcal). For example, the mean per capita consumption in one district was found to be 5.8 ± 1.5 MJ (1,400 ± 360 kcal) per day, which implies an intake of less than 50% of the daily requirement by some members of the community (about 16% of the population, assuming a normal distribution of intake). On the other hand, Tanzania's hardworking communities take in well over 8.0 MJ per person per day. One area had a mean intake of 10.4 ± 1.8 MJ (2,500 ± 192 kcal) per day. Distributed normally, this means hardly anyone with less than 8.0 MJ consumption and only 2.3% of the community with less than 8.8 MJ intake per day.

Studies on pregnant and lactating mothers[2] indicate that 10-25% of these mothers take only 50-75% of their daily energy requirements. As a result the percentage of small-for-gestational-age neonates is as high as 5% in some parts of Tanzania. The next most severely affected group includes primary-school children, who often go without breakfast and lunch except where school meals have been started. Another small group affected by protein energy deficiency is that of old persons, especially those living alone.

Other widespread malnutrition problems in Tanzania calling for strong action include anemia, avitaminosis A, goiter, and fluorosis. All these combined, however, do not cause as much morbidity, mortality, and economic depression as protein energy deficiency alone.

Risk Factors and Their Contribution to Malnutrition

Age determines one's ability to utilize available foods. The ability to obtain food may sometimes depend on one's physique. Chewing and the capacity of one's stomach determines how much one can take at a time.

In Tanzania, infants are lucky that most mothers, especially those in rural Tanzania, still practice breast feeding (table 4). In towns, artificial feeding plays a major role in the causation of early malnutrition. During later childhood and adulthood, food availability becomes more favorable, and, except for avitaminosis and mineral deficiencies, adults generally do not suffer from severe malnutrition. In certain areas with poor staple diets, however, the stresses of pregnancy and lactation often push mothers into clinical malnutrition.

Table 4
Breast feeding in rural Tanzania

Age (Months)		Karagwe	Tabora	Kisarawe	Kilimanjaro	Morogoro
0-6	No. examined	40	44	45	77	108
	No. breast fed	39	43	45	77	101
	% breast fed	97.5	98	100	100	93
7-12	No. examined	44	69	72	104	121
	No. breast fed	43	66	71	95	109
	% breast fed	98	96	99	91	90
13-24	No. examined	70	79	58	171	222
	No. breast fed	68	45	45	114	141
	% breast fed	87	57	78	67	63
25-48	No. examined	—	—	—	331	281
	No. breast fed	—	—	—	43	30
	% breast fed	—	—	—	13	11

Poverty presents itself like the problem of the chicken and the egg, with
low income, low education, and poor food availability following each other
cyclically. Taking poverty as a conglomeration of all these factors, it can be
said to coexist with malnutrition in over 90% of the cases. It has been calculated that T Sh2,000-4,000 per year* is the minimum income required by a
Tanzanian household to maintain satisfactory nutritional status. It can be
seen in figure 2 that over 70% of all Tanzanians spend less than their minimum requirement.

HEALTH SERVICES IN RELATION TO AT-RISK GROUPS

Organization of Personnel and Services

Although the number of fully qualified Tanzanian doctors is still low (603, or
1:25,000), the heavy burden of maintaining a comprehensive medical service
is not left to these doctors alone. Tanzanian physicians are aided by the presence of volunteer doctors from various friendly countries. Assisting the doctors, and often replacing them in rendering medical services, are 14 other
types of medical personnel ranging from Assistant Medical Officers to Rural
Medical Aides and from the community nurses to rural Maternal and Child
Health Aides, and, right at the bottom, the 10-house cell leader who is sometimes used in distributing prophylactic drugs. Although doctors from other
countries argue that a medical assistant cannot replace a doctor, we have been
quite successful in using these lower level workers instead of highly trained
doctors. In fact, most of the work which is required in the rural areas does
not require the advanced skills of a doctor.

Almost all of the 603 Tanzanian-trained physicians are in the government
services. A small group of 75 are in private practice which is likely to be abol-
ished soon. The next level is the four-year trained and experienced Assistant
Medical Officer, of which there are 163. Some of these take further training
at the university level. The next group are three-year trained Medical Assistants, who now number 485 with a target of 1,200 by 1980. The training of
this cadre had lagged behind for years, but two more schools have been
opened recently and the training has almost doubled. Further down the line
come the two-year trained Rural Medical Aides, who act as "doctor" at the
lowest level, the dispensary. There are at present 706 aides, and the aim is to
train about 2,000 by 1980. New schools for training this group have also been
opened.

Assisting the doctors at all levels are the 4,850 nurses, 1,000 of whom are
"state-registered." Current plans are to train about 2,000 MCH Aides to work
at village level by 1980. In addition, we have the usual range of health personnel, such as public and community health nurses, dentists, pharmacists, labo-

*T Sh1 = US$0.145.

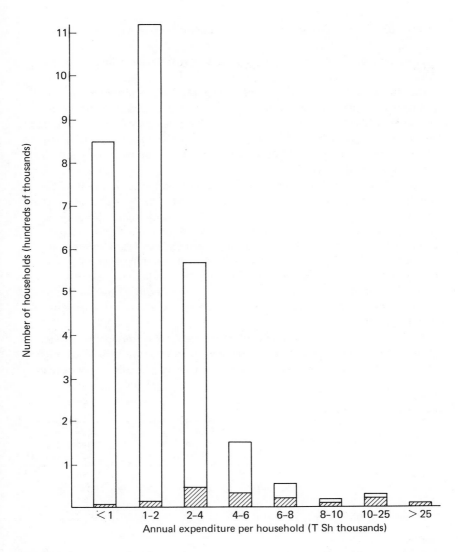

Figure 2
Household expenditures, Tanzania mainland, 1969. Hatching indicates urban households.

ratory specialists, radiologists, laboratory technicians, and hospital administrators.

The health care delivery system is organized strictly according to the administrative system (table 5).

Due to a recent increase of regions and districts, some of the new units do
not have a completed health infrastructure. MCH clinics and medical aide
posts are not, as yet, widely located. The MCH aide courses have just started
in about six regions, but will be held in each region where school buildings are
already under construction. Table 6 shows the health service availability in
different areas of the country.

Since 1972, 60 health centers have been built and the total is now 152
functioning and 7 under construction. By the end of 1976 the total will stand
at 159 or 94,000 people per health center. A strong immunization service
with a central organization has outreach to all medical units down to. the
clinics. Coverage of the child population is variable, but few districts have a
coverage as high as 80% or as low as 20%. Most succeed in covering about
50%. Similarly, prenatal visits and professional deliveries cover only 10-50%
(average 30%) of mothers. With the introduction of both mobile and static
MCH clinics and MCH aides, however, the picture is going to change very
rapidly (figure 3).

Medical plans aim at providing comprehensive medical services to all Tanzanians, but in actual fact the coverage reaches from a low of 50% to a high
of 90% of the population, depending on the district. The utilization of medi-

Table 5
Health services organization, Tanzania

Institute	Number of Institute	Doctors	Medical Assistants and/or RMA	Nurses	Assistant Nurses and MCH Aides, etc.
National hospital	3	20 - 40	10 - 20	50 - 150	50 - 100
Regional hospital	1 in each region (20)	4 - 10	4 - 8	20 - 30	15 - 30
District hospital	1 in each district (over 90)	1	2 - 4	6 - 15	10 - 20
Health centers	2-3 in each district	0	2 - 4	2 - 4	approx. 5
Dispensaries	10-30 in a district, 1-2 in each division	0	1 - 2	1 - 2	approx. 5
MCH clinics (mobile and static)	1 in two or more villages	0	0	2 - 5	approx. 5
Medical aide post	1 in each village	0	0	0	1

Table 6
Distribution of medical facilities, Tanzania, 1972

Region	Population (Thousands)	Population Per Hospital Bed	Population Per Rural Health Center (Thousands)	Population Per Dispensary (Thousands)
Arusha	714	740	143	10
Coast	914	623	457	9
Dodoma	790	1,225	99	8
Iringa	800	825	267	9
Kigoma	504	1,079	168	7
Kilimanjaro	761	732	127	9
Mara	632	1,360	126	9
Morogoro	750	714	125	7
Mbeya	1,141	1,024	228	11
Lindi	499	882	125	8
Mtwara	721	919	120	17
Mwanza	1,209	937	93	11
Ruvuma	448	446	224	7
Shinyanga	1,016	1,868	122	10
Singida	488	823	122	8
Tabora	620	687	125	9
Tanga	806	581	90	7
West Lake	731	559	183	9
Total/Average	13,547	820	137	9

Note: Figures are given to the nearest whole number

cal services by the vulnerable groups has increased greatly, however, because services are now being taken nearer or into the villages.

The Health Budget: 1975/76

The Government of Tanzania allocated US$3.15 per capita for health services and about $0.7 per capita for health services development in 1975/76. For the first time, considerable attention was paid to the development of preventive services (table 7).

DIET, FOOD PRODUCTION, AND AGRICULTURE

So far the agricultural data at hand is very crude and may be misleading if taken individually on a regional basis. Regions differ widely in their ability to produce food and feed their populations (figure 4). Food production data

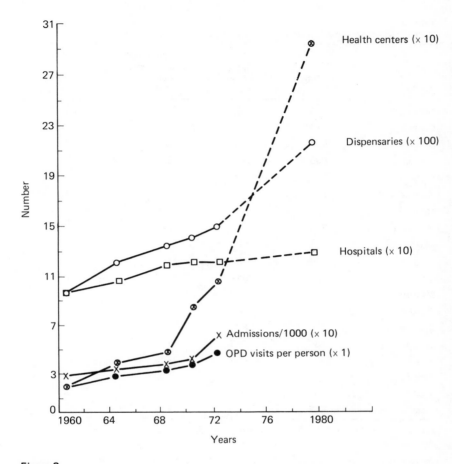

Figure 3
Development of medical services, Tanzania, 1961-80. Source: See ref. 3

Table 7
Distribution of the health budget, Tanzania, 1975

	Percent to be Spent on		
	Manpower Development	Preventive Medicine	Curative Medicine
Development budget US$10,490,756	70	23	7
Recurrent budget US$47,069,733 (incl. administration)	19	7	74

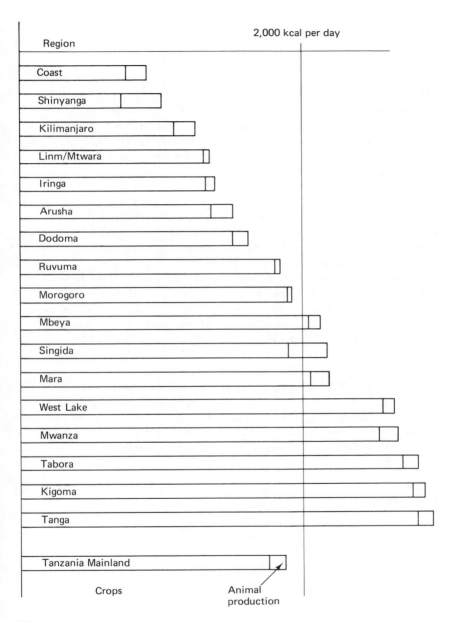

Figure 4
Food production per capita per region, 1970-72.

show only the amount grown within a region but do not indicate how much
was exported or imported.

Diet Patterns

Nutrition and dietary surveys and food balance sheets indicate that, on the
average, Tanzanians consume about 8.0 MJ (2,000 kcal) of energy per day.
This level is shown on figure 4 as the dividing line between areas with adequate production and those with inadequate production. A rough extrapola-
tion of food intake for the whole country can be constructed from a combination of several surveys (table 8).

Crops Cereals are by far the most prominent food items. These include
maize (*Zea mays*), rice (*Oryza sativa*), millets (*Pennisetum typhoides, Eleu-
sine coracana*), sorghum (*Sorghum spp.*), wheat (*Triticum spp.*) and barley
(*Hordeum vulgare*). Due to the large amounts consumed, cereals are a very
important source of energy as well as proteins.
   A second important source of protein are the legumes: varieties of beans
(*Phaseolus vulgaris, lablab niger*, etc.), peas (*Vigna spp., Cicer arietinum,
Pisum sativum, Cajanus cajan*, etc.), lentils (*Lens spp.*) and cashew nuts (*Ana-
cardium occidentale*), coconuts (*Cocos nucifera*), bambara nuts (*Voandzea
subterranean*), peanut (*Archis hypogaea*) and oyster nut (*Telfairia occi-
dentalis*). The production of soya (*Glycine max*), once an important export
crop, has declined; however, combined efforts to increase productivity over
the last 5 years by the Ministry of Agriculture, UNICEF, and FAO may be
succeeding, for the crop is just beginning to increase. This time the crop is not
intended for export, but rather for internal consumption through an oil-pressing plant and full-fat soya flour production. Efforts are also being made to
retrieve edible cake as a byproduct of the oil-pressing process. The oil-pressing

Table 8
Food intake in Tanzania (interpretation
of 5 regional surveys)

	Amount (Per Capita Per Day)
Energy	6 - 10.5 MJ
Ref. protein	24 - 35 g
Calcium	very low (310 mg)
Iron	adequate (16 mg)
Vit. A	very low (220 µg of retinol)
Vit. C	adequate (55 mg)
Thiamine	low (1.0 mg)
Iodine	low
Fluorine	low/high

plant is designed to handle various oil seeds such as sunflower (*Helianthus annuus*) and simsim (*Sesamum indicum*). In fact, cotton seed (*Gossypium spp.*) is already extensively used for oil extraction, but processing of the cotton seed press-cake into an edible form is still too expensive and difficult.

Tanzanian starchy roots and fruits include two very widely eaten crops: bananas (*Musa sapientum* and *Musa paradisiaca*) and cassava (*Manihot esculenta* and *Manihot utilissima*), which form staple dishes for several ethnic groups. Cassava is grown widely, especially in the drier parts of the country. These two crops are very important in determining the nutritional status of Tanzanians. Because of their low protein content, their consumption is often closely associated with childhood and sometimes maternal protein deficiency diseases.

Other common crops in the starchy tuber group include: round potatoes (*Solanum tuberosum*), sweet potatoes (*Ipomoea batatas*), and yams (*Dioscorea spp.*). Except for bananas and some species of yams the leaves of all these plants make popular side dish vegetables. Tanzania also produces a considerable quantity of sugar, which is consumed locally.

The common tropical, and some Mediterranean, fruits are often seen in farms and markets: citrus fruits (*Citrus sinensis, Citrus limon, Citrus aurantifolia*, etc.), pawpaw (*Carica papaya*), pineapple (*Ananas comosus*), mango (*Mangifera indica*), guava (*Psidium guajava*), avocado pear (*Persea gratissima*), apricots and plums (*Prunus spp.*), as well as the wine grapes of Dodoma (*Vitis spp.*), granadila (*Passiflora spp.*) and apples (*Malus spp.*) are available.

The most important cash crops according to the revenue obtained annually are shown in table 9.

Animal Products   Animal products are also common in Tanzanian diets. Beef is especially popular and is also an important export product, earning T Sh42 million in 1972. Milk, milk products, poultry, eggs, and fish are also common,

Table 9
Cash crops, Tanzania

Crop	Annual Growth of Production 1965-72	1972 Value of Production (T Sh × 10⁶)
Cotton	2.1%	417
Coffee	2.1%	364
Cashew nuts	7.6%	184
Sisal	−3.2%	149
Tobacco	20.5%	97
Tea	10.0%	76
Pyrethrum	−6.5%	22

Source: IBRD Report No. 541a-TA

but expensive. The consumption of milk and milk products far exceeds production, so Tanzania imports considerable quantities of these foods.

Production and Marketing of Food

Rainfall Water is a major economic factor in an agriculture-dependent country. In Tanzania, irrigation systems are just being developed, and, therefore, rainfall is the only water supply for agricultural use (table 10). During the two years 1973-74 the total rainfall was low, resulting in poor crops and food shortages.

   Although Tanzanians did not starve to death as a result of this drought, the government spent a lot of foreign reserves to import foods from other countries and a further T Sh16 million to start irrigation projects.

Food Storage and Food Loss Food wastage through poor storage is a great problem in Tanzania. Crude agricultural studies indicate that on the whole almost a third (30%) of the harvested food is wasted, but some foods are more affected than others. For example, legumes stored in local houses lose between 30 to 50% in weight. Cereals, under the same conditions, suffer highly variable losses, from 15-80% per weight from one harvest to the next planting season (9 months to 1 year). Occasionally, crops must be stored where there is no shelter at all, and then they rot completely in a short time. Some losses also occur because of deficiencies in transport to market, which must often be done entirely by hand. The commonly eaten maize flour suffers a 10-40% loss in refining. A further quantity is lost in cooking (ugali

Table 10
Land use and rainfall in selected regions

| Region | Land in Use (%) | | Area with Adequate Rainfall (Over 750mm/yr, %) |
	Medium to High Fertility	Low to Medium Fertility	
Arusha	7	10	3
Dodoma	10	15	2
Iringa	29	21	54
Kigoma	5	27	41
Kilimanjaro	13	18	24
Morogoro	20	33	61
Mtwara	3	34	5
Ruvuma	17	14	66
Tabora	—	21	3
Tanga	11	34	30
West Lake	—	56	44

crust), estimated at 10-15%. So, if we also include storage and transport losses, we find that the food eventually reaching the table is from a shocking
10%, to at best 60%, of the harvested maize!

A number of projects are now being initiated to study and improve local
food storage techniques (table 11).

Land Tenure   Land is owned in Tanzania on a community basis rather than
by individuals. There remain only a few individual farmers on large farms, and
eventually all such farms will be owned by government organizations, cooperatives, or Ujamaa villages. This system works strongly in favor of the at-risk
groups.

Price Control   A price control commission is at work to control price changes
all over the country. The regulations are often quite strong, but the country is
large, and demand and price sometimes get out of the commission's control.
Occasionally, one can find food in the black market at illegal prices. Luxuries
have gone up in price fantastically: four to five times what they were two to
three years ago. The prices of the essential items, like food and clothes, have
risen much less. I believe that the government has had more success with
clothing than with food, where the prices have really been controlled by the
inflation that is taking place all over the world. The current general policy is
to increase prices of luxury goods and lower the prices of essential goods like
food and clothes.

Table 11
Harvested and marketed production, Tanzania, 1972

Food	Harvested Production (Thousands of Tons)	Marketed Production	
		Thousands of Tons	Percent
Maize	881	227	26
Millets	128	56	44
Sorghum	191	38	20
Wheat	98	62	63
Rice	171	72	42
Beans (all)	153	46	30
Cassava	793	181	23
Round potatoes	113	52	46
Sweet potatoes	234	92	39
Groundnuts	29	5	17
Sesame	9	6	75
Castor seed	17	13	76
Bananas	1,206	229	19

Use of New Techniques Tanzania is fairly quick in adopting new techniques and tools, provided they aid in development geared toward the people of Tanzania. In choosing what to adopt, it is our experience that many emerging techniques are not applicable to our circumstances. New technology must be suited to the rural areas for the obvious reason that about 85% of our population lives there.

To assist in developing new techniques for our needs, Tanzania has created a large Small Industries Development Organization (SIDO) for the purpose of encouraging small-scale or cottage industries. Several other organizations have been created to deal with new technology, new equipment, foods, and chemicals, including drugs.

OTHER FACTORS AFFECTING NUTRITION

Income Distribution

As in many developing countries, there is a wide gap between rural and urban income. Rough estimates put rural worker's income at T Sh400 (about US $57) of which up to three-quarters is derived from agriculture and one-quarter as cash from wage labor. Urban dwellers, on the other hand, earn three to four times as much (i.e., T Sh1,200 to 1,600 annually).

For the past ten years, and even more so in the last five, the government's egalitarian policy has tended to freeze urban income and increase rural income potentials. The low income group's salaries in towns have also been raised considerably. Almost all fringe benefits for high salary earners have been pruned, and opportunities for earning more than one salary or owning shares in private companies have all disappeared. These measures have narrowed the gap between high and low socioeconomic groups. Although rural income has not changed remarkably, the provision and utilization of social services has increased considerably. One could go further and say that the rural sector is now ready for development. This year's agricultural crop may indicate a trend to be expected in the coming years: food crop production is improving. Cereal production increased by about 35% as compared to 1972.

Primary Education System

The Tanzanian government's goal is universal primary education before 1980. At the moment, the program proceeds slowly because of lack of teachers. A system has been designed, however, to use the higher primary school students as teachers for part of the day: in the morning, they attend classes; in the afternoon, they become teachers for the lower primary classes!

Coupled with this difficult task, but equally essential, is adult education originally aimed at 100% literacy by 1976. It may sound impossible to educate all adults, but if one thinks of all the other aspects of Tanzania's development formula, the picture becomes clearer. For example, people in Ujamaa villages can arrange their hours for working, resting, and literacy classes to cover every individual in the village. Similarly, literacy classes can be organized through the 10-house cell leaders who are in contact with every person in the cell.

GOVERNMENT ACTIVITY AFFECTING THE NUTRITION OF THE PEOPLE

Background

The problem of malnutrition has been recognized in Tanzania for a considerable time. First, in 1910 medical officers of the German colonial government reported extensive incidence of malnutrition and suggested ways of combating the malady. The Germans' stay in Tanzania was short, and the British colonial rulers who took over encountered the problem while using Africans in World War II and, later, on their farms. Action, in the form of government laws or campaigns, was initiated to improve food intake among laborers, prisoners, and, to a much lesser extent, schoolchildren and hospital patients. The aim of these efforts was to increase labor output in settler farms and other government projects. The most vulnerable group, mothers and children, remained basically untouched until well after independence. Although little was done in the way of programs before independence, the colonial rulers left a functioning Nutrition Unit (started in 1947) attached to the Ministry of Health. This unit has been the nucleus of nutrition activity development up to the present time.

It requires both effort and zeal for leaders to get down to the people and make a community diagnosis of malnutrition. Then, it requires even more skill to talk to a community or nation about the problem. Well-prepared analyses and possible solutions to the problem must be presented in order to avoid the risk of confusing the masses. Tanzania is fortunate to have a president who takes immense trouble to get at the root of community problems and, from his speeches, it appears that he is our best nutrition teacher. Through the TANU policies, many nutrition interventions, suggested repeatedly for years but not attempted, can now be applied effectively.

General Government Activity Which Affects Nutrition

National Five-Year Plans   Tanzania is now putting final touches on her third Five-Year Plan and, in each of the three, nutrition has been given very high priority. In the second Five-Year Plan, for instance, medical nutrition programs (including maternal and child health services) were given top priority and this service is now expanding widely. In the current plan, efforts are being made to include the formation of the nutrition institute and its many projects, as well as primary appendages of a nutrition policy.

Mass Education Several nutrition-related campaigns have been organized and executed fairly successfully in the last five years. Except the recent anti-famine campaign *Kilimo cha Kufa na Kupona* ("Life and Death Farming"), organized and run by TANU, all the other campaigns were organized by our Adult Education Institute which also produces a number of books and pamphlets for literacy classes. A nutrition campaign designed to reach about 3 million adults through the radio and special books is currently underway, supported by government policy through rural activities.

The radio, the press, and group teaching in large political meetings or in small groups are commonly used in teaching the masses. Some problems do arise, however: first, it is difficult to control and harmonize the methods of teaching, let alone the content of the lessons. In nutrition, this problem creates lots of confusion as the number of "experts" and community advisers increases. The second problem is evaluation of the various methods used in teaching. Almost no progress has been made on this front.

The *Literacy Campaign* is a pioneering multipurpose project aimed at enabling illiterate adults to read and, hence, educate themselves for development. About five million adults, all over Tanzania, have sat for literacy examination—i.e., have been tested in reading, writing, and arithmetic. In order to use the literacy acquired, the Adult Education Institute conducts several correspondence and evening courses for adults who are already literate. Educational books and pamphlets are also produced on various subjects relevant to development. Nutrition education books for literacy classes have also been produced in large numbers.

Agricultural Extension Agricultural extension is a well-known and well-accepted project, but recent investigations revealed a need for more specific emphasis on food crops. In the past, training of extension officers tended to be specific for cash crops (cotton, sisal, coffee, tobacco, tea, etc.) and general for all the other crops. Agricultural extension officers with good training were actually cash crop extension officers. These people were taught very carefully how to grow coffee, cotton, sisal, and so on, and were sent out to the rural areas to teach farmers. The rest were inferior types of extension officers, left to do *everything* else. They were masters of nothing, and often they did almost nothing. Essentially no attention was paid to food crops at all, a ridiculous situation in an agricultural country like Tanzania. This situation continued until 1972, when we got into trouble—quite serious trouble—because the country almost went into a state of famine.

Our Ministry of Agriculture is now training agriculture (nutrition) extension staff to concentrate on food crops, with specificity according to region served. The extension officer is expected to link his activities with a counterpart on the medical side. In this way more and better food will be produced and, I hope, *utilized.*

Health Services   For many years doctors have been concerned and have spent large sums of money in treating protein energy deficiency cases in hospitals. This was rightly called a "malnutrition program," because we were actually dealing with malnutrition *cases* alone, a mistake because in treating cases already *in* hospitals, you attain no lasting success whatsoever. In fact, in some of the areas, instead of a decrease, there may have been actual increases in the number of cases, especially after the project ended. In any event, the people lost faith in the hospital services mainly because the children who went back either died in the village or came back to the hospital again and again. In other words, our work in the hospital had not been of help at all.

In 1965, the Ministry of Health Nutrition Unit, after conducting a nutritional status survey in one district, came to the conclusion that in that area alone, there were over 2,000 clinical cases of protein energy deficiency requiring hospital admission. Mobile teams were set up to conduct child welfare clinics in every subdivision and transfer all severely ill children to hospital. In the following year 695 PED cases were admitted and many more milder cases treated in mobile clinics.

Eventually, it became obvious that the problem was not that of children alone: mothers were also affected. In 1970-71 a detailed study of pregnant and lactating mothers was carried out in the same district and from the results obtained and other reports, the need for a unified MCH nutrition service became clear. In the meantime, mobile clinics had become popular and established in almost half of the country. The Ministry of Health staff are now setting up a more comprehensive MCH service headed in each district by one community nurse (Medical Extension Officer) supported by other nurses and MCH aides. The whole team is supervised by a doctor, who may also have other duties. In addition to the medical work, the team coordinates activities with agriculture, education, and rural development workers.

Educational System   Integration of nutrition education into schools and teaching institutions is accepted in theory, but not much has been done, because of mistakes either in colonial policy or in our own. A Tanzanian agricultural nutritionist once remarked that many Tanzanian agricultural graduates know the details of feeding animals and poultry right from birth, but they know almost nothing about feeding their own children. One could also contrast the vast knowledge doctors have gathered on the pathology and treatment of kwashiorkor vis-à-vis the ignorance of doctors on the prevention of the disease.

In many developing countries—Tanzania not excepted—"civilization" has often meant the abandonment of local foods and food habits and the use of foreign items. For the majority of Tanzanians this type of "civilization" leads to misuse of money, improper or deficient feeding, and malnutrition. There is, therefore, a need for educating the young Tanzanians on traditional foods and food habits. This is an ambitious project requiring many nutrition teachers and is one of the tasks to be undertaken by the Tanzania Food and Nutrition Center, to be described below.

Government Projects Dealing Specifically With Nutrition

Any government activity leading to better nutrition for a community could be termed a "nutrition project," but a narrower definition of a nutrition project would only include those projects dealing with food production, food utilization, and the cases of malnutrition. This is the present concept in Tanzania, a great improvement over the still narrower definition of nutrition as dealing with the malnutrition cases alone. It is important to note that the further away from actual malnutrition cases a government manages to apply preventive measures the better the results are likely to be. The least effective project is the curative approach of treating malnutrition cases in hospital, although for ethical reasons it cannot be abandoned.

The TFNC   Until recently, in Tanzania, nutrition activities were the concern of almost any group that was interested, be it a national ministry or international voluntary agency. Naturally, there was a problem of coordinating the different agencies and they often came into conflict. Now, the Tanzania Food and Nutrition Center (TFNC) formed by an Act of Parliament in 1973, is the main initiator and coordinator of all nutrition projects carried out by any ministry, government agency, or voluntary organization. TFNC is a semi-autonomous agency controlled by a board of directors and chaired by the minister of health, its link to the cabinet. The center is organized under a general director, who may be an agriculturist or a medical person, under whom come the specialist directors of the departments of (1) Planning, (2) Manpower Development, (3) Medical Nutrition, and (4) Food Science and Technology. Projects planned for the next five years deal with the following broad areas:

- administration and planning of the center food and nutrition projects
- training, including a new nutrition school
- food development and standards control
- agromedical extension work

At the moment TFNC is faced with very serious difficulty in recruiting staff, as only a few Tanzanians have adequate training in the necessary fields. The major nutrition projects of the center will be described in the following sections.

Schools of Food Science and Nutrition   Two schools under the Ministry of Agriculture give training in agriculture, food science, and nutrition for two years, ending with a certificate. Nutrition constitutes 50% of the training, and agriculture the other 50%. An equivalent school on the medical side will train general nurses in nutrition, maternal and child care, and public health. Although planned, this school has not yet opened. Graduates of these schools will be responsible for running the agromedical extension project. The TFNC and the University of Dar es Salaam are, in addition, planning to start training for diploma and/or degree in Food Science and Applied Nutrition.

Nutrition Campaign A Nutrition Campaign is underway, designed to teach 3 million adults to recognize the problem of malnutrition and practice some of the possible solutions. Campaign arrangements were started over two years ago, and a national coordinating committee was formed. This committee carried out the training and equipment of personnel, as follows:

a   All regional heads (i.e., health, education, adult education, the organization of women, cooperatives, religious groups) were assembled in seminars and briefed on the problem of malnutrition, possible solutions, and the procedures of the campaign. After discussion and distribution of literature, the participants were instructed to return to their regions and conduct district seminars.

b   All district heads were briefed and instructed to call all their divisional heads to similar seminars. At all regional and district seminars at least one national institute member attended to answer questions and give advice. At this point, the main problem was getting the top leaders to participate. In most cases they participated only part-time or through representatives.

c   About 700 divisional seminars took place throughout the country between March and April 1975. This was far too many for national institute participation in each one. Instead, the radio, the press, and pamphlets were utilized and sample areas were visited.

d   The final seminars were held in the villages of each division followed immediately by the formation of discussion groups of not more than 25 adults. A total of 120,000 groups were formed throughout the country. Each adult is provided with a simply written book on the subject and once every week, as the groups meet, a lesson is read on the radio and discussed by experts for 15 minutes. After the radio session, group members reread the lesson in their books. Each lesson ends with questions and suggestions for action. Members of each group, directed by their leader, discuss the subject and decide on what to do in their own homes or villages. If assistance is required, there is a chance for requests to the central government level. Special evaluation teams have been set up centrally and in the regions to record the effect of the campaign.

Agriculture Campaign Following the recent widespread drought, Tanzania was pushed to the brink of famine, but, thanks to the rural development system adopted by the government, no one died. To save life, the government spent T Sh1,148 million in two years to buy cereals (maize, wheat, and rice).

At the same time the whole nation was called on for intensive agricultural development at all costs. Vast areas of hitherto uncultivated land were put into production, more fertilizer was used; and best of all, it rained. This year a bumper crop is expected in many parts of the country. The emergency campaign included several other campaigns on irrigation, fertilizer use, and special food crop programs for rice, maize, cassava, millet, and so forth.

Fortification of Salt with Iodine   The government sponsors a project aimed at iodizing all commercial salt. At present, many Tanzanian communities use locally obtained salts, but with the movement of people into Ujamaa villages plus our nutrition teaching, it is hoped that most people will use commercial salt.

Food Distribution   Food distribution has been and still is a major food problem in Tanzania. Not infrequently, food is found rotting at one corner of the country while another is starving. To combat this, the government has set up several organizations to deal with food distribution, especially of maize flour, vegetables and fruits, fish and meat, and sugar according to the specific needs of different populations. Under-five clinics also distribute donated and allocated foods to malnourished children on a small scale. Some primary schools, nurseries, and refugee camps also distribute foods.

New Food Development   This new project aims at making better use of available foods that have received little or no attention. At the moment, four programs are being studied:

a   *Commercialization of millet and sorghum flour.* To date, the crops are used only by the farmers themselves either as food or for beer: any excess produced finds little or no market. As a result, production is gradually falling and millet farmers are changing to the more popular maize. Since millets are more resistant to drought and pests, it is wise to encourage continued planting. Test production of flour has already been started by our national millers.

b   *Soya Bean Production.* For most of the 1960s, Tanzania produced considerable quantities of soya beans for export. Production has fallen, however, and the government is now starting a project to reintroduce soya, not for export, but for local food. The project is already in full swing, and some farmers are already producing the crop. Beans will be used for full-fat soya flour and oil extraction.

c   *Cassava flour utilization.* Cassava flour is an energy food and Tanzanians lack energy. It is highly important that this crop be fully utilized at all times instead of being left for famine emergencies. In addition, creation of a market system for cassavas will help the farmers. Currently, since there are no market channels, all the cassava grown must be eaten on the farm or simply left to rot. Enrichment of cassava flour and/or composite flours is planned. Plain cassava flour has recently been put on sale to the public.

d *Commercial weaning food.* A formula for a new product has already
been developed. We hope to be able to sell it in addition to distributing it
through MCH centers for needy children because, if a food is produced *exclu-sively* for the malnourished, there is a tendency for this food to be rejected
by everyone. The project will depend partly on the soya project and/or a fish
protein concentrate project, already underway. In addition, we are trying to
develop and improve traditional weaning foods.

Oil Extraction From Oil Seeds We are interested in producing edible oil
from oil seeds and at the same time produce a cake that can be used for hu-man consumption. The planning stage of the project is complete and work
should start soon. However, we are finding it difficult to achieve both goals—
oil and cake—at the same time. Available oil seeds include sunflower, sesame,
and groundnuts as well as soya beans. Cotton seeds are already being used.

Nutrition Rehabilitation Unit (NURU) These are training centers which
admit malnourished children and their parents. In these centers, parents re-ceive lessons on nutrition, home economics, agriculture, child care, and family
care. Mothers with malnourished children may be admitted at such centers
for more comprehensive courses after the child is discharged from the hospi-tal. The practice of making NURU a center for malnourished children alone
has been abandoned.

Because of our previous experience with hospital care programs, we now
believe that hospital cases are more the concern of the doctor, while the nu-trition center, at the moment, has very little direct input from this particular
group. When children are discharged from the hospital, we take over. In the
village, the nutrition team works together with the medical people in the
Maternal and Child Health Clinics. These clinics are located right down at the
village level, using very junior personnel.

Day Care Centers At day care centers, young healthy children are cared for
while mothers go to work. While at the center, disease prevention measures
are taken and children are properly fed. This system is planned for every
Ujamaa village.

School Feeding Program Feeding, particularly in primary schools, has been
recommended. Some schools have successfully established a feeding program
while others have not been successful. Quite a number of schools are still
trying to establish such a program. Many of these latter schools depend on
donated foods which are never in constant supply. The aim of the present
project is to establish a standard procedure for school feeding programs.

Food Laws Until recently, the Food and Drug Ordinance of 1947, with
several amendments, was adequate protection because of the low level of

processing and handling of food. Today things have changed partly because the importation of some foods has stopped, and locally manufactured foods are beginning to flood the market, carrying with them all sorts of defects. Labeling is one of the most obvious problems. Some products are not labeled at all, and others bear false or inadequate labels. Proper sealing of bottles and lacquering of tins is another problem facing many manufacturers. An even more serious problem is the use of unknown colors and preservatives in foods. Finally, the introduction of "false foods" (for example, colored and boiled starch sold as tomato puree) or foods with improper nutrient composition pose serious hazards. For these reasons, Tanzania's food law is now being revised. An expert committee recently presented its report to the Ministry of Health. This report is intended for publication towards the end of 1976.

Proposed Solutions Rejected by the Government

1 Donated foods are unacceptable, in principle, as a means of solving the malnutrition problem. We believe in the Chinese saying: "Give a man a fish and you feed him for a day, but teach a man how to fish and you feed him for life." There are, however, times when donated foods are essential: while one is learning the art of fishing, one must eat.

2 Theoretical research on malnutrition, such as its effect on brain development or specialized treatment of PED cases, is rejected as being mainly academic.

3 The introduction of hammer mills in all rural villages to grind a maize and bean mixture was proposed and rejected. This would use a lot of foreign exchange for a recommendation which was based on a casual, small-sample survey and trial.

4 The manufacture by foreign agents within Tanzania of high protein foods for children may not be undertaken now. Several foods have been proposed, such as full-fat soya flour, fish protein concentrate, beef or game flour, DSM, Supro, and high protein biscuits, but all present a problem of high production cost together with lack of local raw materials.

5 Pure nutrition projects were organized and run for several years, but almost none proved successful. As soon as the central unit staff handed the project to the local people, it died off. In the 1960s, techniques of making nutrition projects multipurpose and local from the start were tried and proved successful. This led to the formation of the multipurpose Nutrition Center to coordinate all aspects of nutrition projects.

FACTORS OBSTRUCTING EFFECTIVE ACTION

The biggest obstacle to effective action is ignorance on the part of the educated leaders of a community. The milk bottle is a typical example of a malnutrition problem brought to the world by the educated people and fully supported by most leaders in the world. Once the parliamentarians, the district leaders, the village leaders are educated, however, and know what should be done, the parents in the villages are only too keen to follow. In fact, in Tanzania, the problem today is not convincing people; it is keeping up with the demand in the villages! The second serious problem is lack of funds, which has escalated tremendously in the last few years.

A third factor should be discussed: the role of external experts, advisers, donors, and often foreign government views on how a project in a developing country should proceed. Very frankly, one of the greatest problems a person like myself faces is the sieving out of mountains of advice coming in from all the outside organizations! This is extremely difficult. Just as we talk of one national nutrition organization, we should talk of one international nutrition organization. It would be helpful if the international community could design such a thing. Obviously, this problem touches on a number of intricate political and professional aspects of nutrition, which I am not qualified to tackle.

DISCUSSION (TANZANIA)

Maletnlema

In opening the case study for discussion, let me thank Mr. Mellor for his very
kind remarks about Tanzania. Remember, however, that whenever you hear
that a football game was very good, you can be sure that the players were
sweating!

Winikoff

The country seems to have done quite a remarkable job of political, administrative, and even physical reorganization. Does this affect your ability to
handle nutrition problems?

Maletnlema

We have, in fact, been able to make our population accessible to interventions, including nutrition. In the past, the population in Tanzania, as in many
developing countries, was scattered all over the country, and it was extremely
difficult to reach the people. So, the present government decided to move the
scattered people to planned areas developed into "Ujamaa villages." The
villages are planned as required by villagers and with the advice of district
leaders. Each village has a living area with houses and a farming area with
cultivated and grazing areas.

The government took the very drastic step of actually, physically, moving
people from their traditional homes to these villages. This was an enormous
task. Some people didn't like it; others tried to play tricks to avoid it, but the
government has, in fact, managed to move a very large percentage of the
people. Some areas, like the Dodoma region, are 100% moved to these communal villages.

As you can imagine, looked at theoretically, this is a very good move, and it
has already paid off in the last two years of famine or near famine conditions:
it was then possible to reach almost everybody with a distribution of foods
because regular administrative organizations cover all the villages and each has
a road.

Winikoff

You mentioned that you had managed to educate the leaders on the importance of nutrition. Did you have any political inducements such as were mentioned in the Philippines?

Maletnlema

I can relate a very interesting story about that. We produced a booklet for our
nutrition campaign. The booklet was supposed to be used by the local people.
Its publication happened to coincide with elections, and, when parliament
assembled for the last time before the election, the people who used up a lot
of our books were the parliament members! They felt they had to know the
nutrition campaign inside-out for their own political campaigns. To be successful at all in the elections, they had to speak about nutrition projects to

their constituents because everybody in the country now knew something about the program and was interested. I wasn't even able to supply all the books they needed, because every member wanted several books to distribute in turn, and wanted to show that he was at the forefront of the government's activities!

Sai
Could you explain how you do your regional studies? When they are done in different years, are they done at roughly the same season, as related to food?

Maletnlema
Yes, we try to do them when the people are planting, at the time of greatest shortage of food. We haven't been able to repeat the studies in several seasons, but we know that they are better off during the other seasons. We deliberately pick the worst season.

In some of the remote areas, where there are no buildings to hold a clinic or a nutrition survey, we have to use the home of the 10-cell leader or the village leader. This is a place acceptable to all the people in the area, and they come. We carry out our examination or survey or give out our information right there. Sometimes, the farmers are extremely difficult to contact. If you want to question them on their diet or on their health, you may have to follow them to the fields. Nurses sometimes interview while helping with the harvesting.

Winikoff
After several surveys in Tanzania how would you summarize your main findings? Did you find any difference in the incidence of malnutrition between the various regions of the country and, if so, did you find out why differences occur?

Maletnlema
We do find major differences by region, and sometimes the results surprise us. One group we looked at is in a fairly sophisticated and fairly well-educated area. Their main diet is banana, however, so they do not do too well nutritionally. The Dodoma area is very dry and very often famine-stricken. We thought this would be the worst area, but the diet there is mainly millet and milk, so, they are, in fact, better off. Except for marasmus during actual food shortage, they do not suffer so much, nutritionally speaking.

The area with the lowest rate of malnutrition is one which had been previously surveyed, in 1969. We covered the area completely at that time with a team of nutrition workers, took all the bad cases to the hospital, and treated them. The second survey showed a percentage of severe cases down from 7% to only 1%.

Tabora is a millet area where cattle are raised. Their main diet, especially for children is also millet and milk. Our studies showed this to be the best area. The children deteriorate later on, unfortunately, at school age, when schistosomiasis and malaria begin to affect them. In this area, school-age children are much worse off than the under-fives.

If you look at the mean birthweights, you will find that in some areas they are well below the standard of 3.30 kg. It is particularly important to compare the birthweights of different economic classes. In Dar es Salaam, the higher class group has a mean birthweight of about 3.3 kg. The Dar es Salaam lower class has a mean of about 2.9 kg., similar to the rest of the population outside the city. The Moshi area has an average of 2,500 kcal (10.4 MJ) in food intake and it has a correspondingly higher mean birthweight. The birthweight is also on the higher side in Kisarawe, representing a higher class of mixed diet. In other words, diet alone has a lot to do with birthweight, and, thus, birthweight is one of our indicators of nutritional status.

Montgomery
Is birthweight, then, correlated with daily calorie intake in the area?

Maletnlema
We have correlated it with calories and with protein. There is stronger correlation between the average protein intake and the birthweight than there is between average caloric intake and birthweight, but both have a correlation which is significant.

Antrobus
One small point. I find it surprising that there is such a high percentage of severe malnutrition when "all forms" is only 30%.

Sai
It's not surprising in the context of the diet there. If you look at an area in Ghana which is dependent on cassava, you will get exactly the same figures. The problem is that weight has questionable validity as a major indicator in cassava-staple areas. For some reason, a malnourished child will maintain its weight for a long time, and then suddenly sicken and die. The period between the change of weight and descent into death is quite a short one. Thus, it is not unusual to see very few moderate cases in relation to a lot of bad cases if weight alone has been used as the indicator.

In fact, I am a little worried about the cassava question, and believe it requires real consideration. As with sugar in Jamaica, this is a food which is almost exclusively a source of energy, yet the population in the area of production uses it as a complete food. How, exactly, do you propose to handle this particular cassava flour program so it does not act adversely?

In addition, about ten years ago, when I was in Tanzania, there was a lot of exportation of the non-flour fraction of the milling industries. What has happened to that export?

Maletnlema
The non-flour fraction is used for poultry, within the country, now, and, in

fact, we are importing some. What we produce locally is not enough because we have reduced the production of non-flour residue considerably. The government emphasized that if any individual was interested in eating highly milled flour, he could go ahead and get it somewhere else. The nation, however, could not afford it and would use high extraction flour. We are now using almost 85% extraction flour.

As for your first question, cassava is certainly a problem but it can be a blessing in disguise if used properly by mixing with other foods or enriching. The higher class can certainly afford to eat more.

Montgomery

I'd like to talk about the law governing the food processing industry that is being revised because I think this relates to a more general problem. I remember reading a Pan-American Health Organization report that said that every Latin American country had a law requiring iodization of salt, but, in nearly every Latin American country, most of the salt that was available in the markets was *not* iodized. The question is really not what you have on the law books but what happens after the law gets passed.

Please forgive me if I go back to my decision-order paradigm, but, using that scheme, the first-order decision is the law, and the second-order decision is how you organize and oversee the enforcement, and the third-order decision, the most important, is how you make it worthwhile to the food processors to comply. Is there a way of developing a constituency for these interventions in the food processing industry?

I gather, in Tanzania, the producers are very small and are scattered throughout the country. Is there some way that you can standardize the responsibility for enforcement without going to complicated bureaucratic structures? In other words, it may be that it is not that the *law* needs changing in Tanzania, but you may have to change the whole system by which the processing of food is tied in to the consumer demands.

Maletnlema

First of all, note that industry in Tanzania is almost entirely in the hands of the government.

Montgomery

Which doesn't entirely protect the people.

Maletnlema

It does to some extent, but at the moment we are failing to meet peoples' demand. In fact, industry requires not only the law but a definition of what is mandated. Most of these industries, except for a few unscrupulous individuals, are quite prepared to comply with changes.

The really bad foods are made by individual vendors, not true manufacturers, but people who literally produce food in their kitchens and bring it into the market because there is a demand for it. Unfortunately, government industry, either due to lack of knowledge or technology, has not entered the market sufficiently to produce some of these popular foods. Right now, this is true of tomato products. But machinery is coming in for manufacture of almost all of these items which, I hope, will eventually mean better nutrition.

Solon

I find it very timely that Lema's paper dealt with the teaching curriculum. Concern for training curricula should be a component of any nutrition program because we will continue to have nutrition problems in the future if we don't do something about the training of teachers, midwives, nurses, and doctors.

In the Philippines, we have created an expert committee on curriculum for the midwifery and nursing schools. I think we should stress that the way to solve our future problems is with new graduates so that we will not be spending so much money on in-service training or pre-service training. Employees will be conversant beforehand with the nutrition program.

Second, I suggest that it is better that we address ourselves to the youth. We will have continuous problems if the parents of tomorrow are not educated today. We have something like 5 million youth in the Philippines, and we must reach them now, in a fashion so that two things can happen: (1) give them knowledge and information, and, having that, (2) the spill-over will be service. They will want to help once they understand the problem, and you must have a ready package of tasks for the energy of these young people.

Wray

In addition, the serious need for biologically sound, but locally appropriate, nutrition education for all reponsible people out at the village level has been apparent for a long, long time. We have known that teachers should be better educated; we have known that the midwives should be better educated; we have known that we should be teaching children appropriately.

What can be done at the international level, if anything? Dedicated people have written very sound textbooks that incorporate the basic principles. It has been there and available for a long, long time, but obviously something is lacking. Does it come back to the local versus foreign input equation? Is it just that you need a core of people on the local scene who have the awareness and who can then take Michael Latham's book or Maurice King's book and translate it into local terms? What can be done to help this process?

Solon

Local publications should be explored, and the rights on books should be relaxed. WHO allows excerpts to be taken from its books as long as it is for the good of the community. It is time international agencies developed a format which could be used according to the needs and the conditions of the community. Doing this locally, in each area, is difficult because every worker is busy, and it requires time even to excerpt sections from a general book into a local book.

Antrobus

That is not where the bottleneck is on this issue in the Caribbean context. The concept that nutrition education is an essential part of teacher training has been accepted there. What has happened, for example, in one particular Caribbean country is that, at the level of the Teachers' College, they say, "Look, it just is not possible for us to fit in an extra two hours or six hours for nutrition because of our already full curriculum." So, the will from above is there, but, when it gets down to the reality of fitting it into the program, it competes with other teaching priorities.

Wray

That, then, is a failure in the education of the leaders of the schools.

Latham

The rigidity of the professionals has always caused very major problems. Looking at the Tanzania health plan now, you see a willingness to use very low level health workers. In the colonial days and the early days of independence, we are told, agricultural work dealt entirely with cash crops. In the educational system, teachers resisted having a good farmer come in to teach the agricultural classes. In addition, doctors, school teachers, and agricultural extension workers were so rigid and so struck with their own professional capability that they felt nobody else could teach them anything or take over any of their teaching. This difficulty is beginning to break down in Tanzania today.

11 NUTRITION AND GOVERNMENT POLICY IN THE UNITED STATES

Kenneth Schlossberg

Kenneth Schlossberg is President of Schlossberg-Cassidy and Associates, Inc., a Washington-based government relations consulting firm specializing in food and nutrition issues. Mr. Schlossberg has lived and worked in Washington for almost two decades as a newspaper reporter of national affairs, as a civil servant evaluating the effectiveness of domestic antipoverty programs, and as the staff director of the US Senate Select Committee on Nutrition and Human Needs for a period of six years. During Schlossberg's tenure with the Senate committee, major reforms were enacted to establish national nutrition programs for families and schoolchildren in the United States.

PROLOGUE

[Editor's note: The ideas in the Prologue were presented during the informal discussions of the United States experience.]

Winikoff

It may seem odd to include a case study of the United States in this context, since the rest of the discussion has referred to developing countries. In a sense, all countries, including the United States, are developing countries. All have to develop institutions and political processes to handle the economic, social, and health problems of their populations, and all must evolve a process of negotiation whereby society can meet the differing needs and balance the varying interests of subgroups within the population. So it is not altogether out of line to include a study of the United States here.

Schlossberg

I have, perhaps, the most unusual assignment of the meeting: to make the domestic nutrition experience of the United States relevant to the problems facing less economically developed countries.

In fact, as I listen to the other case studies, it seems to me that there are many strong substantive comparisons between what has happened in the United States recently and what is taking place in less developed countries today.

In many ways, Ewen Thomson's enumeration of what it takes to implement a national nutrition policy (first, a governmental commitment; second, a policy and program; third, the administrative machinery to put that policy and program across) mirrors what has taken place in the United States and what *is* taking place in many of the other countries. In later discussion we can make more explicit the analogies in the development of a national commitment, the process of translating that into programs and into policies, and then, according to what we have heard, the single most difficult part of building a successful program: translating the commitment and the policies and programs into effective action. That is where success depends on many human beings, all working together, and that is the most difficult part of any government action.

Certainly there are some factors in any success that have nothing to do with various stages of national development, whether you are the most developed country in the world or the least developed country in the world. Personal qualities of energy, initiative, enthusiasm, common sense, and good humor may be the keystone of successful programs in any locale.

As somebody with an interest in the history of the United States, I have always been surprised and disappointed to hear that less economically developed countries find so little of the US experience relevant to their problems. Perhaps I am wrong, but it seems to me that there may be great relevance, not just in terms of what is going on today, but in the *process* the United States went through to arrive at its present stage of development.

If I have understood John Mellor's message, it is that a prerequisite to dealing with less economically developed nations' malnutrition problems must be an aggressive rural and agricultural development program. In the final analysis, if malnutrition is ever to be wiped out, people must work, must grow food if the resource capacity exists to do so, must build a sound agricultural economic base as well as an industrial base. If that is so, surely the United States should serve as an example because, for most of its history, small farmers and agricultural production formed the base of its economy.

When the waves of western European immigrants came to the United States, most of them arrived with the dream of owning a farm. Most of them did end up in rural America, if not as farmers, then as shopkeepers or tradesmen intimately connected with the agricultural economy. Once the nation's industry and cities began to grow, of course, millions of immigrants were drawn into the factories, but the pattern of agricultural and rural development was by then firmly established. Thomas Jefferson fervently believed that the economic, social, and political health of the United States depended upon the agrarian base of small farmers. He was deeply suspicious of the Hamiltonians, who favored industry over agriculture as the primary method by which the United States should develop. The suspicion of cities and industries persists to this day in the rural United States. The conflict between farmers and labor was most recently evidenced by their dispute over the issue of further sales of grain to the Soviet Union.

The historical symbol of the commitment to agricultural and rural development was the Homestead Act enacted in the mid-nineteenth century. The Homestead Act gave millions of Americans the right to settle land and, simply by working it for a period of time, gain legal title to it. Lest you think that this occurred uneventfully and peacefully, let me remind you of the dramatic stories of pitched battles between the small farmers and those big ranchers who were opposed to this piece of land reform.

Even in the United States, many people do not realize the struggles that were involved. They think that change happened without a contest, but social reordering does not take place that way. Frederick Douglass, the great nineteenth century abolitionist, said, "Only fools think that change can take place without the roar of the wind, the crash of waves, and the trembling of the earth." Until the United States became a world power and maintained a large Defense Department, the Department of Agriculture was the largest in the federal government.

Near the end of the nineteenth century, the agricultural sector faced continuous boom and bust cycles. American farmers felt that they were selling their products cheap to the industrial East and being charged dear for industry's products in return. The less economically developed countries, who are engaging in just such a debate with the developed countries today, should find that particular piece of American history quite interesting.

The great crisis of US agriculture in this century, of course, occurred during the Great Depression of the 1930s. That crisis led to an array of formal government efforts such as price supports, subsidized credit, insurance, rural electrification, irrigation projects, housing assistance—all to safeguard the nation's agricultural base. Despite this intensive government effort, the depression and drought in the 1930s broke millions of small farmers, beginning what later became an enormous internal migration from rural to urban areas.

People were fleeing farms, banks were foreclosing, farmers were dumping milk on highways and shooting cattle in troughs rather than sell the products for nothing. The federal government, for the first time, agreed to buy farm surplus products directly. Once it made the commitment to buy those products in order to protect the agricultural sector, it had to do something with them. Given the hardships of the period, the answer was obvious.

If things were bad on the farm, they were worse in the city. Upward of 16 million people were unemployed. Families could not afford to buy food, so the government initiated two basic programs. The first was for families, a distribution of food packages not unlike the packages that have been discussed in other countries. The second was for schools, which received commodities with which, for the first time, to provide lunches for schoolchildren.

This was a critical development, not just in terms of nutrition policy but of social welfare policy in general. Until the 1930s, the federal government in the United States had almost no responsibility whatsoever for the social welfare of the American people. Welfare assistance was a state or local responsibility. In fact, it was often nongovernmental altogether, with voluntary societies caring for the poor or the sick.

The extent of the economic crisis was so severe in the depression, however, that the federal government finally moved into the welfare field. The Social Security System was established as a federal assistance program for children, poor families, the old, the blind, and the disabled. In addition, the first tentative steps were taken towards a federal nutrition program. These steps remained tentative for some years, but as the Chinese proverb says, "A journey of a thousand miles must begin with one step."

World War II did two things to advance the federal government's involvement with nutrition. First, it stimulated the economy, including the agricultural economy, ensuring that there would be continued food surpluses. Following the war, food surpluses assured the continuation of a program to supply commodities to the poor, at that time serving about 2 million families. Second, it provided firm evidence of nutritional need from military physical exams, and thus related that need to national defense.

During the 20-year period after the war, the United States underwent enormous changes, the most significant of which was the growth of general affluence of an unprecedented nature. It is very hard for people to appreciate the radical difference between the United States of today and the United States of just 30 to 35 years ago. At that earlier time, there were probably many

more poor Americans, certainly many less wealthy ones. The difference between poverty and middle class simply did not seem as great. Somehow, general affluence makes isolated poverty appear more severe and less acceptable,
just as general poverty makes isolated affluence appear less acceptable.

A significant factor in this burst of affluence was increased agricultural
productivity as a result of research breakthroughs in the use of seed, fertilizer,
and mechanical harvesting. Output per acre shot up, labor input dropped
down, and one of the results was further acceleration in rural to urban migration, raising unemployment in the cities while leaving many of the old and
the young behind on the farms. The twin problems of concentrated urban
poverty and isolated, but significant, rural poverty were brought into sharp
focus in the 1960s.

In expectation of large budgetary surpluses in the early 1960s, the Kennedy
administration began planning an ambitious national effort to reduce poverty
through programs of community organization, jobs, health centers, and so on.
When Lyndon Johnson succeeded to the presidency, he expanded on this
plan by announcing a grand "War on Poverty" and the creation of a new
federal agency, the Office of Economic Opportunity (OEO), to coordinate
the effort. Initial funding was about $2 billion which was projected to rise to
$4 billion and beyond. Unfortunately, the "War on Poverty" was probably
ill-conceived to begin with: much too ambitious, much too much in conflict
with other agencies of the federal and local government. Finally, it was fatally
undermined by continuing involvement of the country in the Vietnam War,
which soaked up the additional funds the War on Poverty was to receive.

In a way, the OEO is itself an example of failure, demonstrating how any
new bureaucracy attempting to force the rest of the government to do something that it has not been doing will run into resistance and eventually wither.
But it is also an example of success, showing that, if one is willing to engage
in confrontation, that process in itself can result in constructive change on
the part of other agencies.

The publicly stated national commitment to eliminating poverty did bring
forth enormous intellectual effort and involvement by millions of professional and middle class Americans. It was this energizing of a leadership group in
society that eventually led to the identification of insufficient food and malnutrition as a major problem of the poor. The government's previous commitment to provide food to families and schoolchildren, originally based on the
desire to dispose of surpluses, became an opportunity to maintain the momentum of a national commitment to eliminate or alleviate poverty.

The history of this major shift, with food and nutrition programs as leading
tools in fighting poverty in the United States, is detailed in the case study on
the food stamp program. Let me sum up these remarks by saying that the
acceptance of a major food program, a nutrition approach to intervening
against poverty in the United States, is now leading to a renewed and serious
discussion of an even more direct income redistribution approach to solving

that very same problem. The basic point is that, without the precondition of an agricultural base, the productivity of that base, and the general environment that that productivity created, there would not have been *any* initial nutrition commitment by the government in the first place, and there certainly could not have been a *major* commitment in the second place.

BACKGROUND

The US government recognizes a multiplicity of nutrition problems affecting both the minority of its citizens who are poor and the great majority who are either middle class or affluent. The poor, of course, are endangered by malnutrition from insufficient diets, while the middle class and affluent encounter problems of malnutrition from poor food choices or overnutrition from excess consumption. To date, the government is making considerably more progress in dealing with the malnutrition problems of the poor than with the malnutrition/overnutrition problems in all strata of society. This is, in large part, because the intervention on behalf of the poor is significant and direct, while that on behalf of the rest of the population is limited and indirect. There is a consensus regarding the cause of undernutrition among the poor— low incomes resulting in insufficient diets—that leads to agreement on government programs to provide poor families with the ability to purchase adequate diets. There is less consensus regarding the malnutrition problems of the middle and affluent groups in the country, and, therefore, government action is hampered.

The government clearly recognizes that certain groups are especially vulnerable to nutrition problems. These groups include all low income Americans, but particularly minorities such as Indians and migrant workers living in very isolated or difficult conditions. Additionally, special attention is paid to low income pregnant women and their infants, as well as aged citizens.

Certain specific nutritional deficiencies have been identified in these groups. Anemia seems to be widespread among the poor, and a significant number of low income children are apparently low in vitamin A and C intake. There are isolated cases of goiter and protein calorie malnutrition. Among the aged, osteoporosis which may be related to problems of calcium balance and loss of mental acuity associated with a lack of sufficient vitamin B12 are problems. Low income pregnant women often suffer from insufficient levels of folic acid.

For some time it had been argued that the cause of malnutrition among the poor was not insufficient income, but lack of education and knowledge regarding nutrition. Opponents of significant government programs to provide the poor with more food—either directly or by raising income and thus purchasing power—argued that nutrition education was a more appropriate solution. Government studies showed, however, that income levels were the most reliable indicator regarding malnutrition. Education levels generally, and nutrition knowledge in particular, were not an important factor. In fact, some evidence indicated that low income families tended to purchase more nutrition for their dollar than high income families, but where income fell below an adequate level, dietary levels became unsatisfactory.

One cannot deny that poor nutrition education and lack of knowledge are problems in the United States, and proposals are pending to establish national nutrition education programs in the public schools, probably as part of a national program of health education.

During World War II, the government was actively involved in nutrition education, encouraging families to plan meals around seven basic food groups. Posters and booklets were produced and distributed to millions of homes. Since then, however, the government has, more or less, abandoned the field. Most nutrition education is now provided by private industry through advertising in print publications, radio, and television. The heaviest proportion of this advertising is for processed and "fun" foods such as soft drinks and candy. Food products sold more or less as they come from the farm, such as milk, cheese, fruits, or vegetables, are the least advertised. Increasing concern about this trend is leading to increased government interest in public education programs. Compared with commercial advertising, however, the level of interest is still discouragingly low. Individual states, however, sometimes take the lead in these areas, and Massachusetts, for example, has made nutrition education mandatory in its public schools. In addition, certain producers' associations are making a concerted effort to advertise the nutritional value of some traditional foods such as juice and milk. In general, however, educational deficits remain problems of lower priority than incomes insufficient to purchase adequate diets among the poor.

In recent years there has been a major effort by government to eliminate income-related malnutrition among the poor through federal programs. In 1969, federal expenditures in this area amounted to less than $500 million annually. In the fiscal year July 1975/June 1976 spending approached $8 billion. The major change is a tremendous expansion of the food stamp program, as well as a significant increase in the school lunch program. The food stamp program now provides increased purchasing power to 20 million Americans. School lunches are served to 25 million children daily. In addition, a school breakfast program, a special supplemental feeding program for women, infants, and children, and a meals program for poor, elderly citizens have all been instituted.

The problems of the middle and affluent groups are more difficult for the government to tackle. Overnutrition and the attendant problems of dental caries, heart disease, hypertension, obesity, and diabetes affect many more Americans than undernutrition as a result of poverty. Yet appropriate government response is more difficult to devise. There is continuing scientific disagreement as to the exact relationship between diet and disease, for one thing. Proposals that the government issue positive laws or regulations warning against overconsumption of certain foods such as sugar, salt, eggs, and meat, have been rejected. Such proposals have generally been modeled after government rules which require that cigarette packages carry printed health warnings and that televised advertising of cigarettes is prohibited. Instead, the government has issued regulations permitting the disclosure of food contents, such as cholesterol, sugar, and salt, while, at the same time, prohibiting any health claims associated with such disclosures. The major roadblocks to more effective action in this area are lack of scientific concensus and the conflicting interests of industries which would be affected by a more direct approach.

The government aims to ensure nutritional health for the population as a whole by a widespread effort at fortification and enrichment. Bread, rice, milk, salt, cereals, and drinks are enriched with iron, B12, A and D, iodine, thiamine, niacin, riboflavin, and C. This policy is not mandatory at the federal level. However, if manufacturers wish to use standard phrases for advertising—such as "enriched white bread"—certain requirements have been mandated. Some states, individually, do have mandatory fortification laws. In recent years, there has been a trend toward less fortification of basic products such as salt and milk. In the case of salt, the government has responded by requiring positive disclosure of whether it is fortified with iodine or not.

The American consumer is being inundated by new foods. The food industry is both shaping and responding to a lifestyle that values convenience foods. The government does not play a significant role in the development of these foods, but it is attempting to ensure that they fulfill a sensible nutrition role in the national diet. For instance, regulations are being issued to require that imitation fruit drinks approximate, in nutritional value, natural fruit drinks. TV dinners are being required to provide serving portions comparable to home-prepared dinners. Textured vegetable protein products are being required to achieve a nutritional profile comparable to natural meat products, if possible. Concern about chemical additives in processed foods has led to a comprehensive review of additive safety. This is an area of enormous concern to consumer groups in the country, which fear that both individual additives and the total number combined may be connected with the increasing incidence of certain health problems such as allergy and cancer. Recently, and with much publicity, cyclamates were taken off the market because of alleged cancer-causing properties. Both new and old foods now carry fairly comprehensive nutrition and additive labeling on the theory that the consumer needs this information to make intelligent food choices.

On the production side, the United States has, for many years, had an intensive agricultural development program from the federal down to the state and local levels. Billions of dollars are invested annually in research to make farming more efficient and productive. There are special loan, insurance, and price support programs to protect farmers, and there is an extensive system of agricultural colleges throughout the country.

Various nongovernment groups also deal with nutrition issues in the United

States. Among the most prominent are the national organizations of nutritionists, physicians, nurses, and dieticians—for example, the American Institute of Nutrition, the American Medical Association, and the American Dietetic Association. In addition, specialized groups such as the American Academy of Pediatrics or the American College of Obstetricians and Gynecologists play a role in developing nutrition policy. The Academy of Pediatrics, for example, has focused attention on the problem of anemia among both poor and middle class children. This effort, added to other evidence of anemia in the population, led to a government effort to increase the iron fortification of bread. The College of Obstetricians and Gynecologists engaged in extensive research on optimal weight gain in pregnant women generally, while highlighting inadequate weight gain among low income women. Recently, a number of professional organizations constituted an association—The National Nutrition Consortium—to direct government attention toward nutrition problems.

The nutrition-health organizations, in their quest for funds for research, professional training, and education, have been less effective in securing government help than have other groups advocating programs to increase food purchasing power or to provide food directly to the poor and middle class. The American School Food Service Association, representing educators and employees in school feeding programs, is extremely effective at lobbying the government to increase funding for these programs. The food industry, processors, and retailers, represented by the Grocery Manufacturers of America and the National Association of Food Chains, exert pressure on behalf of the Food Stamp Program.

Additionally, until recently, the nutrition-health organizations failed to compete successfully with other health groups for government attention. Medical research funds allocated to diseases, such as heart disease, hypertension, or cancer, did not include specific nutrition components. Health insurance for hospitalization and home visits did not include nutrition counseling or assistance as a covered service. Medical schools, often supported to a significant extent by government funds, did not include nutrition in their curricula.

In fact, however, the single greatest obstacle to creation of national policy in the area of nutrition has been the absence of a clear locus of responsibility within the government for that subject. There is no national nutrition council or committee. Within the executive branch of government, responsibility for nutrition policy exists in both the Department of Agriculture and the Department of Health, Education, and Welfare. Additional responsibility lies in independent agencies such as the Federal Trade Commission and the Federal Communications Commission.

The closest approximation to a national council is the Food and Nutrition Board of the National Academy of Sciences. The academy, situated in Washington, is government-sponsored but also receives private funds for research. Its function is to provide the best scientific judgment on important matters affecting public policy. The Food and Nutrition Board establishes the official Recommended Dietary Allowances for nutrients. These then become the basis for government policy in the area of family and school feeding, as well as consumer policy on nutrition labeling. But the Food and Nutrition Board operates on the fringe of government policy, rather than right in the middle of it at a high level.

In December 1969 there was a White House Conference on Food, Nutrition and Health, at which experts from around the country came together to make suggestions for an improved national policy. The conference recommended the appointment of a Special Assistant to the President for nutrition and the creation of an Office of Nutrition in the Department of Health, Education, and Welfare. Neither recommendation was implemented.

The situation in the legislative branch is slightly better than that in the executive branch. In 1968, the Senate created a Select Committee on Nutrition and Human Needs. While this committee is limited in the sense that it has no direct legislative authority, it has served as a continuing national forum to focus public attention on nutrition problems. It has also prodded other legislative committees into more action than they otherwise would have taken in government food programs, nutrition, and health. In 1974, the Senate committee sponsored a legislative National Nutrition Policy Study Conference, following up on many of the unresolved issues from the 1969 White House conference. There is, however, no counterpart to the Senate committee in the House of Representatives, and this impedes really effective legislative action. Responsibility for the actual legislation which deals with nutrition is, in fact, divided among a half dozen permanent committees of the Congress.

EVIDENCE OF MALNUTRITION IN THE UNITED STATES

Rather than attempt to deal with the entire nutritional situation in the United States, it will be more fruitful to deal with case studies of well-established nutrition interventions whose histories may provide raw material for further analysis. In this context, it will be appropriate to look at the events leading up to the Food Stamp Program and the School Lunch Program.

Need for a Food Stamp Program

More is at stake here than the health and well-being of 16 million American citizens who will be aided by these programs. Something very much like the honor of American democracy is at issue. It was a half century ago that the "fruitful plains" of this bounteous land were first called on to a great work of humanity, that of feeding a Europe exhausted and bleeding from the First World War.

Since then, on one occasion after another, in a succession of acts of true generosity—let those who doubt that find their counterpart in history—America has come to the aid of one starving people after another. But the moment

is at hand to put an end to hunger in America itself for all time. I ask this of a Congress that has already splendidly demonstrated its own disposition to act. It is a moment to act with vigor; it is a moment to be recalled with pride.
—President Richard M. Nixon, Message to the Congress, May 7, 1969

In the space of about 6 years, "Hunger in America" moved from an idea arousing skepticism and doubt to a major national effort to combat its existence. President Nixon's 1969 Message to the Congress was the verbal expression of the turning point in this evolution.

The difficult struggle to bring the problem of hunger and malnutrition among America's poor to national attention began in April 1967, with a hearing by the United States Senate Subcommittee on Employment, Manpower, and Poverty in Jackson, Mississippi. The subcommittee had planned the hearing as part of its routine oversight of government antipoverty programs. To the surprise of the subcommittee members, the major issue presented by witnesses at the hearing was that of hunger among the people living in the Delta area of the state. The day following the hearing, two subcommittee members, Senators Robert F. Kennedy (D-NY) and Joseph S. Clark (D-Penn.) conducted a personal tour of the Delta and were shocked to see the truth of the reports of acute hunger and malnutrition.

The findings were immediately reported to Secretary of Agriculture Orville Freeman who dispatched an investigative team to Mississippi. Within days, Secretary Freeman reported to the Senate subcommittee that the investigative team found "evidence of malnutrition and unmet hunger."

Firm medical evidence also began to accumulate. A team of physicians, under the auspices of the Field Foundation, a private philanthropic organization, publicly reported findings from a field trip to rural Mississippi. Their report titled, "Children in Mississippi" said in part:

In Delta counties we saw children whose nutritional and medical condition we can only describe as shocking—even to a group of physicians whose work involves daily confrontation with disease and suffering. In child after child we saw: evidence of vitamin and mineral deficiencies; serious, untreated skin infections and ulcerations; eye and ear diseases; also unattended bone diseases secondary to poor food intake; the prevalence of bacterial and parasitic disease, as well as severe anemia, with resulting loss of energy and ability to live a normally active life; diseases of the heart and lungs—requiring surgery— which have gone undiagnosed and untreated; epileptic and other neurological disorders; severe kidney ailments, that in other children would warrant immediate hospitalization; and finally, in boys and girls in every county we visited, obvious evidence of severe malnutrition, with injury to the body's tissues—its muscles, bones, and skin as well as an associated psychological state of fatigue, listlessness, and exhaustion.

These medical findings generated skepticism, however, because of the isolated nature of the evidence. This skepticism was reinforced by a report from the Surgeon General that the true extent of malnutrition in the United States was not reliably known and, furthermore, no governmental agency was responsible for assembling such information.

As a result, the Congress in December 1967 enacted PL 90-174 authorizing the Secretary of Health, Education and Welfare to:

. . .make a comprehensive survey of the incidence and location of serious hunger and malnutrition and health problems incident thereto and . . . report his findings and recommendations for dealing with these conditions within 6 months from the date of enactment of this section.

The controversy regarding the actual extent of the hunger problem in America increased considerably during the spring of 1968 with the publication in April of *Hunger—USA*, a thoroughgoing study of the origins and failure of the major government family feeding programs. *Hunger—USA* was produced by the Board of Inquiry into Hunger and Malnutrition, a group of private citizens—lawyers, physicians, nutritionists, social activists—financed in great measure by the nation's large union of auto workers. The study found:

• Hunger and malnutrition exist in the United States, affecting millions of Americans and increasing in severity and extent from year to year.

• Hunger and malnutrition take their toll in the form of infant deaths, organic brain damage, retarded growth and learning rates, increased vulnerability to disease, withdrawal, apathy, alienation, frustration, and violence.

• There is shocking absence of knowledge about the extent and severity of malnutrition—a lack of information and action which stands in marked contrast to our recorded knowledge in other countries.

• Federal efforts aimed at securing adequate nutrition for the needy have failed to reach a significant portion of the poor and to help those they did reach to any substantial or satisfactory degree.

• The failure of federal efforts to feed the poor cannot be divorced from the nation's agricultural policy, the congressional committees that dictate policy, and the Department of Agriculture that implements it. Hunger and malnutrition in a country of abundance must be seen as consequences of a political and economic system that spends billions to remove food from the market, to limit production, to retire land from production, and to guarantee and sustain profits for the producer.

In May, airing of the CBS Television Report "Hunger in America," magnified the impact of malnutrition described in the report while dwarfing the comprehensive analysis contained in the original document itself. What most citizens of the nation had been reading about from time to time in their newspapers was now brought dramatically into their living rooms. The CBS documentary began with the narrator speaking the following lines while the picture on the screen showed a severely malnourished baby:

Hunger is hard to recognize in America. We know it in other places like Asia and Africa. But these children, all of them, are Americans. And all of them are hungry.

Hunger is easy to recognize when it looks like this. This baby is dying of starvation. He was an American. Now he is dead.

The reaction to the documentary was immediate and angry. Agriculture Secretary Freeman wrote CBS that the documentary was grossly inaccurate, attaching a list of particular errors as proof.

The chairman of the House of Representatives' Committee on Agriculture, W. R. Poage (D-Tex.), a conservative, inserted a detailed refutation of the documentary in the *Congressional Record*. Based on an investigation of the documentary by the Agriculture Department as well as a national survey of public health officials, Chairman Poage concluded that ". . . the [CBS] program was deliberately calculated to avoid outright technical misstatements but was intended to convey misunderstandings to the listeners."

Chairman Poage also summed up his own judgment regarding the extent of the hunger problem in the country:

As I see it, the basic premise in each case is political, not factual. It has always been "politics" to talk of "feeding the needy." I believe in feeding the needy. I believe in helping all of those who need help. I believe in providing work for those who want to work, but I don't believe in feeding those who could but won't work. Most of the difference of opinion about "feeding the hungry" seems to actually revolve around the question as to who are unavoidably hungry.

That there is some hunger might be admitted for the sake of argument. That there is rather extensive malnutrition seems to be well established, but that the malnutrition exists because of inability to secure a better balanced diet does not seem to be established, and there seems to be little evidence that any substantial hunger in this country is the result of the refusal of assistance agencies, public and private, to give needed aid to those who are unable to work.

As a result of this heated debate, Senator George McGovern (D-S. Dak.), a liberal, introduced Resolution 281 into the Senate. The resolution called for the Senate to create a Select Committee on Nutrition and Human Needs to investigate thoroughly the issue of hunger and malnutrition among America's poor, to determine its actual extent and causes, to look at the operation of the major federal feeding programs, and to make comprehensive recommendations for solving the problem. The resolution creating the Select Committee was approved by the Senate on July 30, 1968.

The Select Committee began public hearings in December, taking testimony from the nation's leading nutritionists and the Secretaries of the Departments of Agriculture and Health, Education, and Welfare, as well as from the head of health programs for the Office of Economic Opportunity. Then, on January 22, 1969, the Select Committee received the first report from the nutrition survey that the Congress had ordered conducted by the Department of Health, Education, and Welfare in December 1967. The National Nutrition Survey, as the study came to be known, was headed by Dr. Arnold Schaefer, who had conducted similar surveys in many other countries. The initial results of the survey, based on the preliminary statistics from Texas, Louisiana, New York, and Kentucky, were summed up by the Select Committee staff in the following manner:

Dr. Schaefer's report presents preliminary findings on malnutrition among 12,000 individuals living in low income areas in Texas, Louisiana, New York, and Kentucky. The nutritional status of the families and individuals examined was evaluated through clinical and dental examinations, biochemical measurements, and food intake studies.

Discussing the survey's findings Dr. Schaefer reports: "The preliminary data clearly indicate an alarming prevalence of those characteristics that are associated with undernourished groups. Even though these findings come from a small subsample of the total National Nutrition Survey, it is unreasonable in an affluent society to discover such signs as those seen to date."

"In general," Dr. Schaefer states, "the most widespread nutritional problem is one of multiple nutrient deficiency of a combination of one or more nutrients such as protein, vitamins, minerals, and calories. It is important to bear in mind and perhaps shocking to realize that the problems in the poverty groups in the United States seem to be very similar to those we have encountered in the developing countries."

Among the Nutrition Survey's specific findings in that subsample,* Dr. Schaefer cited the following:

Growth Retardation In the sample we have studied thus far, the children between 1 and 3 years of age fall below the average height reported for children in the USA . . . 3.5% of these children have retarded bone growth.

Marasmus and Kwashiorkor To date in our studies we have found 7 cases which the physician diagnoses as severe malnutrition using such terms as kwashiorkor (severe protein and multiple nutrient deficiency) and marasmus, primarily a caloric deficiency. We did not expect to find such cases in the United States.

Anemia One-third of the children under 6 years of age had hemoglobin levels in the unacceptable range . . . The cut-off level for hemoglobin was set at that level considered by physicians to need treatment . . . 15% of the population studied had hemoglobin levels less than acceptable, which means that they are candidates for medical treatment . . . In the impoverished population this problem may actually be on the increase.

Goiter Five percent of the total population examined to date exhibits an enlarged thyroid gland associated with low iodine intake. . . . . In Texas 40% of the local markets failed to even stock iodized salt although there was no price differential.

Dental problems Eighteen percent of all subjects 10 years of age and over reported it was difficult and painful to bite or chew food. Ninety-six percent of the sample had an average of 10 teeth either decayed, filled, or missing, with five of these needing immediate attention . . . only 15 out of each 100 decayed teeth had been filled.

Vitamin A deficiency Thirty-three percent of the population less than 6 years of age were at unacceptable levels. These findings are characteristic of those reported from areas of the world where vitamin A deficiency is a major problem . . . In advanced vitamin A deficiency permanent blindness occurs. We did not find such cases. However, here our concern is the fact that we have such a large proportion, 13% of the entire population studied, that had

*The subsample was drawn from the lowest income quartile of the states based on 1960 census data. The majority of families had annual cash incomes of less than $3,000. Approximately 80% of these families had incomes of less than $5,000.

levels which we consider places them in a high risk category. We do not know how long these people have had these low levels or whether their vitamin intake is now being increased or decreased. We can't afford the risk that any of these persons will develop the severe deficiency.

Vitamin D deficiency Three and seven-tenths percent of the 0 to 6-year-old subjects show evidence of vitamin D deficiency: 18 cases of rickets have been diagnosed . . . The fact that we have discovered cases of rickets again alerts us to the reality that we cannot ignore public health nutrition programs once they have started. This disease was virtually eradicated over 30 years ago through the simple mechanism of fortifying milk with vitamin D at no cost to the consumer.

Discussing the Survey's findings, Dr. Schaefer said, "Our studies to date clearly indicate that there is malnutrition, and in our opinion, it occurs in an unexpectedly large proportion of our sample population." These findings, preliminary as they were, represented the scientific breakthrough necessary to establish beyond doubt the reality of serious and widespread hunger and malnutrition in America.

The Growth of the Food Stamp Program

Due to the aforementioned publicity generated about the hunger issue in early 1969, the Urban Affairs Council, the principal domestic policymaking group of the Nixon Administration, established a food and nutrition committee chaired by the new Secretary of Agriculture, Clifford Hardin. This committee was charged with making an independent review of the hunger issue, and making recommendations for action to the president. On March 17, 1969, the food and nutrition committee completed its task, noting:

There are two Family Food Assistance programs—Food Stamp and Direct Distribution.

A *The Food Stamp Program.* Food stamps provide a bonus for food purchases which varies with the income and family size of the recipient. Current schedules provide an average bonus of $6.90 per person per month in food purchasing power. A family of four with a monthly income under $30 ($360 annual) pays $2 per month and receives $58 in food stamps. At the other end of the schedule, a family with a monthly income of $250 ($3,000 annual) pays $76 and receives $100 in food stamps. Thereafter the monthly bonus for such a family ($24) remains constant up to the eligibility cut-off point, which depends upon State eligibility standards, the highest being $4,140 a year.

Stamp purchases may be made on a monthly, semimonthly, or sometimes, a weekly basis, and participants must be certified as eligible by local welfare agencies. The program is operated by State welfare agencies, while the approval and supervision of participating retailers and wholesalers is done by the Department of Agriculture (USDA). Presently about 1,200 counties operate Food Stamp programs, with about 2.8 million program participants.

B *Direct Distribution Program.* An agency of the State government is responsible for operation of the program within the State, under a Plan of Operation approved by USDA. The State agency orders and accepts shipments of commodities from USDA (usually in carlot quantities) and arranges for their subsequent distribution to local centers operated by the officials of participating areas. Families come to these centers to pick up their monthy allotment of commodities. Staff and facilities must be available at the local level to certify families as eligible for the program by state standards.

USDA is currently offering 22 foods to states for donation to low income families with a value of approximately $13 retail per person per month. The complete package of 22 foods offers adequate amounts of 6 nutrients and less than adequate amounts of energy and vitamin A, compared to the Recommended Dietary Allowances. Few participating counties, however, accept 20 or more foods and many recipients are unwilling to accept some of the foods offered.

The program operates in about 1,400 counties, cities, and territories, as well as on Indian reservations, reaching about 3.7 million individuals. There are 480 counties or independent cities, whose population includes 10% of the US poor, that have no family food assistance program and no present plans to initiate one.

In program areas about one-third of those with incomes below the poverty line receive food assistance. Over 6 million people now receive food stamps or free commodities, among them 40% of the nearly 9 million public assistance recipients.

In the judgment of the committee the Food Stamp Program is preferable to direct distribution. There are, however, a number of flaws in the present Food Stamp Program. Current payment and value schedules are inadequate and appear to discourage participation. The schedule requires payment of up to 47% of income to participate in the program, whereas middle class families pay on the average of 17% of their income for food. The program is therefore inadequate for those whose income is too meager and too erratic to make periodic bloc payments. For those with incomes below the poverty line—over 90% of the participants—the schedule provides stamps insufficient to purchase food for an entire month under minimum USDA criteria. Those in extreme poverty receive stamps which meet only 60% of minimum needs. Finally, State eligibility, requirements, which range from $1,920 to $4,140 for a family of four, are inequitable and have no relation to geographic differentials in food prices.

The food stamp schedule should be revised to provide food incomes sufficient to purchase adequate diets, to permit more of the poor to participate, and to focus government resources on the very poor.

1 The value of stamps issued to all participants should be sufficient to purchase an adequate diet. The recommended standard is the Economy Food Plan, the minimally adequate food budget calculated by the Agricultural Research Service of the Department of Agriculture. . . . This budget varies with age, sex, geographic location and changes in food prices. The current average cost for a family of four with school-age children is $100 per month.
2 The cost of food stamps should be not greater than 30% of income, and should be less than this for the poorest families.
3 A uniform maximum eligibility standard should be used to eliminate inequities between States and to insure that government funds are focused on the very poor.

The president's hunger message closely followed the recommendations of the Food and Nutrition Committee. In speaking of the food assistance programs, the president said that, though these programs have provided welcome and needed assistance, both programs were clearly in need of revision. Furthermore, he proposed revision of the Food Stamp Program in order to:

Provide poor families enough food stamps to purchase a nutritionally complete diet. The Department of Agriculture estimates this to be $100 per month for a typical family of four.

Provide food stamps at no cost to those in the very lowest income brackets.

Provide food stamps to others at a cost of no greater than 30% of income.

Ensure that the Food Stamp Program is complementary to a revised welfare program.

Give the Secretary of Agriculture the authority to operate both the Food Stamp and Direct Distribution programs concurrently in individual counties, at the request and expense of local officials. This will permit the Secretary to assist counties wishing to change from direct distribution to food stamps, and to meet extraordinary or emergency situations.

The requested appropriations will then permit the establishment of the revised program in all current food stamp counties before the end of the fiscal year, as well as a modest expansion into direct distribution counties, and some counties with no current programs.

While our long range goal should be to replace direct food distribution with the revised Food Stamp Program, the District Distribution Program can fill many short range needs. Today there are still over 400 counties without any Family Food Assistance program and this Administration shall establish programs in each of these counties before July 1970.

Shortly thereafter, the administration introduced a Food Stamp Reform bill, which provided for a food stamp allotment at a minimally adequate nutritional level, defined as the Agriculture Department's Economy Diet Plan. The bill authorized expenditures for the program of $315 million for fiscal 1970, $610 million for fiscal 1971, and open-ended authorizations. Senator Herman Talmadge introduced a second bill to leave unchanged the allotment level existing in the program but to authorize $525 million for fiscal 1970 and $900 million for fiscal 1971.

The Food Stamp bills were referred to the Senate Committee on Agriculture and Forestry which held public hearings and developed its own Food Stamp Reform bill in July 1969. This bill set the allotment level at the Economy Diet and authorized $750 million for fiscal 1970, $1.5 billion for fiscal 1971, and $1.5 billion for fiscal 1972. The bill came to the Senate floor for consideration, at which time Senators George McGovern and Jacob Javits offered a substitute bill containing authorizations of $1.25 billion, $2 billion, and $2.5 billion for fiscal 1970, 1971, and 1972, respectively. The substitute bill also contained national eligibility standards, greatly increasing potential participation in the program. The McGovern-Javits substitute was adopted by the Senate. The House of Representatives did not adopt its own bill until December 1970, and a final reform bill did not become law until January 1971.

Part of the president's message had called for a White House Conference on Food, Nutrition, and Health to be convened in December 1969. At that Conference, the administration announced significant changes in the Food Stamp Program that it planned to implement pending the passage of final legislation by the Congress. These changes included a uniform increase in the food stamp allotment, regardless of how poor the family happened to be, and a general reduction in the cost of the stamps to purchasers. The allotment was raised to the Economy Diet level, $106 monthly for a family of four, and the purchase price was reduced to no more than 30% of a family's income. The president subsequently requested a supplemental appropriation of $120 million for fiscal 1970 to cover the increased cost of the program.

Following the announcement of these administrative changes, participation in the Food Stamp Program began rising steadily. Between January and February 1970, participation increased from 3.8 to 4.4 million. By June, participation had risen to 6.5 million. The increase was encouraged by the administration's pledge to bring new counties into the program during this period. Also, during this period, the expenditures of the government in bonus stamps went up from $26,873,101 to $86,493,273 monthly. Total food stamp spending for fiscal year 1970 finally totaled $578 million.

In December 1970, the House enacted its own Food Stamp Reform bill, setting the allotment level at the Economy Diet, providing for open-ended authorizations, and establishing a national eligibility line at the poverty standard. In conference with the Senate, the final bill directed the Secretary of Agriculture to provide a "nutritionally adequate diet" (which he subsequently set at the level of the Economy Food Plan) with a cost of living adjustment, provided for an authorization of $1.75 billion for fiscal 1971 and open-ended authorizations the following 2 fiscal years, and authorized the Secretary of Agriculture to set a uniform national eligibility standard at the poverty level.

By the time the president signed the law in January 1971, participation in the Food Stamp Program had reached 9,727,200 persons, and the monthly bonus expenditures were $129,844,125. By June participation reached $10,567,240, and expenditures were $140,907,077.

In 1973, several additional food stamp amendments were passed, making the program mandatory nationwide and eliminating the commodity distribution program, as well as adding a cost-of-food escalator increasing the food stamp allotment automatically. In 1974, a four-person family was eligible for food stamps if its income fell below $6,480 a year. The benefits for a family with little or no income amounted to over $1,900. In the next two years, under the pressure of recession and inflation, food stamp participation rose to over 19 million persons who received stamps worth over $8.7 billion at an annual cost to the government of approximately $5.3 billion.

The National School Lunch Program

In the early 1940s several surveys furnished statistical evidence of poor child nutrition in America. In Vermont, 85% of children examined showed signs of healed rickets; in a New York City examination, 21% of the high school students in low income families had less than two-thirds of the daily caloric requirements; and in North Carolina, 24% of children examined had swollen gums, accompanied by a low vitamin C level. This was followed by a surprisingly high Selective Service rejection rate during World War II for young men with poor nutrition histories. This situation was very embarrassing, indeed, and the correlation between "adequate nutrition and full production, full production and adequate nutrition" impressed itself on booming postwar America.

Postwar surpluses led in 1946 to a formal institutionalization of the national lunch program. The National School Lunch Act states:

It is hereby declared to be the policy of Congress, as a measure of national security, to safeguard the health and well-being of the Nation's children, and to encourage the domestic consumption of nutritious agricultural commodities and other food, by assisting the States, through grants-in-aid and other means in providing an adequate supply of foods and other facilities for the establishment, maintenance, operation, and expansion of nonprofit school lunch programs.

The act represented a substantial step forward in attempting to deal with the nutritional problems of America's children. An open-ended fund authorization, reinforced by a national policy declaration, theoretically provided sufficient money. An apportionment formula, together with a sliding matching scale, was an attempt to deal with the fact that some states would need more aid than others. A nonfood assistance provision helped needy schools which lacked the equipment required to establish even a small-scale lunch program. Since 38 states had passed laws excluding state aid to private schools, the new federal law brought these schools within the scope of the act so that their students could also receive the benefits of the lunch program. Finally, the Congress attempted to counterbalance any social stigma attached to being poor by banning any lunchroom discrimination between the needy children who were to receive free or reduced-price lunches and their more affluent classmates.

It is important to keep in mind that, at the time, the primary purposes of the programs were, first, to support the farm economy, second, to dispose of surpluses, and only thirdly to protect the nutritional status of schoolchildren. While the law governing school lunch programs clearly stipulated that poor children should receive lunches free, there was no requirement that poor children be given priority over middle class children in terms of where program funds could be allocated. In fact, in all of the next twenty years, the program primarily served to benefit middle class children, making it enormously popular politically but of dubious nutritional value for the poor.

Finally, the National School Lunch Act failed because, for many years, actual government funding was very limited. By 1968, the National School Lunch Program was feeding over 18 million children, with an increasing percentage receiving free or reduced-price lunches. The efficiency of the program, however, remained an open question.

In 1968, "Their Daily Bread," sponsored by five women's organizations—

Church Women United, the YWCA, the National Council of Catholic Women, the National Council of Negro Women, and the National Council of Jewish Women—conducted a thorough study of the lunch program. On the basis of a 35-page questionnaire and extensive personal interviews, the procedures and progress in the lunch programs of 40 communities in rural and urban areas were studied.

The project aimed to determine (a) why more children did not participate in the National School Lunch Program; and (b) why the program failed to meet the needs of the needy children.

The results confirmed what many who had worked in the program strongly suspected: the goal of the program was unattainable due to limitations built into the system. The problem areas were:

• The USDA knew that only 18 million eligible schoolchildren participated in the program. Yet, the rate of federal financing advanced at an incredibly slow rate, although large increases each year would have had a tremendous effect on the participation rate. Many school administrators, moreover, rather than face a constant worry over the program and an annual fight for lunch funds, chose not to participate at all.

• The matching formula requiring $3 of state and local revenues for every $1 of federal money was in fact met by payments from the children. Under these conditions, when the costs could not be met, the price of the lunch to the child rose. This caused the poorer children to drop out and, as their contributions were lost, the price rose again. Those states that did contribute on a substantial scale found that the extra money allowed a phenomenal increase in participation and more importantly, in the number of free and reduced-price lunches that could be served. Louisiana and South Carolina, both heavy investors in their lunch programs, had participation rates of 73% and 61% respectively. Their rates of free lunches stood high above the national average—25.6% for South Carolina and 18% for Louisiana.

• The lack of uniform national standards for determining eligibility for a free lunch created inequity. With no guidelines, local officials were often influenced by extraneous factors such as the child's conduct or attendance record. At the same time, administrators failed to connect hunger with lethargy or poor performance. With varying guidelines, children from the same family attending separate schools were judged and fed by different standards. Hence, a child might be "poor" in one school while his sister was considered "not poor" in a different school, a few miles away. This lack of national standards denied to many children the lunch that the Congress had guaranteed them.

• The lack of appropriations for nonfood assistance resulted in a program of de facto economic discrimination against the poor. Many of the slum area schools did not have the facilities to serve lunches even if money was available to buy food. Since the poor attended these schools, they were the ones denied lunches under the program.

The findings of "Their Daily Bread" documented the vast discrepancies

between the goals of the 1946 National School Lunch Act and its programs as
of 1968. The financing of the program was woefully inadequate; the administrative procedures were, at best, marginally acceptable; the discrimination
between paying children and nonpaying children was disgraceful and frequently in violation of the specified provisions of the act.

The main recommendation advanced by "Their Daily Bread" was the adoption of a Universal Free School Lunch Program in the United States. The
committee believed that food at school was an integral part of a sound education, and that, indeed, without it there could be no educational system in the
true sense of the word.

Until this could be implemented, seven short-term recommendations were
made:

1 increase federal, State, local, and community contributions to decrease the
price of the lunch
2 change USDA regulations to establish the school district, and not the individual school, as the contracting unit, so that all the children in one family,
though in different schools, would receive the same benefits
3 higher reimbursement rates and increased Section II special assistance
funds to needy schools
4 a uniform, national standard of need to determine the eligibility requirements for a free or reduced-price lunch
5 strict prohibition of discrimination, segregation, or identification of needy
children in the lunchrooms
6 consolidation of all school food programs at all levels under one administration for uniformity in funding, eligibility standards, record-keeping, and
reviews
7 more aggressive implementation of the objectives of the National School
Lunch Program by USDA and the States

"Their Daily Bread" served as a much-needed stimulus for the demand of
more effective administration and greater coverage in the lunch program. It
emphasized that the act was not intended to establish a welfare system and
should not be administered as such. The philosophy of the program was
voiced by the president of the American School Food Service Administration: "We use the food to get the child into the school; we use the school to
get the child out of poverty." By underfinancing the program, particularly for
the hungry and the poor, the government was, in reality, shortchanging the
future health of the nation.

The White House Conference on Food, Nutrition, and Health further advanced the school lunch issue. The 3,000 delegates met for three days in
Washington, representing the academic, medical, industrial, and agricultural
worlds, together with approximately 400 poor people who were involved in
the panel discussions and recommendations. The panel on school feeding
recommended a sweeping overhaul of all programs.

Foremost among the long-range recommendations was the call for a univer-

sal, free school lunch program for every American schoolchild regardless of
family income. In addition, nutritional supplements for the needy, particularly free breakfasts, were thought necessary to compensate for long years of
malnutrition. Comprehensive and imaginative "outreach" programs were
recommended for preschool children and school-age children in child service
institutions and summer programs.

The panel also recommended: complete federal financing, except for construction costs, of the nutrition program; the establishment of a Child Nutrition Administration to administer all the school feeding programs; incentive
grants to bring schools into the program and federal sanctions to ensure their
adherence to established, minimum nutrition standards; funds for annual
evaluation, research, and development; and the establishment of a National
Citizen's Advisory Committee to encourage citizens' participation in the
program.

In the short term, the panel urged: a crash program to feed the 5 million
needy children entitled to a free lunch but not receiving it; a national standard of eligibility for a free or reduced-price meal; a simple self-certification
process free from any humiliating stigma; the development of breakfast programs complementing, not substituting for, the lunch program; and a concentrated effort to reach those poor urban schools without lunch facilities.

On December 24, Dr. Jean Mayer, the conference director, announced
President Nixon's pledge to provide free lunches for all needy children by
Thanksgiving Day 1970. This was the strongest and most direct pledge ever to
come from any administration on the school lunch issue. The executive
branch for the first time went on record in agreement with the proposition
long known to millions of poor Americans: "A hungry child cannot learn."

In July 1965, the chairman of the Senate Agriculture Committee introduced a bill to extend benefits to more children, called for increased appropriations, and proposed an administrative overhaul in the National School
Lunch Act and the Child Nutrition Act. The chairman of the House Labor and
Education Committee introduced a similar bill in the House during January
1970.

Directed primarily to reaching hungry children too poor to afford participation in The School Lunch Program, the Senate bill provided for the following:

1 All appropriations for the National School Lunch Act and the Child Nutrition Act were to be authorized 1 year in advance of the fiscal year they were
designated for, and funds appropriated but unspent would be carried over
into the next year. This would provide the local school authorities with a
greater degree of certainty about type and size of program they could plan.
2 Funds for nonfood assistance to needy schools were to be increased, and
states would match such funds on a 25% basis.
3 Funds available for direct federal purchase and distribution of commodities
were fixed after certain specified limited expenses, such as: (a) a maximum

3.5% for federal administrative expenses; (b) a maximum 1% for nutritional
training and education programs for workers and participants, and for the
surveys and studies needed for a more efficient program.
4 State funds (other than revenues derived from lunch payments by the
children) would be required to match the federal contribution at a 4% level
for fiscal years 1972 and 1973; 6% for fiscal years 1974 and 1975; 8% for
fiscal years 1976 and 1977; and, at least 10% each fiscal year thereafter. This
change would mean an influx of more than $30 million to the program by
1978. The matching provision was designed not only to increase the number
of free and reduced-price lunches served but also to encourage more careful
state administration.
5 Local authorities would be required to announce publicly and apply equitably a plan for determining the qualifications to receive a free or reduced-
price lunch. As a minimum, consideration had to be given to the level of
family income (including welfare grants), the number in the family, and the
number of children in the family attending school or a service institution.
Furthermore, any overt identification of those receiving free or reduced-price
meals was strictly prohibited.
6 The bill provided an apportionment formula based on the number of 3 to
17 year-old schoolchildren in a state, in families with incomes less than
$3,000 per year plus the number of such children in families receiving more
than $3,000 per year from federally assisted public assistance programs.
Funds were to be used to assure access to the School Lunch Program by
needy children; hence, the money followed the "need of the child," not the
school. Financial assistance up to 80% of the operating costs of the program
was allowed in circumstances of severe need.
7 States were permitted to transfer funds among the various child feeding
programs, provided plans to do so received federal approval. A maximum of
1% of the funds might be reserved for special development projects.
8 A National Advisory Council on Child Nutrition composed of representatives from the various fields involved in the child feeding programs was to
study the programs and recommend actions needed to improve administration and implementation.

In response to the announced aims of the White House conference and in
light of President Nixon's pledge of free lunches for all the needy by Thanksgiving Day 1970, five amendments were offered on the Senate floor by a
bipartisan group led by Senators McGovern and Javits.

One amendment called for the establishment of national uniform eligibility
standards for free and reduced-price lunches, with the states determining who
qualified for free and who qualified for reduced-price lunches. Some national
standard clearly was required, since utter confusion had prevailed when standards varied from state to state, district to district, and school to school.
Furthermore, evidence indicated that many areas ignored USDA regulations
calling for a publicly announced eligibility policy. All children from house-

holds eligible for the Food Stamps or Commodity Distribution Programs, or from families of four with an annual income below $4,000 would be eligible. The $4,000 per-year income level matched that established for the Food Stamp Program; however, it remained below the Bureau of Labor Statistics' index of $6,000 in yearly income necessary for a family of four to maintain a "low standard of living." The amendment further stipulated that only an affidavit by the parent was necessary to prove eligibility, thus eliminating long, inquisitive, and frequently embarrassing interviews.

The same amendment also required that no reduced-price lunch could cost more than 20¢. "Their Daily Bread" had demonstrated that the lower the price, the higher the number of students who bought the lunch. In schools where the price was 20¢, participation was 100%; at 25¢, participation dropped to 80%; at 30¢, only 27 to 37% of the students participated. The opposition to the 20¢ limit on a reduced-price lunch claimed that this was an unreasonable restriction and unenforceable unless full and adequate funding was assured. According to the USDA, both the national eligibility standard and the 20¢ lunch would force many schools to drop out of the National School Lunch Program, thereby depriving the needy children of their free lunch. Furthermore, the USDA pointed to the lack of provision for regional differences, for example, 26.2% of the families in the North fell below the annual income of $4,000 figure, while in the South, 46.5% of the families were below the index. Despite strong opposition, the amendment was finally passed by a margin of one vote: Amendment 508 passed the Senate 41-40.

Yet another amendment applied the national minimum eligibility standards of the prior amendment to the School Breakfast Program. Emphasis was focused on needy children because witnesses before the Select Committee on Nutrition and Human Needs had pointed out that many poor children subsisted mainly on the free lunch from school. All too often, children came to school hungry and were unable to learn. Because of the evidence of the value of breakfast in the educative process, increased authorizations were proposed: $25 million for 1971, $50 million for 1972, and $75 million for fiscal year 1973. Provision was also made for federal reimbursement up to 100% of the operating costs in the very poorest of the schools. Under the amendment, 3 million children would be eating breakfast free by 1973.

Opponents of the amendment felt that it might violate the Equal Protection clause of the Constitution. Since only $25 million was asked for (as opposed to $250 million for free lunches) and only the neediest children would qualify, rigid economic means tests would have to be applied to select the participants. The amendment, however, clearly implied a yearly expansion of benefits, and it, too, passed by a very narrow margin.

A third amendment proposed as the basis for the new allocation of funds, the number of schoolchildren from households with an income of $4,000 or less per year for a family of four, where the original bill had proposed an index of $3,000 annual income. The amendment also proposed a reimbursement rate up to 100% (the bill offered up to 80%) for schools not able to provide the number of free lunches to which their students were entitled. Several Senators objected to a 100% reimbursement rate, claiming that it destroyed state and local initiative. On the other hand, despite the best intentions, the most depressed schools just could not manage their programs and cover all of the needy children if they were forced to pay 20% of the costs.

Another provision of this amendment sought to correct the most glaring deficiency in the National School Lunch Act—the lack of accountability on the part of local school districts and states to the USDA. Each state would be required to file an annual plan of its school feeding programs stating:

- how the available money for free lunches was to be spent
- how the state intended to extend the National School Lunch Program to every student
- how the needs of the poor, in particular, were to be met

Cash and donated commodities would not be given to those states failing to file a plan, but failure to achieve the goals of the program would not mean a loss of federal aid. In addition, local school districts would be required to file monthly reports to the state on the number of children entitled to a free lunch and those actually receiving them.

Critics of this amendment contended that the plan asked the impossible, and that many state education agencies did not have the competence to require their school districts to submit plans. Proponents of the amendment pointed out that the amendment was constructed not to place an onerous requirement on the state, but to focus the state's attention on meeting its nutrition priorities and to inhibit it from misallocating its child feeding funds. This amendment was also accepted.

President Nixon's Thanksgiving Day deadline was a mere 9 months away, yet the administration requested only $44 million for the school feeding program. The Agriculture Committee itself had projected $712.8 million as the sum necessary to feed the 6.6 million children it estimated as "needy." Even with a normal 10% absenteeism reduction, more than $640 million would be needed. The Bureau of the Census, however, placed the number of needy children at 8.4 million. Since the combined federal-state-local contribution for free and reduced-price lunches in fiscal year 1971 would reach only $400 million, a minimum deficit of $240 million remained, even using the administration's figure of 6.6 million needy children. It seemed clear that President Nixon's pledge could not be attained without a vast increase in funding; $44 million would be totally inadequate to meet the need. An amendment was submitted to remedy this defect by increasing authorizations to $250 million for fiscal year 1971, an increase of $206 million over the USDA request. To cover the census bureau's estimate of 8.4 million needy children, authorizations were to increase to $300 million and $350 million for fiscal year 1972 and fiscal year 1973. The Senate, however, rejected this amendment by a vote of 36-35.

The final legislation, a compromise bill between both houses of Congress, included the following:

1 Instead of a $4,000 annual income index as the national minimum standard, the Secretary of the Department of Agriculture was to establish a national standard.

2 The Conference Committee deleted the provision of up to 100% reimbursement of operating costs at the neediest schools, and retained merely a maximum *per-meal* reimbursement rate to be determined by the Secretary.

3 The 3-year breakfast program funded at levels of $25 million, $50 million, and $75 million for fiscal years 1971, 1972, and 1973 was reduced to a 1-year pilot program with an authorization of $25 million.

4 The provision requiring submission of state plans for extending free lunch programs was modified slightly.

The fundamental revisions of the National School Lunch Act and the Child Nutrition Act proposed by the Senate were retained intact. With effective implementation, millions of additional children would be covered by the lunch and breakfast programs.

The crucial language of the legislation, that "meals shall be served without cost or at a reduced cost to children who are determined by local school authorities to be unable to pay the full cost," meant that each needy child had a *right* to a lunch. This, together with the president's pledge to provide every needy child with a free lunch by the end of 1970, meant that the legislative structure existed to establish a truly effective child feeding program. Many of the more general activities of government, of course, are directly and indirectly responsible for ensuring the nutritional well-being of the American people. The government has been involved for some time in regulating the food industry to ensure a safe national food supply. The various divisions of the Department of Agriculture, as well as the Food and Drug Administration of the Department of Health, Education, and Welfare, have conducted inspection programs for both processed and unprocessed foods. Many of the laws giving national agencies the power to conduct inspection programs were passed over the vigorous opposition both from those who believed the power should remain at the state level and from the industries whose operations would be affected.

Except for laws governing fortification, and the effort at nutrition education during World War II, the government's involvement in nutrition per se has been, historically, rather limited. The expansion of this involvement has been a relatively recent phenomenon. The Department of Agriculture, for instance, is now responsible for managing major feeding programs and has also established a Human Nutrition Research Institute in response to criticism that it was more interested in the nutrition of animals than people. The department's Extension Service, nationally oriented toward rural families, offering advice on farming and canning produce, is now more urban-oriented, supplying information on how to cope with the modern food supply. The Food and Drug Administration has shifted from dealing only with food safety to attempting to guarantee nutritional quality through production and labeling requirements. The Federal Trade Commission is following suit by insisting that food companies, advertising companies, and the mass media play down fantasy and fun in food and emphasize nutrition. The Federal Communications Commission, responsible for regulating television, is bringing pressure to bear on networks to be more responsible in advertising food to children and to reduce the number of minutes during an hour used to promote soft drinks, candy, cake, and so on. Joint efforts between government and private agencies in the field of nutrition have also been growing. In recent years, the government has provided both food and funds to charities and churches within the country to provide meals for the poor, and much of the nutrition assistance abroad is channeled through charitable organizations.

Often, policy decisions in the agricultural area have important nutritional side-effects. For example, agriculture research and production programs intended to improve efficiency caused sudden and mass unemployment in the cotton industry. When cotton picking was mechanized in the southern United States in the early 1960s, hundreds of thousands of families lost their means of support. This caused the hunger that led to the fight for an improved food stamp program. It also caused migration from the rural south to the urban north, increasing the demand for social services in the cities. Additionally, many families experienced difficulty adjusting to the modern food marketing system when they had been accustomed to growing their own staple foods. A similar upheaval is about to occur in the tobacco industry, and, more slowly, in the fruit and vegetable industries.

Another policy with unintended nutritional results was the government practice of practically unrestrained food export sales, especially to the Soviet Union. The 1972 sale kicked off an inflationary food price spiral that has still not stopped. High food prices deepened the national recession, forcing more families to use food stamps. High food prices also led middle income families to change their diets: most have reduced their meat consumption considerably and rely more heavily on bread, cereals, rice, and beans. This "buying down" had the effect, unfortunately, of causing even more rapid price increases in the staple foods upon which the low income families had been dependent. These trends put the poor under tremendous pressure, and also increased the cost to the government of supporting feeding programs for families, schoolchildren, the aged, pregnant women, and infants.

While the country is undergoing great changes in diet as it shifts from a once simple and unprocessed food supply to a very sophisticated and highly processed food supply, these changes are not unexpected. They are the result of a rapidly changing lifestyle in which traditional meal patterns are disappearing and fast-food preparation is at a premium. The food industry seeks growth by providing built-in service for which more affluent consumers are willing to pay. Until recently, there was minimal interest in the nutritional impact of this changing life and dietary style. Now, a greater effort is being made, both within and outside of government, to relate this change to nutrition and health.

CONCLUSIONS

In this history of the United States, it seems to me, are examples of many of the things that we have described as desirable: local initiative, local government participation, and agricultural development in particular. Development was "planned" only in a sense: there was a plan to give people the resources and to let them work, but, beyond that, it was up to them. Obviously, the end result was that the American farmer was enormously successful, with considerable government assistance, and created the economic base upon which the industry of the country developed. Even today, as people are reminded, agriculture is enormously important: the sale of agricultural surpluses has partially offset the greatly increased cost of oil.

Thus, we had an economic base to work from, and we had what I would describe as a deeply ingrained food ethic. We also had evidence that, if we did not insure adequate nutrition, no matter how else we might attempt to break the cycle of poverty, there could be no assurance that people would be able to take advantage of the opportunities open to them.

As a result and, I might add, with great difficulty in overcoming very, very serious opposition, a large program developed within six years. The law was written, the administrative regulations were spelled out down to the local administration, and the federal government's commitment to nutrition programs was increased from less than $5 hundred million to over $8.5 billion. The number of families receiving family food assistance through a food stamp program increased, and the number of individuals reached went from 3 million persons to about 20 million persons by the 1975/76 fiscal year. The number of low income children receiving free or reduced price school lunches went from 3 million to over 10 million. A breakfast program was started that went from 0 to about 3 million participants and, on top of that, a special supplemental feeding program for low income pregnant women, infants, and children was added. That program began three years ago at a $10 million level, and the funding in fiscal year 1977 will be $250 million, serving about 800,000 women and children. Thus, in an unplanned way, the enormous agricultural success in the United States laid a base for a commitment to food and nutrition which at this point is still developing and expanding.

DISCUSSION (UNITED STATES)

Latham

It's very surprising to hear Ken Schlossberg talking in these terms because I have heard him be most critical of what the United States has done. I will admit, however, that a great deal has been done in the last six years.

In painting this rosy picture I regret the lack of emphasis on how sad it is that very little had been done until six years ago in the United States. Certainly there had been an agricultural and economic success before six years ago. How did it come about, then, that the wealthiest country on earth, with a vast amount of surplus food, had 20 million malnourished people six years ago? At the same time this wealthy country was saying to the rest of the world that "all you need to do is have an economic and agricultural success, and you will have gotten rid of malnutrition"!

The other point of concern in the United States is that, while it is admirable to have a food stamp program providing aid to 20 million people, the other affluent nations in the world (e.g., the Netherlands, Sweden, Britain, the USSR) do not seem to require a food stamp program or a food commodity program. They are relatively successful in dealing with the problem of nutrition without specific nutritional programs, simply by providing adequate income to their low income people!

The difference, I think, between the food commodity program you describe and what Solon and Sandoval described for their countries is that the United States food commodity program was entirely based on surplus foods in the beginning. Until the Senate Nutrition Committee got under way, it was not at all based on nutritional needs, and therefore was often very unbalanced in the commodities provided. The program was entirely a subsidy to get rid of farm surpluses and to help poor Southern farmers. It was not designed as a nutrition program.

To look at the other side of this thing, it really took politicians and concerned laymen in the United States, rather than physicians and nutritionists, to spot the existence of a serious problem and to insist that surveys be done and that the country look at its nutritional problems. The United States, despite the successes that you cite, is still 16th or 17th in world infant mortality rates. In fact, infant mortality rates among black Americans are still almost twice what they are among white Americans, similar to the level in Barbados and some other islands in the Caribbean, which are one-tenth as wealthy as the United States.

Antrobus

Is the program in the United States conceived purely as a supplemental feeding program or is it conceived as part of a total social development program, including such other components as day care, skilled training, employment opportunity, self-help, and so on? If it is the former, isn't this purely "symptomatic treatment"? How far is this going to lead the United States and these 25 million poor people? Are they going to live perpetually on welfare?

Schlossberg

The United States for many years has had maternal and child health centers
for low income people. The supplemental feeding program was started first as
the delivery of a food package to low income women and children who qualified. After several years of experience, it was decided that that was entirely
unsatisfactory, and it was converted into a coupon program, operating
through health programs. When a woman is pregnant or has just delivered, she
has to enroll in the health program in order to receive the food coupons. The
coupon is thus an incentive to get the women and the children into the health
program, to ensure that there is appropriate prenatal care and postnatal care.
This program is not, in itself, related to anything else. It's not related to
whether the woman is employed or not employed or any other factor. I cannot tell you what the relationship will be between the assistance received
through this program and the future of the recipient family.

I *would* like to say something about the serious misconceptions of welfare
in the United States. There was some evidence, developed in the 1960s, that
there existed in the United States a large, large number of permanently poor
people. There is some truth to that, but, for the most part, it is not true. In
fact, the poor population in the United States is very fluid, and, within that
population, there are families who move in and families who move out, sometimes depending on the state of the economy.

Secondly, there is a misconception about the work ethic among those
people who are poor in the United States. In fact, many of them *do* work,
but their wages are so low that they are still unable to take care of their basic
human needs. So, the problem of breaking out of the poverty cycle, in many
cases, is not related to work or training. It could be related to the state of the
economy or a person's health. There are many factors in unemployment that
are not easy to deal with.

Maletnlema

I am surprised to hear of a program in the United States which has not analyzed why these people are poor but instead assists people in a way which will
not necessarily help their poverty. From the questions and answers, it looks
as though they are going to remain poor perpetually. What will happen eventually if the government fails to provide help? It seems as though the help is
coming from the success of certain farmers. Why shouldn't there be a kind of
redistribution from those who are successful to these people who are unsuccessful? Why shouldn't the two programs go together?

Schlossberg

The first answer is that it is not appropriate to think of these families as permanently poor, each one requiring a total package to lift it out of poverty.
Many are families which, as I said before, may not have been poor previously
but may be poor now for reasons that have nothing to do with what the government can do for them.

There *are* families in the United States that are welfare families from generation to generation, but the size of that problem is greatly overstated—overstated, in some cases, to make a particular point. Where it is true, the families are usually located in isolated areas, such as Appalachia, where there is endemic poverty and, often, limited employment possibility. On the other hand, such families may be located in large urban ghettos. But, you know, we are talking here of one or two generations in the context of an extremely dynamic society.

There has been, in recent years, great skepticism about efforts by the government in personal assistance programs, in setting up bureaucracies to teach people trades, give them appropriate health care, and so on. There is a feeling that personal services are not the real answer to the poverty cycle, and that, in fact, the way to help is simply to provide in-kind or cash assistance so that poor families can live like other Americans. If they do, it is felt, the children growing up in those families will have the opportunities to enable them to take their rightful place in society.

We have spent billions of dollars over the last thirty years to provide all kinds of social services directed towards the poor, and, yet, the poor are still there. If we could redistribute the money a little bit, raise the levels of income, and put these people on some sort of equal footing with the rest of society, they can take care of themselves. Many people do not want bureaucrats or social workers to show them the way to a better life.

Wray
This reminds me of an account of just such a problem family. The mother was from one of the American "poor" families, unemployed, with many social problems. She had many children, and, because of welfare policies and the lack of enough income to hold the family together, the children, one by one, became wards of the state in one form or another. Sometimes they were in jail, sometimes in special hospitals, sometimes in special schools. The point was that, ultimately, this woman's children were costing the government $100,000 a year for care in various special facilities. The proposition was offered, and I think with some validity, that, if the mother had been given the cash to keep the children together and take care of them, much of this money could have been saved. This is one type of argument in favor of direct cash income support for families in contrast to social services.

One of the things that Ken has left out, about the United States, is the widespread popular sentiment that anybody who is willing to work can make a decent living. The assumption remains that anybody who is poor is therefore not willing to work, or is stupid or immoral. I think this has been one of the major obstacles to any kind of direct assistance welfare program. Specifically, some people feel that if you simply give people money, they will just sit back and enjoy it. There is exactly the same kind of sentiment in many other countries, very specifically with regard to food programs, when there are large masses of people who cannot find jobs. Some people passionately resist giving food to the children of these people because they feel it is morally debilitating and will make the parents permanently dependent.

Schlossberg

We tried to deal with those arguments in the Senate discussions, and I think we did so rather successfully. First, we provided as much proof as possible that the idea that poor people do not work is wrong. In fact, some of them are the hardest working people in the United States, but the wages they receive are not high enough. A classic example is the migrant worker. These workers travel thousands of miles, from the South to the North, in several streams on the East Coast, in the Midwest, and the West. They work the longest hours, live in the worst conditions, and make the lowest wages. Nobody can say that those people, who are very poor, do not work or do not want to work.

Second, the idea that the welfare mothers have been on welfare all their lives and never work is also false. I personally met many women, when I was with the Nutrition Committee, who had worked for years, but, who, for one reason or another, simply could not continue to work. It was not that they didn't want to work. I remember one woman, in particular, who had worked for something like 20 years and then developed diabetes, was unable to work, and was forced to go on welfare.

Once you deal with these two arguments, you take away the notion that assistance should depend on whether people work or not. In fact, I think we made a fairly good case that, if you provide assistance to needy people, you increase the possibility of their working as opposed to diminishing it.

Solimano

I would like to emphasize that often we incriminate people because of their malnutrition or poverty, without attempting to analyze the system in which those people function. I think if you want to be fair, you have to look not only at the people, but at the system and whether, without changes in the system—minor, moderate, or large—the problems can be solved. This is very relevant to the problem of nutrition. We talk about the problem of the malnourished population in terms of the third degree cases, the second degree cases, and so forth. On the other hand, if you gave a family with children suffering from third degree malnutrition only *part* of the money that you are already spending on hospitals in the care of those children, the whole family would probably be better off.

The people that have been concerned with nutrition have made the same mistake by looking at the malnourished population as an isolated group that needs some kind of welfare. Of course you have to give food, but you must realize that sometimes it is inevitable that the malnourished exist. Some systems work in such a way that it is not possible for them *not* to exist. That point needs to be taken into account.

If you really want to solve the problem, you must examine the national and institutional factors that are determining all social problems, including malnutrition. A nutrition problem is no more than the consequence and expression of the fact that a certain society is malfunctioning. This comment is not related particularly to the United States, but, in a more general way, it applies, I think, to every society.

Schlossberg

We know what is wrong with the system in the United States in this particular area. The main problem is that we are politically willing to accept an *un*acceptable level of unemployment. We seem to believe that we cannot have unemployment at a lower rate without creating a problem of inflation. If we could embark on a full employment policy as a national commitment, we could include a fairly sizeable program of public service employment. We could well invest billions of dollars in the isolated poor rural areas and the depressed urban areas, hiring many of the people who live in those areas to restore them. We would then be providing people with employment and income and, in the process, probably eliminating much of the malnutrition problem that we are attempting to deal with in other ways.

Unfortunately, we have not yet been able to reach that point. Given the economic block that we are facing, we are attempting to deal with the problem in other ways and devise other measures, though they do not go to the root of the problem. Basically, we are attempting to provide services or income in an in-kind way which effectively redistributes resources and raises the people who we keep at the bottom at least to a point where the problem of malnutrition will no longer exist. What we are pushing for is, first of all, some commitment to do something about the problems of these people, and two, to do it in a way that makes sense. Now, if that means accepting, for the moment, an $8.5 billion investment in in-kind nutrition programs, we will take it as the best we can do.

If the expenditures in that area become sizeable enough so the difference between doing it round about, in terms of in-kind nutrition programs, and doing it straight, in terms of income maintenance, becomes small, we might well be able to make a bridge from the nutrition service approach to the income approach. If we do finally make the bridge to the income approach, it would then become apparent both to the politicians and to the public that, if we are going to spend all that money to raise people's incomes, maybe we should think of providing employment instead and getting some benefit in return.

Sai

I worry about this kind of discussion because, in a simpleminded medical way, I understand that most of life's things are distributed in a Gaussian curve, with a certain proportion of the population at the two ends of the curve. One of the questions is: what percentage will be acceptable at either end if, indeed, wealth and everything else get distributed along this curve?

Solimano

And there is also the question of what *level* will be acceptable for the two ends.

Sai

Yes, but basically there has to be a certain core problem group. Do we know what would be an acceptable core problem group?

Mellor

What is missing in that analysis is that we have, in the United States, a number of people who are below an absolute level of welfare, at a level considered unacceptable on a worldwide basis, in a world in which incomes generally are a great deal lower than the average in the United States. Yet, even given the substantial number of people below this absolute level and the extremely high incomes in our country, we are still unwilling politically to meet that problem on a welfare basis.

Some of us think that it need not all be met on a welfare basis if we make some other changes in society. As long as we don't change society, however, we find we cannot even guarantee a minimum absolute level that people in much poorer countries would also consider a minimal level. It is not simply a matter of always having to worry about the bottom 10% of the scale, which continually goes up as incomes go up.

In fact, I have been impelled by this discussion to comment on the whole question of foreign aid. It seems to me that foreign aid, at its best, can play a very useful role in influencing policies in a country, not so much by forcing countries to follow policies which they don't want to follow but by forcing countries to face up to conflicts in policy. A little leverage from the substantial funds involved, I think, can serve a very salutary purpose if there is intelligence in use of foreign assistance.

Turning that around and looking at the United States, I have the feeling that it's unfortunate that we are not a major foreign aid *receiver* because I think that would bring the right light to bear on policies in this area. An excellent expert panel could be put together to look at questions of poverty in the United States, and, I think, if they looked intelligently, they would have a good deal of sympathy for much of what Ken has had to say. On the other hand, I have a suspicion that they would find something in the rather simple point that Michael Latham made, and that is that there seem to be some other countries in a similar income bracket that have a smaller base of hard-core poverty. I think the conclusion of such a panel would be that the United States shows some interest in understanding the nature of the problem and in dealing with its symptoms but shows no interest whatsoever in getting at the root causes of the problem and finding out how much of the root cause can be ameliorated and how much cannot.

The conclusion might be that there are some difficult political problems to be dealt with if we really look at the bases of poverty in the United States. On that basis, aid might be denied, with a statement that, following this pre-appraisal mission, there would be an appraisal mission later if the country showed some interest in putting together a sensible statement!

This process is often stupidly done with respect to Asian, African, and Latin American countries, but it *can* be a very useful process. As I say, I regret that my country is not going to have the benefit of that exercise for the foreseeable future.

12 ZAMBIA'S NATIONAL FOOD AND NUTRITION PROGRAM

A. P. Vamoer

A. P. Vamoer has been involved with nutrition in Zambia over a time spanning the transition from British colonial administration to Zambian national policy planning. In his capacity as a nutrition advocate, he has worked closely with local, regional, national, colonial, and international agencies and thus brings a broad historical perspective to the issues discussed in his paper. Currently, Vamoer serves as Executive Secretary of the National Food and Nutrition Commission, a key post for nutrition activity in Zambia.

HISTORY

In Zambia, malnutrition has, for a long time, been recognized as a national problem: attempts have been made to combat it, and the need for action has been recognized at the highest level. Because the subject is so vast, most of the following remarks are confined to an account of the historical background and evolution of the Zambian nutrition program. It was started by a very few interested medical doctors in the '30s and has now evolved into what is being called the Zambia National Food and Nutrition Program.

Indications from investigations going as far back as the early '30s to the most recent food consumption and nutrition status surveys, confirm the grim conclusion that malnutrition and undernutrition are widespread in Zambia. Lack of food is not the major problem; much worse is the hidden hunger of malnutrition caused by poverty and ignorance. As recently as 1966, an FAO team concluded that "malnutrition is a major limitation to the life and welfare of Zambia. Unless firm action is taken promptly, the situation will worsen and become more intractable."

Zambia (then Northern Rhodesia) was colonized by Britain in 1920, and, for the first ten years of the British colonial rule, nothing was done in the field of nutrition except famine relief work and orders to plant root crops in areas subject to locusts.

Nutrition awareness began in the early 1930s when Richards and Widdowson kept daily records of foods eaten by selected families in a tribal village in Serenje District, made estimates of total supplies, and maintained a record of various environmental and sociological factors which influenced total intakes. They also sent samples of foodstuffs to England for nutrient analysis and made calculations of the chemical composition of the diet. Their research work even attempted a comparison between intake of food and output of work. Their main conclusions were:

• There is a striking seasonal variation in African diets and a real food shortage during two months of the year.
• Compared with European standards
  1 the African diet is little more than half in calorie value
  2 the diets are strikingly deficient in fat
  3 the amount of animal protein is very small and may be entirely absent.
  4 Intake of calcium and phosphorus is considerably higher.
• Vitamins A and B are well represented in the diets. Vitamin C is also present as long as fresh plant foods are eaten. Vitamin D appears to be entirely absent from the diets.
• The calorie intake is insufficient to provide energy for the work required.

Although such a telling report should have stimulated government response and action on the problem of nutrition, it was the League of Nations and not the Northern Rhodesian Government that provided the next impetus for nutritional research. At the Sixth Assembly of the League of Nations in 1935, it was resolved that, "Having considered the subject of nutrition in relation to public health," the League "urged the Government to examine practical means for securing better nutrition."

Subsequently, the League set up a "Mixed Committee" charged with the responsibility of studying the health and economic aspects of nutrition as a world problem. The subsequent report of the committee was an unbalanced document, concerning primarily the conditions and problems in Europe and other Western countries. With regard to nutrition in Africa, Asia, and other tropical countries, the committee only reported that the problem was acute! "Hundreds of millions of persons dwell in these parts of the world. It is notorious that a large proportion of them live in a state of continual malnutrition."

Probably stimulated by the League committee's report, the British Secretary of State for the Colonies issued a directive on April 18, 1936 "that there should be a comprehensive survey of the position in each of the Dependencies," with the following terms of reference:

- a review of the present knowledge of human nutrition in each Dependency
- a review of the further studies and researches on the subject which appear desirable
- a review of the practical measures which have been taken in the past to apply scientific knowledge to the improvement of nutrition
- a review of such further measures which appear desirable to be taken in the future
- a review of the consequences which improvements in nutrition may have upon the economy of the Dependency

In its directive, the Colonial Office also realized the importance of a combined and coordinated approach, stating that the subject "concerns many branches of Government, notably the Secretariat, the Administration, and the Educational, Agricultural, Veterinary and Medical Departments; *and if a proper plan of action is to be laid down and effectively carried through, there must be close cooperation between them all.*"

Following this, the Northern Rhodesian Governor set up a Standing Committee to deal with the nutritional status of Africans under Sir Stewart Gore-Brown, which, as one of its first acts, developed a questionnaire and distributed it widely. Only 60 replies were received. The most startling reply, perhaps characteristic of the prevailing attitudes of some European settlers towards African nutritional problems, read as follows:

I hold the view that the fuss about vitamins will die away . . . I do not think that green vegetables can be of much consequence in human food. The African natives certainly do not appear to require any.

Fortunately, the Standing Committee held different views and "accepted that there was an accumulating body of general evidence that malnutrition and effects of dietary deficiency were common." The committee also noted that "very little serious and effective effort had yet been made in Northern

Rhodesia to apply existing scientific knowledge to the improvement of nutrition."

One important contribution of the committee was its recommendation that the government amend the Employment of Natives Regulation. The recommendation took into consideration the practice of the Rokana Mine Corporation to provide food rations to its workers. Rokana Corporation had noted that feeding its workers resulted in improved nutritional status and increased efficiency, and the committee, therefore, recommended that "agricultural, domestic and casual laborers should be fed according to nutritional scale requirements already in force on the Copperbelt. Employers should be under a clear legal obligation to supply their employees with meat and fresh vegetable foods." In other words, the proposal was for what are currently known as workers' feeding programs or workers' canteens. For British expatriates who employed domestic servants, there was now a new demand, above the monthly salary: a supplement for food. This recommendation was accepted by the government.

The committee also noted that improvements in nutrition meant improvements in health and improvements in health meant a more productive working life. The committee listed the probable consequences that better nutrition could have in the economy:

- certain diseases would be lessened or eliminated entirely
- resistance to all diseases would improve significantly
- better continued health as well as less ill health would result
- infant mortality would be reduced
- physical fitness would be improved
- greater earning and purchasing power would be ensured
- improved interest in and output from agricultural work would ensue
- improved educability of children would result, with an attendant increase in their eligibility for occupations now practically closed to them

Dr. Richards submitted the following recommendations to the committee, all of which were endorsed:

- greater encouragement of maize growing
- encouragement of poultry keeping and native butcheries in townships
- introduction of European vegetables and fruit trees in villages
- proper organization of the fish trade and institution of greater fish markets
- improvements in methods of storage and cooking of food
- research in infant feeding
- education in agriculture and marketing

Other reports submitted to the committee emphasized the fact that grains (millet) were available only for a period of about 10 months of the year and for the other two months the people depended mainly on foods like sweet potatoes, pumpkins, caterpillars, flying ants, and so on. On the average the staple food (millet) provided 6 lb per day per household.

While the Standing Committee was still gathering available information on the nutrition status of the people in Northern Rhodesia, a Committee of the Economic Advisory Council in Britain was already considering reports received from 48 other British Dependencies. In July 1939, it reached the following conclusions:

• "We have no doubt [of] the great importance of the subject [nutrition]. We are confident that improved nutrition will bring very great benefit to the Colonial Empire. At the present time, the effects of malnutrition are seen not only in definite disease but also in general ill-health and lowered resistance to infection, inefficiency of labor and industry and agriculture, maternal and infantile mortality, and a general lack of well-being."

• "An important but often overlooked criterion for the drawing up of dietaries is that the food prescribed, its cooking, and its serving should conform as far as possible to the dietary habits of those to be fed."

• The main causes of malnutrition were that:

   1 the standard of living is often too low

   2 there exists great ignorance coupled with prejudice, both in regard to diet itself and to the use of land

   3 there exists an influence of other diseases, especially parasitic infestations, which react upon the state of nutrition of the individual

The British group made the following recommendations:

• family production of food to meet family needs, especially with reference to protective foods

• careful drying of green foods, to counter the effects of seasonal fluctuations

• development of better storage facilities

• development of early maturing or drought-resistant varieties of the main staple food or the planting of special famine reserve crops

• improvement of the yield per acre by the use of better seed and of better methods of husbandry

• diversification of staple foods by the increased consumption of animal products

The first nutrition survey ever attempted in a British Dependency was done in Malawi (then Nyasaland) under the direction of the late Dr. B. S. Platt, who visited Northern Rhodesia in July 1939 and discussed the possibility of a similar survey. Unfortunately, the start of World War II prevented any follow-up along these lines, and no nutrition work was done in Northern Rhodesia for the duration of the war.

A new phase of nutrition awareness in Northern Rhodesia began in 1946; this laid the groundwork for the present program. On the recommendation of Dr. Platt, nutrition officers within the Department of Health were posted to various Dependencies to coordinate the activities of all the departments that were developing plans for improving nutrition. Although this recommendation seemed a logical solution to the problem of coordination, it mistakenly assumed that junior professional officers could influence the attitudes and activities of various departments and mold the policy of government. It later proved, however, that no matter how competent the junior professional officers were, their lack of local experience coupled with their low status in the civil service hierarchy made any such impact impossible. All their influence had to be exerted indirectly.

For example, practically all the work on nutrition in the country had been done in rural areas and none in urban areas. Betty Preston, Northern Rhodesia's nutrition officer, therefore undertook a survey of food consumption in Chilenje Suburb, Lusaka. This was the first attempt at bridging the information gap between rural and urban nutrition and drew attention to the problems in the cities. Results showed that

At present wage levels and prices, no more than 30% of the families in the Location and 56% of the families in the Township could manage to maintain a reasonably adequate diet throughout the month; but these percentages only apply when the monthly expenses are reduced to a minimum and there are no purchases of sundry goods such as clothes, furniture, or household utensils. The money available for food depends on other requirements during the month, and if they are extensive the diet will naturally suffer.

The following recommendations resulted:

• Wages should be paid weekly instead of monthly to assist in budgeting.
• Improved government price control was essential, since all foodstuffs sold by African traders in the markets exceeded the controlled price.
• A milk drink, such as cocoa, should be supplied to schoolchildren, since many went to school without having had any breakfast.

Although this study contained no medical evidence of nutritional deficiencies, it is generally believed that it played a big role in the government decision to introduce a subsidy for maize meal and roller meal.

In April 1947 a much more ambitious "Nutrition Survey in Serenje District" was started by five members of the Friends Ambulance Unit. The team kept records of the quantities of foods eaten and also took account of the social and economic background of the household; agricultural work done throughout the year; the types of foods eaten and cooking methods used; livestock and animal products used as relishes; and food consumption throughout the year including feeding in schools.

The survey report said "the number of meals cooked each day seemed to depend as much on chance variables as on inadequate stocks." The survey reported also that practically all protein in the diet came from vegetable sources and that only for a few weeks of the year could it be considered reasonably satisfactory. Vitamin deficiencies were noted and fat was reported as being "sadly lacking in the diet."

Nutritional studies were also carried out in other parts of the country: the Bangweulu Swamps, Namwala District, and Ndola Rural District. In 1948 both a qualitative survey and a clinical survey were done in the Luapula area. Coupled with other quantitative work done previously, a fairly clear pattern of food consumption in Luapula emerged.

THE NUTRITION PILOT PROJECT

The government, around the same time, sent a team including a nutritionist, agriculturalist, and administrator to the Nutrition School, under the auspices of the Colonial Office at Makerere University College, Uganda. This group produced a work plan for a coordinated food policy in Kawanbwa District, based on a broad medical, agricultural, educational, and economic approach. The work plan won the support of Dr. Dean A. Smith, who was in charge of the Nutrition School, and before the school year ended Dr. Smith was invited by the government to undertake a further clinical survey and to coordinate work already done in Luapula.

Dr. Smith arrived in October 1949 and carried out investigations in Luapula valley, the center of most nutrition activity in Northern Rhodesia, and on the plateau of Senior Chief Mushota.

In early 1950, Dr. Smith submitted his report which included a plan for a pilot project. He envisaged a scheme which would, in three years, produce a revolutionary change in well-being in the area and this would, in turn, create a demand elsewhere for a similar campaign. The plan was approved by the government and an application made for a grant from the Colonial Development and Welfare Funds. At the same time, Smith was asked to lead the team to implement his recommendations. On February 8, 1951, the Secretary of State approved a large grant, but by this time Dr. Smith was no longer available to do the work.

The original plan had included the construction of a hospital and a Development Area Training Center at Kawambwa, but these projects were later omitted. As the facilities were essential to the original health and nutrition scheme, it was decided in 1952 that the project be moved to Mansa District (then Fort Rosebery).

In the later part of 1952, however, a White Paper proposing the creation of the Central African Federation of Rhodesia and Nyasaland was published and provoked angry reactions throughout the country, particularly in Mansa. There, Senior Chief Milambo called for the boycott of all staff in departments of Agriculture, Forestry, and Game and Fisheries. For the time being, then, political problems ended any possibility of a coordinated approach for the scheme.

The Federation of Rhodesia and Nyasaland was, in fact, created in 1953, and the pilot project scheme was revived in August 1955 by the Commissioner for Native Development. At this meeting, it was agreed that a WHO expert be requested and that the Health and Agriculture ministries would make staff available from the outset. The Department of Agriculture, however, considered it most unlikely that a suitable person would, in fact, become available. Another apparent impasse.

In February 1956, Dr. J. M. Bengoa, the WHO expert, visited Lusaka to evaluate the government's request. He concluded that the program

In some ways appears to be a "health demonstration area," but the inclusion of agricultural activities as well strengthens the project immensely. As far as I am aware, there are few programs in the world of this kind and its development will be a matter of considerable interest.

The scheme was given a go-ahead but did not fare too well from the start because of a whole series of problems. There was no teaching included, as originally planned; there were also no preliminary studies, no prior consultation with the people in the community, and no provision for supporting staff from the Ministry of Health. The creation of a new province, Luapula, in January 1958 complicated the project, and the task of coordinating activities now fell on the Provincial Commissioner. Difficulty at the provincial level— when there was no coordination at territorial and federal levels—was an ever-present problem.

The scheme was rescheduled and divided into three phases:

1 *Investigational Phase:* conducting surveys on
   a health
   b nutrition
   c agriculture
   d sociology

2 *Assessment Phase:* initiation of improvement in measures found in Phase 1.

3. *Assessment Phase:* repeating of initial surveys to determine the improvement in health, diet and living conditions, and to estimate the cost of such improvements.

Three localities with differing topographical and economic conditions were chosen: Matanda, a riverine area; Shikamushili, a lacustrine area; and Mutipula, a plateau area. The team held discussion with the chiefs and headmen to explain the objectives and obtain their consent for the project. Later, the chiefs and headmen were invited to a week-long course at the Development Area Training Center where details of the scheme were further elaborated.

At Matanda and Shikamushili the reaction was favorable, but at Mutipula only the health aspects of the scheme and not the agricultural aspects of the scheme were accepted. Apparently, someone had convinced the people that the scheme was devised by the Europeans to steal their land. Mutipula was therefore abandoned and urban Fort Rosebery substituted.

One major problem in implementing the project was the coordination of the various workers belonging to different organizations: officers came from the territorial government, federal government, WHO, and the Rhodes Livingstone Institute. Monthly meetings were instituted to deal with this situation, but other administrative problems arose. Construction of camps at pilot areas, establishing office organization, preparation of contracts for staff employed by the scheme, equipping of the laboratory, arranging payment of salaries, systematizing the delivery of material and the control of transport—all had to be arranged on an ad hoc basis when the staff were already in the field instead of being prepared beforehand.

In August 1958, a major subject was the posting of local medical staff from the Federal Ministry of Health to take over the work of the WHO consultants. The Director of Medical Services said, however, that he would post a Medical Inspector instead of a Medical Officer, noting that enough was known about parasitic infections in the pilot areas, and that their control could be initiated by methods already tested elsewhere in the country. The Director of Agriculture warned of the difficulty of replacing the Agricultural Officer attached to the scheme and due to go on leave. He said, however, that he would post a subordinate African staff member. The Director of the Rhodes Livingstone Institute was the only one who undertook to recruit a suitable sociologist of the required caliber.

At this stage, it was already apparent that the activities of the different disciplines were getting out of phase. To tie up with the scheme, the Development Area Training Center sent teams to teach village women childcare, cooking, sewing, knitting, and general care of the house; and to assist in building better village houses. On the agriculture side, the Livestock Officer cooperated by bringing in improved poultry, goats, sheep, and guinea pigs—the latter a popular food item. In the meantime, discussions were held among the WHO consultants and the Provincial Education Officer on what material to teach on hygiene.

In 1959, the Federal Ministry of Health followed through on its proposals by sending a Medical Inspector, an Anti-Malarial Officer, and a Medical Officer to the field. Their work included provision of protected water supplies, schistosomiasis control with molluscicide, and latrine digging as priority projects.

At Matanda the health team carried out a mass vaccination for smallpox and large scale treatment for intestinal parasites. A similar therapeutic campaign at Shikamushili had to be abandoned because the people refused to cooperate. The digging of latrines proved to be a slow process, with many households unwilling to find time to work.

One interesting, though unfortunate, development prevented success of part of the scheme at Matanda. Word spread that the proposed follow-up medical treatment and vaccination campaigns were aimed at sterilizing the children. Again the accusation of a "white man's scheme." The police advised the medical team that it was not safe to continue with the scheme, and thus, for the time, ended the Implementation Phase of the Health and Nutrition Scheme.

THE HEALTH AND NUTRITION SURVEY

Before the WHO team left, it identified the main dietary problems to be tackled:

Calorie Deficiency The reference scale for calorie requirement was based on the report of the FAO Second Committee on Caloric Requirements, adjusted to local conditions as recommended. The average caloric requirements per capita per day for Fort Rosebery (Mansa), Matanda, and Shikamushili were 2,146, 2,050 and 2,080, respectively. In the Fort Rosebery urban area it was found that households earning over £5 per month had an adequate caloric intake. In Matanda the calorie intake was slightly above the minimum requirement while at Shikamushili it fell below the requirement.

Deficiencies of Vitamins A and C Biochemical investigations indicated that 29% of children examined had vitamin A plasma levels below 20 micrograms per cent, indicating widespread and severe vitamin A deficiency. The nutrition survey showed that vitamin A intake was about 60% of requirement in Shikamushili and Fort Rosebery but almost adequate in Matanda. Clinical examination of 1675 children showed a high incidence of blindness, other eye symptoms, and skin changes, all of which were generally ascribed to vitamin A deficiency. Vitamin A deficiency was also considered a principal factor in the general poor health and the high child mortality rate due to lowered resistance to infectious diseases and parasitic infestations.

Vitamin C determinations were carried out on a comparatively small sample. Results indicated that in Fort Rosebery, 35.5% of children and 89.5% of adults were below requirement; in Matanda 28.6% of children and 100% of adults were deficient; and in Shikamushili 34.8% of children were below requirement.

The report recommended growing spring onions, more peppers (which, in the red stage, have a high content of vitamins A and C), as well as the planting of fruit trees and pawpaws.

Other investigations documented incidence of malaria, hookworm, schistosomiasis, and anemia.

Anemia

	Infant 0-10kg	Preschool 10-20kg	Schoolchildren 20kg
Matanda	97%	97%	78%
Fort Rosebery	97%	85%	69%
Shikamushili	88%	76%	35%

Rates of both anemia and parasitic disease were found to be quite high, but the report noted that infestation by one parasite alone did not play a major role in the etiology of anemia. It considered, however, that coupled with a low dietary intake of iron and protein, the total load of all parasites could be presumed to be the underlying cause of anemia.

Food analysis showed that all diets had an iron content well above 12 mg. In view of the clinical findings, it seemed possible that either the requirement was greater than suggested, and/or the iron was present in a form that could not be readily absorbed by the body.

Deficiency of Vitamin B The team also suggested it possible that lack of B vitamins may have played a part in producing some of the anemia. The team recommended increased consumption of foods of animal origin, pulses, and fresh young leaves.

Inadequate Feeding of Infants Observations in the field confirmed that the feeding of infants after the age of six months was one of the major problems to be tackled and emphasized that the training of women as extension workers was of prime importance to improved nutritional standards. The team recommended that simple cooking be introduced early in schools and that equipment used should be related to that available in the villages.

Economic Factors Important relationships between economic factors and nutrition improvement both in the urban and rural areas were shown. The report quoted the example of a village in which 14.8% of the limited income was spent on fish, 5.0% on salt, and not less than 22% on other food. "Widows and old couples spent an even greater proportion of their incomes on food; for there is a dependence on cash purchases of foodstuffs despite subsistence production. This fact underlies the well-known need for rural economic development."

Changing Patterns The nutrition survey also revealed some effects of urbanization and education on the food consumption pattern. It indicated that "if effective measures to improve economic status and create better living conditions are introduced in rural areas, these will be reflected in a changing food pattern. Imported foods like bread, tea, sugar, and milk become increasingly popular among wage earners."

As a result of these findings the WHO team made the following recommendations:

- Introduction of registration of births and deaths in the pilot areas
- Programs to control malaria, schistosomiasis, tuberculosis, smallpox, diphtheria, whooping cough, venereal disease, and eye problems
- Improvement of infant diet
- Antenatal and well-baby clinics
- Education of women and school pupils in health and nutrition
- Special training of selected families in nutrition, hygiene, gardening, and keeping livestock
- Introduction of a high protein biscuit as a school snack
- Promotion of school gardens
- Better village planning

THE AGRICULTURAL SURVEY

The agricultural survey placed special emphasis on obtaining quantitative details for comparing the pilot areas and clarifying the relationship of production to diet and health. The investigation observed that "improved nutrition will depend to a great degree on improvement in subsistence agriculture." Those engaged in the survey concluded that before initiating full-scale extension work to improve subsistence agriculture, further research was needed on such topics as the work done per day by the men and women and the total man- and woman-days of work required for adequate subsistence production; the price of labor and the various methods of payment; the timing of millet sowing and the effect of providing better seed beds than in the traditional system; the testing of crop strains and species not indigenous to the area, and so forth.

The Agricultural Officer felt, however, that a few obvious needs could be met at once. These included, among others, the eradication of vermin (the biggest single factor in decreasing crop availability), the introduction of disease-free cassava cuttings and educational propaganda on the use of this planting material, the provision of seed supplies for secondary crops, and the planting of fruit trees, as well as the resettlement of overcrowded communities.

THE FIRST ZAMBIAN NUTRITION INTERVENTIONS

The Problem of Blindness

A detailed survey in 1956 estimated the prevalence of the totally blind as 2,365 per 100,000 population. The cause of this extensive blindness was unclear to the government ophthalmologist in charge of the survey, who stated that "malnutrition is definitely not present in the population as a whole, so it can be excluded as a contributory factor. The only conclusion that seems to be feasible is that universal use of native treatment supplied the necessary 'noxious factor.' "

In 1961, however, an investigation of blindness concluded that "the major cause of blindness in the Luapula Province is keratomalacia caused by juvenile malnutrition, especially as regards vitamin A."

An ophthalmologist from Britain stressed the multiple pathology of the blindness cases by noting that "malnutrition (usually in the form of vitamin A deficiency resulting in xerophthalmia) is responsible for the majority of blindness seen and infection, trachoma, and sometimes native medicine are important secondary factors. Measles and smallpox are very often associated with the onset of blindness, usually because they precipitate the child into an acute malnutritional state, and at the same time reduce the resistance to bacterial infection."

The following year, a fellow ophthalmologist stated his belief that opacification of the cornea was due to vitamin A deficiency caused by malabsorption of vitamin A and its precursors from a diet grossly deficient in fat.

However, Mr. C. M. Phillips, a government ophthalmologist, later raised some questions regarding these opinions:

• Why, with roughly 300 children admitted to Lusaka Central Hospital suffering from the grossest form of deficiency and malnutrition, do only one or two cases per year have eye lesions?

• Why do identical lesions occur in adults who use native medicine, without any background of measles or malnutrition?

• Why does the Southern Province, with the worst record for avitaminosis and malnutrition, have the lowest blindness record of any province?

Further studies on the distribution of blindness and on the 1963 census proved beyond doubt that the original rates for blindness were grossly overestimated, although there was a close relationship between the density of population settlement and the incidence of blindness, and the onset of blindness did occur primarily in children under 10 years of age.

Following these studies, the Zambian National Council for the Blind and Handicapped obtained cabinet support for a supplementary feeding program for the Luapula Valley to begin in October 1966. The scheme was dropped after a very short time and was criticized for its performance on the grounds that:

• the supervisory staff was totally inadequate for the area covered
• supplementary food was issued irrespective of clinical need and without nutrition education
• no system for effective evaluation of the scheme's results had been devised

From Mining Companies to National Nutrition Council

Meanwhile, outside of government and international organization schemes, the Rokana Mine Corporation was organizing nutrition interventions among its employees. As far back as 1955, Rokana had established Malnutrition Clinics, under medical supervision, in which all children were under regular medical supervision from birth until they reached the weight of 40 lb. In 1961, a survey of the incidence and severity of malnutrition among Africans at the Rokana Corporation's Nkana Mine revealed that malnutrition occurred in children under the age of three years and that "most of the trouble appeared to commence at weaning." No relationship was noted between the amount of wages earned and the incidence of malnutrition "but [malnutrition] appeared to be closely connected with the character of the mother."

The incidence of malnutrition was higher in the first six months of the year, with the most severe cases and deaths occurring in January and February, or following a visit to the home village. The periodicity of malnutrition results from the fact that the rains begin in November or December, by which time the stores of the previous crops are exhausted. Rains also bring with them a period when intestinal diseases are common, producing conditions favorable to the onset of malnutrition. At the onset of the rainy season, women go out early to cultivate the fields taking with them the small children and little or no food to eat until they return home late in the afternoon. This pattern continues until March or April when the crops ripen, at which time the incidence of malnutrition begins to decline. This Rokana study also produced evidence counter to the common belief that the onset of kwashiorkor in an older child coincides with the birth of a new infant: out of 314 cases of kwashiorkor, 278 were the youngest in the family and only 36 had a younger sibling.

Conscious of the findings from the many surveys and continuing in its efforts to find an answer to the problems of malnutrition, the government sought assistance from international agencies (WHO, FAO, UNICEF) to establish an Applied Nutrition Program in Luapula, Mongu, and Balovale. The three areas chosen represented major population concentrations, a high incidence of diseases, blindness, and vitamin A deficiency, as well as seasonal food shortages. The areas also had few or no facilities for marketing agricultural products, as well as poor communication. These very reasons for choosing the areas for the project later became major contributing factors to the failure of implementation of the programs.

Drawing up of the Plan of Operations began in 1962, and it was finally signed by the government in February 1965. The general goals of the program were "to raise the standards of living and the level of health of the rural population of Zambia and to strengthen the agricultural economy." The program aimed to "promote home production and consumption of adequate food crops to alleviate the nutritional need of the people." Specific short term objectives included training of agricultural, health, and community development workers, carrying out a program of applied nutrition in the three pilot areas, and establishing a National Food and Nutrition Committee to achieve an integrated approach to rural development. The plan of operations, therefore, provided for the establishment of a new coordinating body called the National Nutrition Council.

THE NATIONAL NUTRITION COUNCIL

This National Nutrition Council, designed to achieve an integrated approach to the applied nutrition scheme through coordination of the various agencies, departments, and ministries, represented the most important development in national nutrition policy to that time. It was the first organization ever formed to coordinate nutrition efforts in the country.

Although well-intentioned, properly defined, and carefully planned, the implementation phase suffered considerable delays due to unforeseen circumstances:

• Following the dissolution of the Federation of Rhodesia and Nyasaland, the responsibilities shifted from the federal to the territorial government. The structure of government underwent complete reorganization. New ministries and new policies were formulated and adopted, new priorities were set, and the Applied Nutrition Program, like many other schemes, suffered as a consequence.

• The great distances between the three pilot areas posed serious difficulties for adequate supervision.
• Uncertainty regarding future policy of the new government toward services by expatriates resulted in many expatriate workers leaving, thus creating a sudden shortage of qualified staff.
• The post of full-time secretary to the council, who would coordinate the activities of the scheme, was not filled for about 18 months.

The Executive Committee of the council had its first meeting in December 1964, and the full National Nutrition Council held its first meeting in February 1965. The council was composed of the Permanent Secretary of the Ministry of Agriculture as chairman, with members representing the ministries of Health, Education, Information, Housing and Social Development, and Local Government, and the Zambian Institute of Social Research, and also including the Mayor of Lusaka and the Archbishop of the Anglican Church. Many of these people were so involved in their own high level work that they really did not give the council very much time. In the end, the council met only twice: the first and last meetings. The Executive Committee met eleven times, but on the average each member attended only three meetings and the turnover at meetings was almost 100%. With the exception of the chairman, the membership from the ministries was completely changed three times in 18 months. In addition, the level of representation was normally such that there was no ministerial responsibility for decisions taken. At best, each member would undertake to report to his ministry and urge early and sympathetic consideration.

Finally, the council came into being just at the time Northern Rhodesia became Zambia, i.e., at the time of independence. This brought about a problem of shifting responsibilities. Originally, health matters were the responsibility of the Ministry of Health of the federal government of Rhodesia and Nyasaland. These responsibilities had now to be taken on by the new government. Not only that, but the new government was involved in reconstructing its entire organization, policies, and ministries, once again leaving much nutrition work under local control. Under these circumstances, the council did not work properly as a central body.

In addition, a number of people involved with the program in a decision-making role were expatriates, who, at the time of independence, felt very uncomfortable. They did not know whether to continue working for the government or what their future would be; a number of them left. This meant a shortage of staff to carry out the program by the end of 1966.

REORGANIZING NUTRITION EFFORTS IN ZAMBIA

FAO Recommendations

These experiences led the government in 1966 to suspend the Applied Nutrition Program and request FAO assistance in a search for successful coordination. The FAO team carried out a short term Food and Nutrition Survey, concluding that malnutrition was a major problem in the country, one that was likely to become worse without prompt and decisive action. The team also observed that there was lack of basic data on local and national levels to allow any meaningful planning of either nutrition policies or programs.

The following specific tasks remained to be carried out according to the recommendation of the team:

• To give full national campaign status to the start of a program for nutrition improvement. National campaign status was felt necessary if the program was to have any impact.
• To center the National Food and Nutrition Campaign *directly* under the cabinet in order to formulate policy.
• To appoint a National Food and Nutrition Commission, divorced from all ministries, to implement policy.
• To appoint an Advisory Committee of experts to advise the commission.
• To appoint an Executive Secretary to the commission with ancillary staff.

And, with the help of UN specialized agencies and friendly governments:

• To make statistically representative sample food consumption and nutrition status surveys in order to fill gaps in basic data.
• To build up an integrated program for promotion of good nutrition based on factual data collected.
• To reinforce and expand preventive services against malnutrition.
• To link with the Office of National Development and Planning for incorporation of nutrition improvement policy in overall development planning.

Government Policy

In accepting the recommendations of the team, the policymaking body for the commission laid down some basic principles:

• The program would be national in character, initiated and activated by the Government of the Republic of Zambia with assistance from international agencies and friendly governments;
• Each ministry would be responsible for executive action relating to subjects within its portfolio;
• Priority was to be given to implementation of plans based on current knowledge, rather than research, but the need for research was recognized and accepted;

• The maximum cooperation and understanding of the people was to be ensured at all levels of planning and execution;
• The ultimate responsibility for adequate nutrition was recognized to rest with the family.

This policy included the creation of an independent, statutory body, the National Food and Nutrition Commission, answerable to the cabinet through the Minister of Health. The debate in the National Assembly and the strong supporting speech by the Ministry of Health made public the government's policy and gave assurance of powerful and sustained political support.

Before deciding on the cabinet as the policymaking body and creating the National Food and Nutrition Commission as an independent body, a study was made on the state of the administrative infrastructure in Zambia and other countries regarding nutrition programs. A review of international experience and practices indicated that coordination is the most puzzling problem. Responsibility for nutrition planning and coordination is allocated variously to a national nutrition institute, the individual ministries, or national nutrition councils or commissions. In trying to arrive at a form of organization suitable for Zambia, each of the above solutions was closely examined. Institutes seemed, by definition, primarily devoted to research and training. It was felt that as "institutes" their role would be only advisory and that a further disadvantage would be the tendency to be dominated by one discipline. On the other hand, if a ministry were given total responsibility, nutrition would be relegated to a low priority among many other activities. Where nutrition councils or committees exist, they are usually composed of representatives from the ministries, and, as was experienced in Zambia from 1964 to 1966, the level of representation is often such that there is no ministerial commitment to decisions taken. Under such an arrangement, there is also the tendency to leave all responsibility for a particular project to the ministry which initiated it, thus dashing any hope of successful coordination.

After much study, the ideal characteristics of a coordinating body were defined to be:

• conviction in the soundness and vital importance of the program which it administers, and a determination to carry it out
• authority to carry out the program, with ready access to the source of government policy in the event of obstruction
• the respect of the disciplines and agencies to be coordinated
• unbiased approach in efforts to attain harmonious collaboration
• effective units within each agency capable of being coordinated
• self-effacement, permitting all credit to go to the executing agencies
• capacity to shoulder responsibility for deficiencies and a resilience to be able to remedy them

It was felt that the creation of a corporate body would free operations from the stultifying effects of bureaucratic procedures and increase flexibility to cope with both governmental and nongovernmental organizations. By placing it under the cabinet, the new organization was saved from the ministerial sphere of influence, so often characterized by rivalries and jealousies.

The goals of the commission were spelled out in detail. These included mandates to reduce mortality due directly or indirectly to malnutrition, to improve the nutritional status of vulnerable groups, to create community interest in better nutrition, to make nutritional provision for a rapidly growing population, to collect food consumption and nutrition data on a national scale, to incorporate nutrition improvement in food and agricultural development planning, and to implement the government's food and nutrition policy.

Approved by the cabinet, the Food and Nutrition Commission was formed in 1967. Perhaps the biggest single undertaking carried out by the Commission, with financial and technical assistance from the UN Special Fund and FAO/WHO, was the countrywide comprehensive nutrition survey. Under the maxim, "No survey without subsequent services," the work was regarded as a means to an end: the introduction of measures to improve the nutritional well-being of the population.

The request to the UN Special Fund for financial assistance was made in December 1967 and approved by the Governing Council in January 1969. The survey started in September 1969 and the project officially ended in December 1972. The survey aimed at quantifying year-round food intake for the rural population and identifying variables that influence food intake. Data collected included information on expenditure, sociocultural factors, village subsistence agriculture, food losses, food storage, traditional methods of food processing, and seasonal food variations. The results from the survey showed that cereals, especially maize, were the most important staple in all the provinces, followed by cassava. Consumption of vegetables was also very high compared to items such as fruits, eggs, milk, fats, and oils. Fish consumption in all the provinces was a more important source of animal protein than meat. In effect, the problems identified were the same as those identified from the beginning in the early '30s.

Survey Findings

The FAO estimated that the national average for calorie requirement is about 2,050 calories per person per day. The survey showed that average calorie intake varied from 1,580 to 1,850, an overall calorie deficiency of about 20%. These figures describe household averages and not individual consumption, and the uneven distribution, both on a regional basis and within each household, implies that the percentage of households suffering severe deficiencies must be quite high. The FAO reports conclude that "the general deficiency of food intake in terms of calories is the most serious nutritional problem."

As for protein, surveys showed an average intake of 36.8-38.4 g reference protein per day, a significantly higher level of consumption than the 25 g estimated requirement. Thus, protein deficiency per se is not a serious problem; however, the report concluded that "protein deficiency is present as a result of calorie deficiency, because a portion of protein calories is presumably used to meet energy requirements." In communal feeding, maldistribution of food within the family may result in individual instances of protein deficiency, because, as Thomson notes, "intake varies with the size of hand and manual dexterity, to the disadvantage of the young." The data suggest, furthermore, that variation in protein intake is directly correlated with fish consumption, particularly dried fish, which is not readily available during the wet season. Thus, where protein deficiency does exist, there is a wet-season peak in its occurrence.

A total of 7,550 individuals were examined during the clinical evaluation phase of the project. Malnutrition was found to be widespread throughout the country, affecting all groups, with protein calorie deficiency most prevalent among children aged 0-4 years. Of this age group, 37.3% were classified as being severely malnourished (below 60% of standard as given by Jelliffe, 1966), with growth retardation beginning at about four months after birth.

Of the 5,287 children examined, only 14 (0.2%) had kwashiorkor; 34 (0.7%) had marasmus; and 5 (0.1%) had marasmic kwashiorkor, indicating that these severe forms of PCM were probably not a problem. The report, however, cautioned that the number of children 0-4 years examined may have been too small and that "because of this and the subjectivity of the clinical diagnosis it would not be safe to draw conclusions from these data on the relative severity of PCM . . . nor would it be justified to conclude that it does not exist. . . ."

Although severe forms of protein calorie malnutrition were relatively uncommon in the 5-14 age group, occurrence of some cases was indicative of extensive poor nutrition in the community. Evidence from previous surveys and hospital records supports the view that PCM is still a major problem. Reports from the Schools Medical Services showed that of all primary schoolchildren examined, 25% to 27% showed marked signs of malnutrition with a further 50-60% suffering from some degree of undernutrition or mild malnutrition. In addition, the Ministry of Health Annual Reports for the years 1964, 1965, 1966 listed bronchopneumonia, gastroenteritis, malnutrition, tuberculosis, and measles, all of which are frequently associated with PCM, as the major individual causes of death among children.

Anthropometric measurements and biochemical test (serum albumin levels) showed that pregnant and lactating mothers also suffered some degree of calorie and protein deficiency. The average weight at the end of pregnancy was generally not much greater than that of nonpregnant women. Only in one province (Central) was the average gain in weight in the third trimester at an acceptable level (8.5 kg).

Occurrence of anemia was generally found in association with parasitic infections (malaria, hookworm, schistosomiasis). Using the hematocrit test, deficient values were found in 5.2% and low values in 13.4% of the 6,740 people examined. Although average serum iron levels were not found to be deficient, it was strongly felt (a) that iron deficiency coupled with malarial infection was the main cause of anemia, and (b) that since the diet was based mainly on cereals, absorption of iron was low due to poor ascorbic acid content.

The report considered that a serious level of vitamin A deficiency existed in 15% of the population. Although no cases of keratomalacia were found during the survey, cases were reported from hospitals. Vitamin A deficiency has been designated as one of the major nutritional problems of Zambia because of the possible effects of vitamin A deficiency in growth retardation and poor resistance to infection.

Riboflavin deficiency was widespread and occurred in the same areas as PCM.

HEALTH DEVELOPMENT PROGRAMS IN RELATION TO NUTRITIONAL PROGRAMS

In the past, most medical facilities and budget allocations in the health sector were devoted to curative medicine. Recently, however, the government, with the collaboration of WHO, developed and began implementing a 10-year National Health Plan (1972-81) for Basic Health Services, with emphasis on the construction of more rural health facilities. Under this program activities of all under-5s clinics, Schools Medical Services and Health Education have been incorporated in the Maternal and Child Health Program. Under-5s clinics have been renamed Children's Clinics and will provide care up to the age of 11 years with special emphasis on the improvement of nutrition of infants, children, and pregnant and nursing mothers. In the Basic Health Services program more emphasis than ever is being placed on preventive measures, including nutrition education and demonstrations. Clinics and Health Centers provide a framework for nutrition surveillance through the use of weight charts.

Nutrition Rehabilitation Centers are currently being operated by four nutrition groups and two mission hospitals where mothers, with their malnourished children, are kept for periods up to three weeks. During this period, the mothers are taught nutrition while the children are given medical care. After discharge, the nearest Health Center provides follow-up care.

AGRICULTURAL DEVELOPMENT PROGRAMS IN RELATION TO NUTRITIONAL PROBLEMS

Traditionally, Northern Rhodesia or Zambia has been dependent on the export of copper. We have now come to realize that copper is a depletable commodity. The present policy of the government is, therefore, to reorient the

programs toward agricultural production both for home consumption and
for export.

Agricultural policies and programs are undergoing great changes in order to
achieve the government's goal of self-sufficiency in almost all foodstuffs that
can be locally produced. A seminar was mounted at the beginning of 1974 to
draw up a program of action, and the policies adopted included:

- subsidized farm expenses, such as fertilizer, seed, water supply, fences, and
so on
- assurance by the government that it would buy all the farmer's produce at
a government-fixed price irrespective of the farm's location with respect to
centers of consumption
- free extension service to all classes of farmers

The seminar adopted the slogan "Grow More Food and Feed the Nation."
In staple foods, such as maize, the goal is to grow enough for self-sufficiency
plus 50% above demand as reserve.

Each year prices are declared for a number of crops well in advance of the
planting season. Producer prices of beef, pork, and milk are also regulated and
vary periodically in the light of changes in the cost of production. The producer pricing mechanism is used to encourage or discourage production of
certain crops.

The government also pays a wide range of subsidies to producers and consumers to keep down prices of certain foods such as maize meal and meat. In
the June 1975 "Watershed Speech" by the president, 60% of these subsidies
were to be removed and the cost passed on to the consumer.

In accordance with its policy of rural development, the government is making every effort to carry out an agrarian revolution by making every village a
productive unit for foodstuffs as well as a locus for the secondary industries
based on agriculture. The major production units at the moment are state
ranches, state farms, commercial farms, and various cooperatives.

A new boost to rural development and to food production in particular is
the introduction of "national service camps" in all the districts. This program
with a budget of K17.5 million (US$27 million) for 1975/76 is aimed at
encouraging youth to "go back to the land" and take up farming as a career
in order to increase food production and provide employment. In order to
carry out this policy, the government announced in June 1975 major changes
in the pattern of land tenure. All freehold land was converted into leasehold
for a period of 100 years, with no private buying or selling. For the next
century, all is invested in the president as custodian on behalf of the people.

Under the Female Extension Service Section of the Department of Agriculture, a program has been devised specifically for women to help them produce more and varied foods for their families. The program is coupled with
home economics and nutrition education. The training takes place at Community Development Centers, Homecraft Centers, Farm Training Centers, and
informally in groups at the village level.

The mobilization of the masses to produce more food is in keeping with the Philosophy of Humanism, a policy centered on development programs for the people which calls for production by the masses rather than mass production by the few. Long term improvement in the level of nutrition of the population now living mainly at subsistence level will depend to a large extent on their entrance into the market economy.

To further the aims of this policy, the previous encouragement of foreign investment in the Zambian economy has been changed. Last year, 54 items were deleted from the import list. These food items—tea and tinned things which can be produced locally, such as fish and vegetables—are now no longer imported into the country. Related to this policy, the government is allowing private investment and private enterprise only up to the point that the private firm makes a net profit of K0.5 million (about US$770,000). After that, the government steps in and acquires controlling interest. This is done purposely to prevent anyone from becoming a large scale capitalist within a "Humanistic" society.

The Zambian Food and Nutrition Program is therefore based on having an adequate administrative infrastructure, an effective means of communication, and a systematic method of planning on a national basis. Its approach to nutritional problems is not based on supplementary food disbursement but on integrating food and nutrition policies and programs into development programs of the various sectors, coupled with a strong national nutrition education campaign. The commission's main roles are thus: (1) supervisory in all matters concerning food and nutrition; and, (2) advisory to the government and the administration, providing information on the nutritional needs of the people, guidance on ways and means in which improvement can best be effected, and assistance in the coordination of plans and programs for development involving nutrition.

Table 1
Malnutrition in Zambia, 1970-73

	Hospitals			Health Centers		
	Outpatients	Inpatients	Deaths	Outpatients	Inpatients	Deaths
1970						
Total	26,481	7,851	907	56,715	3,793	132
1972						
Total	15,413	7,570	1,048	50,299	3,354	118
1973						
Province:						
Central	1,872	1,085	228	8,718	131	7
Copperbelt	1,485	2,765	456	7,689	158	8
Eastern	962	637	86	2,352	520	24
Luapula	944	496	89	3,669	278	14
Northern	1,532	979	107	5,659	850	31
North Western	851	401	35	1,649	252	3
Southern	2,212	1,240	113	4,840	265	14
Western	1,354	637	75	1,227	106	3
Total	11,192	7,640	1,189	35,812	2,560	104

Table 2
Six major causes of mortality and morbidity in childhood. Zambia health centers totals, 1973

Diagnosis	No. of Outpatients (New Cases Only)
Malaria	413,493
Measles	65,719
Respiratory diseases	1,164,974
Gastroenteritis	1,154,613
Malnutrition	35,812
Anemia	24,754
Total	2,859,365

Table 3
Six major causes of mortality and morbidity in childhood. Zambia hospitals totals, 1973

Diagnosis	No. of Outpatients
Malaria	151,215
Measles	15,558
Respiratory diseases	348,566
Gastroenteritis	389,668
Malnutrition	11,192
Anemia	11,355
Total	927,554

Table 4
Inpatient case fatality rate (number of deaths per 1,000 admissions), Zambia, 1970-73

Diagnosis	Year 1970	1972	1973
Health Centers			
Malaria	6.0	7.2	8.4
Measles	25.8	30.4	30.1
Respiratory diseases	13.2	15.2	16.2
Gastroenteritis	13.5	17.1	12.9
Malnutrition	34.8	35.1	40.6
Anemia	34.5	43.5	45.1
Hospitals			
Malaria	17.9	14.9	18.0
Measles	68.4	68.9	78.5
Respiratory diseases	51.9	48.7	56.1
Gastroenteritis	57.4	54.7	51.5
Malnutrition	115.5	138.4	155.6
Anemia	49.7	53.7	67.4

DISCUSSION (ZAMBIA)

Wray

Those of us who follow the literature but haven't been to Zambia have heard a lot about the under-5s program. I wonder if you could tell us something about the impact of those clinics on nutrition, especially on PCM in preschool kids?

Vamoer

They have worked and they have not. If a nutrition program has been associated with the under-5s clinics, then the clinic has an impact. In 1968, we had an MCH specialist from Denmark, who was assigned to Luapula province where we had the largest number of under-5s clinics. His duty was to organize nutrition and health education. He worked there for over two years on education and also held seminars and workshops for the paramedical staff. In a 1971 follow-up report in that province, it was shown that the mortality figures had dropped from 43% to 23%—a reduction of about 50% in two years. On the other hand, where under-5s clinics operate as hospitals, offering purely curative services, they do not seem to work.

Wray

From what I read about these under-5s clinics, I thought that the basic concept was that they would *not* operate as hospitals, that they were specifically *not* for curative purposes.

Vamoer

Yes, this was the concept, but the Medical Assistants who run them sometimes act as if they were hospitals. In the new plan, set up in 1971-72, emphasis in all the clinics is going to be on nutrition and health education. There is a demonstration area being tested to organize a center which will serve as a focus for about 10,000 people. There will be a medical assistant, a midwife, a nutritionist, a rural development worker, and an agricultural extension worker, all five working as a team serving that one area.

Sai

What involvement has the university in your programs? I think this will be very important in the long run.

Vamoer

Just a minimum role, at present. We do have plans, of course. In the setup of the commission, there is provision for nutrition research. We did have plans for our own nutrition research unit, but this did not materialize partly because we have a National Scientific Research Council which coordinates and carries out research for the whole country.

As far back as 1968, the commission wrote to the vice chancellor of the University of Zambia to see if they would establish a chair of nutrition so that nutrition research could be done within the university, but nothing has

happened along those lines. We have even promised to provide one nutritionist to teach both in the biochemistry section and in the medical school, noting that this one person probably could provide a core for the eventual establishment of a nutrition research unit. But, again, nothing has happened.

Sai
Well, without waiting for a chair, how about involvement of the medical
students in their communities?

Vamoer
We are not ready for that yet. We are coordinating our work with the National Scientific Research Council, which has a good laboratory.

Wray
Did you have many medical students involved in surveys, for example, or
other activities?

Vamoer
No.

Latham
The problem is, of course, that so few physicians are interested in nutrition.
There isn't anybody available at the medical school.

Wray
But getting the students involved in these surveys is one way around that. It is
not infallible, but if you can catch them early enough, it might make a difference.

Vamoer
A difficulty in using the university students is that the surveys require full-
time workers for a year. A student would not do that.

Latham
One of the success stories, I think, that Zambia has been too modest about is
the public relations aspect of nutrition. I do not know any other country that
has done so well in this area. Right from the beginning, the nutrition people
made the president and the cabinet ministers aware of the nutritional problem. One can now turn on the Zambian radio at any time and, within an
hour, hear some nutrition message coming over the air. There is a huge effort
to put out educational materials coming largely from the Zambian Food and
Nutrition Commission that Alec heads. They produce records, films, and
other material. Again, I do not think that this has been evaluated in terms of
its effect on nutritional status, but, in my view, creating awareness of the
nutrition problems in a country is an essential first step.

   The Zambian Food and Nutrition Commission also, I think, is unusual in
that it has been set up as a separate entity, not a part of any ministry. In
Tanzania, they have only now reached the stage where they are trying to get

such an institution started. In Ghana, they have shifted from one thing to
another. The Zambian Food and Nutrition Commission was established as an
organization to coordinate nutrition; it has been in operation for a good number of years now, and there has been a fair amount of progress as a result.

Vamoer
The public relations aspect came about because we were trying to improve
the survey by running an education campaign simultaneously. This was done
in the belief that if you want to create consciousness, you must use every
possible channel. We started by using radio broadcasts: 50 minutes a week for
the program, 30 minutes in English, and the remaining 20 minutes in the local
languages.

Then we published the posters and pamphlets, which we sent out together
with a description of how to use them. We do not send these things to be
used simply as wall decorations, either in the clinics or in individual homes.
Each one of our posters is tested beforehand in the villages to see whether the
idea being conveyed by the posters is actually being understood by the
people. We have, in addition to this, leaflets that we send to schools and clinics. We hope that, through these activities, changes in the attitudes of the
people will, in the long run, influence adoption of better nutrition practices.

Sai
You did start a periodical or a journal, I remember. Is it still going?

Vamoer
The *Nutrition News* is still going.

Thomson
I have been closely associated with this case, but there is a part that I do not
know. I would like to ask Alec whether the results in this newest survey differ
in any way from the findings of Richards and Widdowson in 1934.

Vamoer
I think the simple answer there is "No." There is not any significant change
from the early surveys to the surveys we did. I think the reason is that, when
the surveys were done, some suggestions for programs were made, but implementation never took place.

Latham
Alec is being very kind to the international organizations that supported
Zambia. The survey was largely an FAO survey with some WHO support,
conducted with a very large effort from Zambia. The belief was fostered by
these groups that this nutrition survey—perhaps the world's largest and most
expensive—would result in the UN agencies' providing some help to solve the
Zambian problems uncovered in that survey. In my view, the international
organizations did not come through adequately afterwards.

This, I think, is a very important issue, and raises a question we can discuss

in general terms: Is a very expensive survey *ever* justified unless the organization which supports it is willing to spend perhaps ten times the cost of the
survey doing something about the problems discovered by the survey? I
would like to be openly critical of FAO in this regard. This is an example,
maybe, of the kind of case worth looking at in regard to the whole question
of surveys. They are useful if they elicit information about nutrition, but the
problem, as Mr. Thomson mentioned earlier, is that, in this survey, they
weighed and measured food in households and did other costly things when
they could have gotten information *almost* as worthwhile in a *much* cheaper
way.

Sai
I would like to underscore Michael's question about when the search for
exact scientific measurement has to stop and some common sense acceptance
has to be used as a basis for planning. When I was in FAO, I was known for
not being very scientific in my attitude because I said that, if you go to the
major markets of an area and the staple food is not available, then the people
are starving. You do not have to go and weigh. One of the things that we need
to consider are indicators: not only scientifically precise indicators, but qualitative indicators that can be used for very rapid assessment of whether a community is likely to be having nutrition problems.

Antrobus
It certainly strikes me that the amount of information being injected into
surveys in general has been increasing exponentially, with an inverse relationship to the practical usefulness to the country concerned. In the Caribbean,
one of the things that we are trying to determine is the minimum data required to provide a useful working diagnosis for formulating food and nutrition policy. The whole theme of nutritional diagnosis is a very important
issue.

   More specifically in relation to Zambia, you mentioned the banning of
import of some 50 or more food items. What these items had in common is
that they were tinned, manufactured products. Was this, therefore, done
primarily for nutritional considerations?

Vamoer
Economic considerations.

Antrobus
Certainly, among many of those tinned items, are some of the most useful
foods for the poor in terms of nutrient cost. Would the Nutrition Council
possibly have some say, as an advisory body, in which foods are no longer
imported?

Vamoer
These items have been banned, first, because of the economic considerations;
second, because of their conflict with the present course of rural develop-

ment. The items which we import as tinned foodstuffs can be easily grown in the country. It is hoped that willfully creating a deficiency of the items will stimulate the growing of some of these foodstuffs. In other words, it is hoped to discourage the importation of foods from other countries and the imposition of foreign habits.

Antrobus

By the same token, does the Nutriton Council have a say in the agricultural policies regarding which goods are grown?

Vamoer

Originally they did not consult us. Now, with the emphasis on rural development, this may change. Work is proceeding on the third national development plan, and we have been consulted on the proposed prices and crops and how agricultural projects should relate to overall government plans.

II COMMENTARIES

13 THE SYMBIOSIS OF SCIENTIST, PLANNER, AND ADMINISTRATOR IN NUTRITION PROGRAM IMPLEMENTATION

Ewen C. Thomson

NATURE OF ACTION IN THE AREA OF NUTRITION

Symbiosis is defined as "the living together in more or less intimate association or close union of two dissimilar organisms in mutually beneficial relationship." There are obvious difficulties in bringing together such dissimilar organisms as scientists, planners, and administrators, but, to achieve positive action and results, on the scale required and in the time available, demands the utmost effort for harmonious collaboration by all of those who should be involved in nutrition programs.

Forty years ago, men of vision recognized the need for action to combat hunger and malnutrition and that such action should be interdisciplinary. In 1935,[1] the League of Nations established a Joint Committee on Nutrition with the stated objective of bringing about the marriage of health and agriculture, but the marriage has existed in name only.* At the international level, rivalry or lack of accord exists between agencies or even between different departments of one organization. At the national level this bureaucratic malady is often intensified.

In January 1967, President Kaunda of Zambia transferred responsibility for nutrition from the Ministry of Agriculture to the Ministry of Health and prepared the way for the National Food and Nutrition Commission of Zambia. The Executive Secretary of the Commission called on the Director of Medical Services, who responded, "This is excellent. Now we can tell those others what to do and your outfit can see that it is carried out." What a basis for collaboration! The reaction of the then Permanent Secretary for Agriculture was even more extreme. "Speaking on behalf of the minister, I am to say that, as instructed, I am handing over the files relating to nutrition, but, from now on, agriculture will have nothing to do with nutrition." Fortunately officials come, ministers go, and situations change. Had responsibility for nutrition been transferred to a coordinating rather than a specialist ministry, as had been recommended, attitudes might not have been so intransigent.

The struggle for control of the subject nutrition in another country in Africa lasted for many years and became well known locally as the "tug-of-war." Appreciating the indispensability of having an integrated approach to solving nutrition problems, the Ministry of Agriculture established a nutrition unit and, through bilateral aid, engaged a medical nutritionist, a biochemist, and others. Within the governmental framework this solved no problem re-

*In the '60s FAO and WHO negotiated a "gentleman's agreement," undertaking not to trespass on each other's spheres of interest.

garding an integrated approach on a national basis. Applied Nutrition Projects in many countries were based on a similar fallacy, but in such cases it was the health ministries that sponsored protein production through animal husbandry, poultry, horticulture, and fish-farming. The awareness of a need for joint action was demonstrated, yet, by ignoring the normal machinery of government, this type of approach was not replicable on a national scale.

The integration of scientific knowledge is an acknowledged need, but all too many regard such integration from the point of view of a dominant discipline, their own, served by other disciplines. The bridging of disciplines—producing nutrition educationists, medical nutritionists, and nutrition programmers—is valuable, but such integration is still limited. Ideally there should be complete understanding in the mind of the individual responsible for action, but the scope of relevant knowledge is too vast and the only solution is to rely on a team, in which there should be precorrelation from the earliest stages rather than an attempted postcorrelation of independent, disciplinary studies. Connections cannot be grasped until there are factors to be connected, and a team's first task is to identify these factors. Thereafter, the integration of a team's combined knowledge is mainly dependent on its members' attitudes of mind. It will be far from easy to find teams which are determined to maintain human benefits as paramount and willing to subordinate self-interest or disciplinary prestige to the objectives of the programs.

A food and nutrition program cannot be considered in isolation, for it should involve a multitude of interests; yet for that same reason programs tend to be the responsibility of none. The fragmentation of science into ever more specialized subdivisions, each with its own esoteric language, is paralleled by the breakup of governments into highly specialized compartments. A Ministry of Agriculture may have a dozen or more different departments, with inadequate communication among them. Another important set of interests, but with other motivations and objectives, is private enterprise, as represented by commercial farming and the food processing and marketing industry. Change in the price structure of food products, or advertising, for example, may have more marked significance than intensive nutrition education.

In addition there are certain relevant characteristics of newly independent countries. There is a general lack of social discipline as instanced by deficiencies in legislation and in law observance and enforcement; failure to accept responsibility and take decisions; lack of obedience to instructions handed down to public officials at various levels; often collusion between these officials and powerful local persons or groups of persons; a general inclination of people to resist public controls and their implementation; and an apathy due to the fear of hope.

Where malnutrition is a national problem, in the sense that there is significant incidence of malnutrition in all parts of the country, it demands nationwide action and a national program. To have a series of small pilot projects at village level, in all provinces of a country, does not mean that all provinces are "covered." Those persons reached may represent a tiny fraction of the population. Nor does a nutrition institute become "national" solely because it is the only one in the country. To merit the title "national," the nutrition policy and program must involve reasonably rapid expansion so that the majority of those in need of help may be reached within a foreseeable future.

The melancholy fact is that effective nutrition programs rarely come into being. There have been projects and programs galore, many attaining good results within limits, but failing to achieve the impact and scope demanded by the magnitude of the problem.

Any meaningful nutrition program must be based on the best available scientific knowledge. The application of that knowledge must be planned, but the most perfectly prepared plans remain a mere paper exercise, unless there are the means to carry them out. Much emphasis on policy planning has been generated by international agencies, but such pressure appears to be premature when related to countries which do not have the administrative machinery to carry out a nutrition program. This is especially troublesome when the international agencies themselves do not coordinate their policies.

ADMINISTRATION

Traditional Role of Ministries

Because poor nutrition is often manifest first as a disease, the whole subject of "malnutrition" has been classified with diseases rather than with social conditions which should not exist. Health ministries have normally been allocated responsibility for dealing with clinical problems, and hence the whole subject of nutrition has often been relegated to the health bureaucracy. In the hierarchy of ministries, the Ministry of Health is comparatively weak and rarely can compete in the struggle for scarce resources with the ministries which deal with the economy and defense of the country. For example, in its Statement of Development Policies, 1971-80,[2] the Government of Malawi asserts: "The Malawi Government's revenue position does not permit expenditure on both the minimum acceptable level of treatment as well as on major preventive schemes: it is for this reason only that preventive health must for the time being be given a low order of priority."

Within the health ministries curative medicine dominates. Probably this priority is inevitable; as one matron-in-chief expressed it, "the sick are with us." Thus nutrition becomes a low priority responsibility of the impoverished partner, preventive medicine, and competes with the claims of smallpox, cholera, tuberculosis, and leprosy for a share of the meager resources available.

Quite apart from being accorded a low priority in a ministry's program, nutrition is further handicapped by being multidisciplinary. There is a natural tendency[3] for ministry officials to prefer objectives which are entirely within their own ministerial sphere of influence and control. Such circumscribed objectives are much less time-consuming and much more easily administered; rivalries, jealousies, and frustrations are lessened; and it is more satisfying to the personal ambition of the ministry staff, as credit for success cannot be in dispute and any lack of success is more easily locked away in the ministry's cupboard. Specialist ministries are notoriously inept in coordinating the activities of other specialists who, in turn, resent and resist extraneous attempts to exercise initiative and leadership over their activities. Thus there is a tendency to set up distinct objectives for each specialist agency, which pursues its own course of action in isolation.

Relationship to Other Administrative Machinery

Effective implementation depends upon the power behind the program, the sustained support from the highest levels of government. Many would maintain that only governments have the power to launch a national program and that, within government, the focal point for nutrition action should be as close to the mainspring of power as possible. This would probably result in putting nutrition within the responsibilities of a coordinating ministry, but there are also other possibilities. In Malawi, for example, there is no appropriate coordinating ministry and nutrition has become the responsibility of the Ministry of Agriculture, a very powerful ministry, whose minister is the Life President.

There can be no universal solution for the optimal administrative machinery. Each country's problems require individual understanding and response, not only because of differences in political policies and procedures, but also to cope with environmental variations and cultural contrasts. Malawi and Tanzania are neighboring countries, with very similar nutritional problems and cultural backgrounds, but with major differences in administrative organization. In a much larger country, Indonesia, which spans one-eighth of the world's circumference, there can be no simple national blueprint. Assuming a five-day week, an indefatigable traveler would require twelve years in order to spend one day on each of the inhabited islands. It is inevitable, therefore, that program planning in Indonesia must be broken down into homogeneous and manageable units, fitting into the existing political and administrative system.

Whatever solution is adopted, little is likely to happen unless the government has the will to work towards the means to achieve adequate nutrition for all its people. Under external pressure, many countries established national nutrition councils or committees. Although such committees may have provided merely a facile facade as a substitute for action, they were welcomed by the international bureaucracy. The National Nutrition Council of Zambia was established in this way. It was chaired by the Minister of Agriculture and its membership consisted of six parliamentary secretaries. At its first meeting it set up an executive committee and eighteen months later a second meeting was convened. At the first attempt only the chairman and his own parliamentary secretary turned up; at the second attempt a quorum decided to recommend that the council be dissolved.

The executive committee of that same national council, save for one representative from the university, consisted entirely of civil servants from the same ministries as were represented on the council. It met on eleven occasions, but there was no continuity of membership; on average, the attendance of an individual was three meetings; one ministry was represented by seven different individuals. The only continuity was the file of the minutes of the meetings, provided that the file could be found. The level of representation was another critical factor. Senior officials attended initially, but the tendency grew to send the officer who could be spared most easily. There could be no ministerial commitment; at best, the members would undertake to report back to their ministries. For most of the time the executive committee was served by a part-time junior official as secretary; the committee was executive only in name.

The Freedom From Hunger Campaign, National Committee of Zambia, had an even shorter active life. It was composed of very busy and influential dignitaries, who met only once, at an inaugural luncheon.

These examples of the ineffectiveness of councils and committees are by no means unique; their inefficacy has been repeated, with local variations, in almost all countries where they have been established. Their failure is easily understood; for membership of such committees is a secondary function of busy people whose primary loyalty is to the power and prerogatives of their own institution or geographic region. The existence of a national nutrition council or committee does *not* mean that government has the will to tackle nutrition problems; nor is it sufficient that ministerial decrees issue from an individual ministry.

Personnel and Administrative Organization

Particular attention must be paid to the personnel who are likely to be involved in the implementation of a national nutrition program. The late B. S. Platt early recognized the need for governments to formulate nutrition policies. At the end of World War II, he persuaded the then Colonial Office of the United Kingdom to support the training and appointment of nutrition officers, who would advise governments on nutrition policy. Selected graduates in nutrition, or its equivalent at that time, were given further training and were appointed to various dependencies, including Northern Rhodesia (Zambia). In this, there was a lack of understanding of how governments work. No matter how forceful and brilliant an officer might have been, there was virtually no chance of young and newly appointed, junior, professional officers having any major impact on an entrenched and stultified bureaucratic system.

There were opportunities, however, for these officers to collect the data which would build up gradually into an issue that claimed the attention of government.

In many countries, the status of the nonmedical nutritionist is very unsatisfactory. They have tended to be posted to do welfare work or advise on hospital diets. Save for the few who enter research institutes or universities, there is no career structure and recruitment is affected accordingly. Hence, although numerically there may appear to be an adequate number of qualified nutritionists, their training and subsequent experience may not fit them for large scale operations. Joe Wray[4] has pointed out that in industrially developed countries, a newly qualified graduate is employed by an established organization wherein there is direction and control, supervision and instruction from experienced senior staff, and recognized procedures and support services. Where no established organization exists, a newly qualified graduate may be thrown into a void, especially difficult if the immediate appointment is at director level.

At a workshop on the Nutrition Intervention Pilot Project, held in Bali during March 1975, the Indonesian participants were unanimous in considering managerial capacity as the prior constraint. It is an art involving ten components: foresight, creativity, planning, organization, direction, motivation, communication, coordination, control, and evaluation. The art of administration or management is the result of a long apprenticeship, through which some, but only some, acquire the instinct of reaching the right decision on insufficient evidence. Although high level training is now available for nutrition planners, no attempt has been made, as yet, to provide courses for nutrition administrators. Let there be no misunderstanding: a nutrition planner or programmer is not the same as a nutrition administrator. In many recently independent countries, technical assistance from expatriate professionals was welcomed, but administrative functions were considered to require no special training. Most countries are now providing intensive training in administration, but, however good the training, it is no substitute for apprenticeship. In launching a national nutrition program, administrative as well as professional aspects will require technical assistance.

Whatever the administrative organization established for a national nutrition program may be, the characteristics of its chief executive are critical for success. Naturally, the chief executive must have drive and determination and a conviction of the benefits to be derived from the program. The job is operational. The status of the chief executive in relation to the whole hierarchy of the civil service is vital, for there must be direct access to the top personnel of all the agencies involved. Preferably, there should be wide experience of high level administration with particular reference to coordination; there should be adequate knowledge of the subject and a thorough understanding of the needs and attitudes of the people and of their likely responses. In addition, there should be the ability to prepare project proposals, reports, and budgetary estimates; to steer motions and argue cases on committee; to persuade doubters and motivate colleagues; to temper urgency with patience and to have the resiliency to try again should there be any lack of success.

Political Will

Greater by far in importance than the will of rich countries to provide financial and technical resources to others is the will of developing countries to accord priority and allocate adequate resources for their own national nutrition programs. Such a will can only stem from thorough awareness and general understanding of nutritional problems on a nationwide basis. From a study of international experience and practice, it thus appears that awareness and commitment are the two prerequisites for governments to initiate and implement a national nutrition program. Furthermore, the governmental machinery must include seven components if there is to be any hope of success. These seven components are:

1 a firm, long-term and unambiguous policy
2 an administrative body with authority and flexibility to coordinate and implement the policy
3 executive bodies, with adequate financial, technical, and manpower resources to be capable of carrying out the administrative decisions
4 a source of scientific and technical advice
5 the means for effective communication and for formal and informal learning
6 facilities for training and research
7 a decentralized organization, which enables people to be involved meaningfully in planning and implementing measures for their own nutritional improvement

The will of a government must be expressed by decisions involving the collective responsibility of cabinet through legislative action: by Act of Parliament as in Zambia and Tanzania, or by Presidential Instruction, as in Indonesia and Malawi. Such a will stems from the realizations that (1) adequate nutrition is as important as education as an input of human resources for development and (2) to achieve the nutritional goal requires that government accord priority and allocate resources for a national effort. Such a will also involves the understanding that only an integrated approach to coordinated action can achieve success. Where, as yet, a government has not taken effective measures to tackle its nutritional problems, the first task would be to motivate the government to have the will to implement a national program. Such motivation would be likely to be based on an assessment of the nutritional status of the population according to available knowledge; an understanding of the strengths and weaknesses of current intervention measures; an analysis of the machinery for implementing these current intervention measures and its relationship to the power structure of government; and an

appraisal of the communications facilities available to influence both decisionmakers and beneficiaries.

POLICY AND PROGRAM

Policy is defined as the broad course of action to be adopted by a government. There are those who maintain that, first of all, policy must be formulated, then a program designed to carry out the policy. Policy, however, is a
course of action, not a pious expression of wishful thinking and, before it can
be determined, prior analysis is required of the problems and objectives,
taking into account the resources, constraints, trends, and other political
objectives. In practice, policy and program planning must proceed in parallel
if a feasible program is to be the result. Without estimates of costs and identified sources of funding, no government can decide on policy; funding cannot
be identified without a program.

In every country some data are available, but much of the data are partial
and obsolete and have been collected for research purposes rather than for
policymaking. However, the collation and analysis of what is available is the
first step and, when considered in the light of experience in similar circumstances elsewhere, there is more likely to be sufficient information to indicate
the incidence and nature of the malnutrition or undernutrition and the dietary deficiencies which are the causes. The factors which cause the dietary
deficiencies, however, are sure to require further study.

Many governments demand action based on available knowledge rather than
on further research. This is understandable, for it is a fact of political life that
once a decision has been made public, there should be speedy and overt action. Baseline studies are essential for evaluation, however, and thus through
this need it is possible to incorporate the further studies required to improve
planning.

Initial action in a nutrition program may include pilot trials of various intervention measures and different delivery systems. These can be compared for
cost and effectiveness so that expansion of the program will be on an improved and tested basis, but they cannot substitute for the broader action
demanded by the importance of the problem. All programs should be dynamic and flexible and adjusted according to the results of trials and experience.

PLANNING

Alan Berg[5] has described the ways in which a conceptual approach may be
applied to nutrition program planning and a number of countries are currently trying to recruit nutrition program planners, but such people are few and
far between. The task of such officers would be: to collate available information on food and nutrition and to quantify, as far as possible, all the factors

which appear to affect the nutritional status of the population; to define tentative goals and target groups and to identify the objectives of the program; to plan the various intervention measures designed to attain the objectives, together with criteria and indicators for evaluation; and to develop a national program which will be acceptable to the development authorities of government and has the promise of success.

Whatever criticism one may have of the postwar worship of economic growth as the measure of development, it is a fact that ministers of finance and planning control the power and resources to deal with nutrition problems. The nutrition program must be presented in such a way that it is acceptable to development planners. While cost-benefit analysis would not be feasible for a nutrition program, cost-effectiveness is possible on the same basis as for educational programs. The program must be presented in a form which can be incorporated into the national development plan and it is only when the nutrition program becomes part of the government's normal, departmental activities, that it can be deemed to have become a national program. It is also important that other components of the national development plan should be studied from the point of view of their impact on the nutritional status of the population and that this aspect should be taken into consideration before final decisions are taken.

All over the world, nutrition program planners are scarce; in tropical countries, where the need is greatest, they virtually do not exist. There is an obvious need to train such personnel. Short courses have been given in a few Western universities; but such courses can form only the prelude to what is required, and there is need for evaluation of the results which have been achieved by these short courses. One director of a health department in an Asian country commented: "He was a good nutritionist before he went on the course; now he has learned of various theoretical alternatives and he can no longer make up his mind." In a South American country, an official who had attended a course on planning became adept at finding reasons for objecting to any proposal.

It would seem much preferable to hold training courses in the regions where the trainees will operate. Not only is it cheaper to transport a few lecturers and instructors rather than numerous trainees, but the content of the course should be more directly relevant to the needs of the region and maximum use can be made of local teaching ability. It would also be simpler to take account of existing projects within the region and, where they consist of directionless activities pursued for their own end, it would be possible to use them as case studies so as to convert them into purposeful action, aimed at defined objectives. The closer one is to the source of the problems, the easier it is to ensure that the objectives are kept simple, consistent, practicable, and attainable, and involve minimal change in cultural patterns.

There is always a danger that planning can become too theoretical and centralized. Experience has shown that unless those who will benefit are involved in the planning process, they may resist the proposed program, however well it may be conceived. Furthermore, it is likely that, when there is adequate consultation at the grass-roots level, the program will be improved by the local knowledge and wisdom of the village people.

Another problem in planning has been the "blanket" utilization of many interventions, providing the benefits of an intervention measure to all, whether they need it or not. For example, a vitamin A prophylaxis project in one country in Asia aimed at providing massive doses of the vitamin by capsule, every six months, to all children between the ages of 12 and 48 months, in the pilot areas. The number of children of this age group at serious risk is estimated to be about 4% of the target group. The operation of the project has been very successful, reaching over 90% of the target group, but there remains a niggling doubt as to how many of the missing percentage are part of the 4% at risk. The cost of the pilot project makes it very doubtful if it can be replicated on the scale required and such prophylaxis can only be regarded as being a temporary measure, pending improved nutrition of the children at risk. Similarly, many supplementary feeding projects have tended to be blanket operations, providing a supplement to all who attend the MCH clinic. Those who make use of the facilities are often the better educated and better-off.

When a project depends on people coming forward, it is often those who are most in need of assistance who stay away. It seems to be essential to seek out those who are malnourished, to determine in what way they are affected, how badly they are affected, and where they are so that they can be reached. Only in this way is it possible to plan for a "target" approach. Recently, for example, in the very same country which has the vitamin A capsule program, an ambitious and comprehensive series of studies has been designed on the etiology and epidemiology of xerophthalmia. As for supplementary feeding, it should always aim at being an educational process, with the supplement being used as a teaching aid for the better nutrition of the child in the context of available foods and the particular cultural patterns.

Data relating to the manifold factors affecting nutrition are lamentably incomplete in most countries; hence policies and programs based on available knowledge can only be imperfect—some might say superficial. The collection, analysis, and interpretation of the extensive data required to create econometric and nutrometric models demands time, skill, and finance, all of which are in short supply. It may be that they entail major expense and achieve dubious success. Evaluation of the results obtained from such models, in terms of improved nutrition status, would be a guide to the usefulness of national surveys.

Unless a survey is directly related to an action program and essential to that action program, its main value may be to delay action and decision, and to be confused with substantive action. In the prevailing situation, there is an urgent need to grapple with the immediate problems; a perfectionist policy must compromise with the current measurement of misery and need for action. At any given point in time, policy and programs can only be based on available knowledge, but the programs must not be inflexible. Far from being a fixed course of action, the best of programs can be improved and refined as more knowledge becomes available.

Planning is not an end in itself. It is a very valuable tool to be used in converting scientific knowledge into practical action. It is an essential process to induce development planners in development ministries to make adequate resources available.

NUTRITION SCIENCE

The vital core of a nutrition program is the scientific knowledge upon which it is based; not just nutrition science, but all the sciences involved in food production and supply, food processing and distribution, food consumption, consumer education, and behavior change. No suggestion should prevail that the administrative aspect is more important than the scientific. It is not so. The administrative aspect is a tool to enable the scientific knowledge to be applied.

In this, scientists have many responsibilities. They must advise the planners on the validity of the available knowledge; they should be expected to determine the baseline data for any project, carry out monitoring during its progress, and be obliged to design dynamic evaluation as well as to carry out the final evaluation. Much research remains to be done on the causes of dietary deficiencies, the optimal means of controlling malnutrition, and simple methods for early diagnosis.

More basic questions must also be resolved. There are grave doubts as to whether the recommended daily allowances of nutrients, based on studies in Western industrialized countries, apply to tropical countries, where centuries of adaptation may affect requirements. Certainly, there appear to be anomalies; the recorded calorie intake of apparently normal, active people is little above their needs for basal metabolism. In Zambia, intake of calcium was found to be far below the recommended allowance, yet the evidence of post-mortems indicated no clinical lack of calcium.[6] Is the measure of intake wrong, or the recommended daily allowance, or perhaps both? Are the figures used inappropriately and taken too literally?

Because the incidence of malnutrition has the most devastating effect on the young child, research and remedial measures have tended to concentrate on this age group, and on pregnant and lactating women, appropriately called vulnerable groups. Schoolchildren and adolescents are often regarded as further age groups in need of prior attention, especially for nutrition education. In the less developed countries, children under 15 years of age represent at least 45% of the population. Taken together with the aged and handicapped, half the population is dependent. It is the other 50% who are the workers and producers, those upon whom the country depends for development. In the interest of development, it could be argued that priority should be given to the nutrition of the workers; at least they should not be ignored. Further study on the interrelationship between nutrition and working efficiency and productivity is urgently required.

NUTRITION EDUCATION

Another field for further study is nutrition education, which, as frequently practiced, seems to reveal that defect of the lecture system in which the notes of the lecturer are transferred to the notes of the student, without passing through the mind of either. At a later date, in another place, when the student becomes a lecturer, the same notes pass on.

David Henry[7] quotes the following meal plan from a booklet "Nutrition for Mother and Child," issued by the Indian Council of Medical Research.

Meal Plan For One to Three Year Old Children

On rising	Breast milk or boiled animal milk	1 feed 4 oz (110ml) ½ tumbler
9:00-10:00 A.M.	1 Cooked cereal-pulse preparation such as Khicheri, dalia etc. or bread with butter	2 spoons
	2 Soft boiled or poached egg or boiled animal milk	1 egg ½ tumbler
	3 Fruit juices	¼ - ½ tumbler
12 noon-1 P.M.	1 Cooked cereal or starchy vegetable or Ragi dumpling ball	1 spoon 1 small ball
	2 Boiled pulse, fish or minced meat, liver, etc.	1 - 1½ spoons
	3 Leafy or green vegetable (cooked)	1 spoon
3:30-4:00 P.M.	1 Boiled animal milk	½ tumbler
	2 Fish liver oil	1 teaspoon
6:00-7:00 P.M.	1 Cooked cereal such as suji, broken wheat porridge	2 spoons
	2 Boiled animal milk	½ tumbler
At bedtime	Breast milk or boiled animal milk	1 feed ½ tumbler

Milk and other preparations may be sweetened if liked.

In many areas, some of these foods would not be available and, even if they were, they would be well beyond the purchasing power of most of the people. Such a meal plan is utterly impracticable when the work pattern of village women is taken into account, not to mention the fact that there may be no clocks available!

Equally irrelevant has been nutrition education based on: "Four Healthy: Five Excellent." In this plan, foods are divided into five categories: (1) carbohydrates; (2) fruits; (3) vegetables; (4) animal protein products; and (5) dairy products. The focus tends to be on the importance of dairy products, which are rarely available, and often culturally unacceptable. Animal protein is normally beyond the means of most families. The main source of protein for most people is the staple cereal, which is classified as a carbohydrate. It is not surprising that this style of nutrition education has been found to be counterproductive when applied to poor families, who resent being told to do what is impossible in their economic circumstances.

At Ilonga, Tanzania, an evaluation exercise on nutrition education carried out in 1973[8] revealed that mothers could quote the correct answers to questions on nutrition, but there appeared to be no change in the nutritional status of their children. In the Luapula Valley of Zambia, a follow-up was done on the effect of school gardens. The home gardens of some of those teaching the subject were checked. The teachers did not follow the improved methods which they were teaching at school; it was the teachers' wives who looked after the home gardens. In the Lower Shire Region of Malawi, a study[9] was carried out on the personal response of recently trained homecraft workers. Few put into practice any of the home economics teaching in their own homes, but they continued to pass on the instruction to others.

Instead of nutrition education, the aim should be nutrition learning; instead of providing didactic instruction on the facts of science, the objective desired is behavioral change. Before devising the strategy to bring about such a change, there should be knowledge of the food habits, patterns, and beliefs of the target audience, the factors which might motivate those learning to change, and identification of the local decisionmakers. Often the change desired would involve no more than emulation of the mothers who already feed their families quite adequately within the particular community. Only when the changes involved in achieving adequate nutrition become part of the culture of the people and are passed on automatically to the next generation can the task be deemed to have been completed.

FOOD SCIENCE AND TECHNOLOGY

During this century, technology has been judged desirable when it adds to the wealth of a country or relieves poverty and hardship; it has been the mainspring for social and economic progress. New products and new techniques dominate the process of growth and the key participants have been businessmen and inventors. International companies have been very successful in marketing their products. It is not surprising, therefore, that food technology has been mainly the servant of the food industry and that relief of poverty, hardship, and malnutrition has tended to be incidental.

Food science and technology could make a very important contribution to improved nutritional status in developing countries. One must, however, escape the idea, expressed by some food technologists, that the appearance, convenience, and sales appeal of the processed food product is of more importance than its nutrient content. Fortunately, there are other food technologists who advocate that courses for food scientists and technologists should include adequate teaching in human nutrition, as many of the results of food technology have been detrimental nutritionally.

An interesting exercise, for example, is to challenge a bottle-feeding sponsor to sterilize a bottle and prepare a feed using only the facilities and utensils available to a mother in a typical village or city slum. Weak, lightly contaminated mixtures are very understandable at the end of the month, when money is short: mothers assume that "if it looks white it looks right." Of even greater concern is the sight in African markets, or among those waiting in line at a clinic, of babies sucking bottles filled with sweet fizzy drinks. One country in Africa considered introducing legislation restricting the sale of feeding bottles to those with a medical prescription only.

Food technology has given excellent service to big business and the profit motive. It also has the knowledge and power to bring about marked improvements at the village level, through the use of intermediate technology for the small operator or for home use. The need is great; the technology can be evolved; unfortunately, difficulties are considerable when it comes to incorporating adequate profit. Studies are required, from the points of view of the food scientist and food technologist, of what happens to food right from the beginning, immediately after harvest or catch. What are the problems; how is the food transported, marketed, processed, packaged, distributed, and retailed? What are the wasteful or inefficient links in the chain? What are the solutions to the problems which are identified?

There are other areas for action, such as the formulation and production of supplementary foods based on locally grown products. However, in tropical countries, there may be no need for food supplements if the estimated wastage of 30% of cereals between farm gate and consumption can be reduced significantly.

Intermediate technology could have a marked, beneficial influence on the work burden of rural women. Although handicapped by endemic parasites and disease, the women are the source of survival and the providers throughout the subsistence sector. In many regions, the mother of the family must keep the home, bear and rear the children, plant the seed, weed and cultivate the fields, harvest and store the crops, thrash and winnow the grain, pound or grind the flour, collect and carry the fuel and water, as well as cook the meal. The importance of women as food producers is beginning to be recognized.

AGRICULTURE

Historically, ministries of agriculture tended to concentrate on cash crops and conservation. Recently independent countries were faced with the need to diversify and expand their production of cash crops and export as much as possible to gain foreign exchange. Agricultural production became the key to progress.

Conservation tended to be ignored and when allegedly objectionable controls imposed by colonial governments were no longer enforced, cultivation often spread to steep hillsides and to the headwaters of rivers such as the Luangwa in Zambia and the Solo in Java. In many countries, soil erosion took place in the hilly areas; then, when the rivers became slow-flowing in the valleys, silt was deposited—partially blocking the river bed. At the season of heavy rain, the flood waters could not flow through freely enough and were forced to overflow the river banks and flood the adjacent agricultural land. Controls continue to be necessary to ensure that, whatever is done in the struggle to grow enough food, the cultivation is not environmentally disastrous.

Agricultural production has tended to keep pace with population growth, so that the food available per capita continues at the same low level, which maintains widespread malnutrition. This increased production has resulted, in great part, from expansion of the area cultivated. In many countries there remains for further expansion only land which would require high investment either to make the soil fertile or for conservation works to make the cultivation permanent.

Population control, land tenure, and income distribution are all factors affecting the application of scientific and technical advances, but, in the context of a food and nutrition program, a matter of major concern is the availability of essential inputs. The small holder is always the last to benefit from the provision of any technological package.

Despite the rapid growth of urban populations, the absolute number of small holders will continue to increase for the foreseeable future. In most of the less developed countries, the vast majority of families will still depend upon what they produce to feed themselves in whole or in part.

There will also be an increase in the number of those living in a money economy without money and many will be seriously affected from lack of food consumption. This is not a situation which can be remedied by nutrition intervention measures alone, but, if there are programs to tackle these socioeconomic problems, it is important that there should be the inclusion of a nutrition component.

Much could be done in the rural areas to increase yields, diversify crop production, improve storage and processing, and enhance understanding. Extension services have naturally concentrated on the politically and socially more important farmers with larger holdings and with title of some sort to their land. The small farmer, whose holding varies in size according to the pressure on land, may own less than 0.2 hectare of paddy land, as is the case in about 50% of the small holdings on Java; or it may be a matter of holding less than 50 hectares to qualify as a small holder as in Northeast Brazil. The factor in common is that these small holders have been neglected by agricultural extension and agricultural credit has rarely been available, except on a cooperative basis. Suitable agricultural packages must be worked out so that there may be increased production by small holders, both for their own consumption and for sale. The yields from unassisted holdings are normally so low, that it should not be difficult to bring about significant improvement.

In those countries where women play a major part in food production, the value of female extension officers has become recognized. Many countries run courses such as the Agriculture and Nutrition Extension Officers Course in Zambia and the Farm Home Instructresses course in Malawi, but many more require training to meet the needs. A subsistence economy is, at best, only a partial money economy and economic intervention measures are likely to have less effect than agricultural measures to increase production and the motivation of the producer to consume the home production.

Any hopes for significantly increased production are related to systems of land tenure. In many parts of Africa there is the system of usufruct, in which an individual retains rights to land only for so long as the individual cultivates that land. Under such a system there is little incentive to introduce permanent improvements on the farm. In the matrilineal areas, where a man's heritage passes to his sister's children, there is minimal motivation to increase the family heritage. Under other systems, absentee landlords, sharecropping, and landless laborers present problems which are very hard to resolve. Where consolidation of holdings and registration of title have replaced customary land tenure, problems are arising regarding transfer of title to the next-generation farmers.

TRAINING

Training of personnel for undertaking nutrition programs involves as much reconsideration as is needed for nutrition education. Initial training of new personnel, retraining of established personnel through in-service courses or more advanced courses, and orientation courses for collaborating staff are all required to mount a national nutrition program. This training is, in fact, a major requirement during the initial phase. Before attempting to design a course and to define its content, there should be a full job description of the work to be undertaken by those trained. The content of the course should cover all the knowledge and skills required to fulfill the job description, a task which will inevitably require multidisciplinary involvement in syllabus planning. It is also necessary to provide established posts and a career structure for those who complete the training.

In many countries, a rehash of what has been provided as nutrition training is unlikely to suffice. An example in one African country is a course given for nutrition instructors. The sole practical work of the trainees was to act as enumerators on a nutritional status survey. There was no practical training in adult education, the task for which they were being trained. There was no attempt to ensure that the trainees recognized that nutrition learning depends on the desire of those taught to learn and their active involvement in the learning process, that the material presented should be within the learners' capacity to understand and accept, and within their ability to put into practice.

Training covers three main levels: professional, technical, and the field. Perhaps the most difficult of the three is the training of the field workers, the contact personnel who are the direct agents to bring about the desired changes. The training of these contact personnel requires the greatest skill and it is not a function to be delegated to junior staff. Of equal importance is the selection of workers, in which personality has more significance than educational level. It is essential to find just the right spark-gap. As in a spark plug, if the gap is too wide there is no spark; if the field worker is too highly educated or too sophisticated, there may be an "us" and "them" relationship, which is a serious blockage to change. If the gap is too close there is an ineffective spark; local workers recruited from the village may participate in the village culture and may share all the local beliefs about food so fully that they are not very helpful in changing food habits. The spark-gap must be not too much, not too little, but just right.

For their training, it would be a mistake to be too ambitious regarding the nutrition content, which should be decisive, fixed, and non-academic, deal with foods and not nutrients, and be directed towards specific local problems and the methods which are the simplest likely to achieve results. Contact personnel should be well supported by tested teaching aids and communications media.

At the technical level, staff will be involved in supervisory duties, for which skills training is often omitted from didactic courses. These duties include nonnutritional aspects of training: minor administration and logistics, organization of work programs, control of equipment and local expenditure, staff supervision, public relations and collaboration with colleagues. The staff must also be able to make good contact with the people among whom they work and exercise tolerance and understanding of the difficulties facing those being helped. Those who come from the higher socioeconomic group may need to apply themselves to gain an adequate understanding. All training and the implementation of a nutrition program depend on the leadership of experienced staff. In addition, well-qualified, adaptable staff are required as directors of field programs, for the organization of preventive and curative services, as instructors and teachers, and for consultation by other services, such as agricultural extension, public health, and social welfare.

SOCIAL COMMUNICATION

All aspects of nutrition programs need the support of a communications system. In many countries traditional information services have been relied on for communication, but they have tended to indulge in a mere outpouring of material. Social communication involves a new philosophy of action demanding a more comprehensive approach. It must not be regarded as action on a limited scale, in selected areas, between specialist teacher and fortunate pupils. The enlarged scope can be illustrated by Alfred Smith's definition:[10] "Communication does not refer only to verbal, explicit, and intentional transmission of messages ... but includes all those processes by which people influence one another." It is concerned with the whole complex of human relationships, through which ideas are exchanged, skills acquired, knowledge increased and behavior changed.[11] The techniques of communication involve a careful appraisal of the recipients' patterns of behavior, the creation of messages based on this, and, in turn, a careful study of the recipients' reaction to the messages.[12] The term social communication has been used to highlight the way in which the concept of communication has been broadened from its popular identification with mass media; social communication is much more than the use of audiovisual aids for teaching purposes.

At best, the application of social communication will be a slow process, involving social diffusion. The first task is to create awareness of malnutrition and the need for good nutrition. From there, the objective becomes the stimulation of active interest in nutritional matters and, when interest is strong enough, to encourage trial of new foods and new methods. Then, finally, to influence acceptance of the trial so that a change in behavior will be adopted.

Ideally, social communication means mounting a comprehensive campaign and creating a systematically designed structure out of an indefinite number of methods, media, agencies, and opportunities. Thus the buildup of each means of communication is an integral part of the total campaign and each means is coordinated with the others, so that the campaign becomes part of the social environment of the recipients. Successful communication is a two-way activity, a circulating flow of information from the sender to receiver and back again. From a study of the recipients' reactions to the message, it can be adjusted, if required, to correct defects or increase impact.

Modern social communication is a highly professional subject, demanding skill and expenditure; and, should the attempt be made to introduce the techniques without adequate staff, with insufficient financial support, or in conditions which are not favorable, the whole exercise will be doomed to failure. This would not be because it was beyond the powers of communication to solve the problem, but because of inadequate application.

Social communication involves five factors, which are closely interrelated:

- "What To Say"
- "How To Say It"

- Pre-Testing Material
- Operational Organization
- Evaluation

"What To Say," the content or topic, is the responsibility of the relevant scientists. Experts within the same discipline frequently differ; between disciplines viewpoints tend to diverge; and there are always individual idiosyncracies. However, when experts from different disciplines have experience of working together as a team, which in itself is a process of social communication, the difficulties and differences diminish, even if they do not disappear entirely. In any given circumstance, a great deal of work and thought is required to reach agreement on content. "What To Say" depends on the results of research, on the vast body of prevailing scientific knowledge which may be applied, and on the facts relating to the way of life of the target population, whose educational level, technical capacity, and attitudes have great bearing on the content chosen.

The technical capacity, or what is feasible, is most important. For example, in some countries of Africa, the politically inspired attempt to leap from cultivation by the hoe to tractorization resulted in rusting relics being scattered throughout the rural areas. It is equally pointless to advocate a pint of milk per head per day for people living at subsistence level in areas infested with tsetse fly. Feasibility depends on the potential will and skill of the people, the capacity of the land and waters to produce, and the financial and material support available. The content must represent a clearly defined and consistent series of messages, varying in form and detail according to the socioeconomic status and educational level of the recipients, but never being self-contradictory.

"How To Say It" is the realm and responsibility of the communications expert, whose strategy should involve the creation of a systematic campaign that is thoroughly planned and efficiently executed. The communicator is responsible for the form and design of the messages and the methods and media to be used. There is no ideal medium: what a method gains in impact, it loses in coverage. Field experience has suggested that personal contact with the target population, giving practical demonstrations using local utensils, facilities, and materials is the most effective means, but economic and practicable reasons preclude the employment of an enormous, well-paid field staff. By using the radio broadcasting system and transistor receivers, it is possible to reach the remotest village, hence coverage can be nationwide, but radio is not a self-sufficient medium. Ingrained ways of life usually cannot be changed merely by radio broadcasts, nor do they suffice for teaching new techniques. Radio is able to reinforce other media and methods and, if coupled with listening groups supervised by extension staff, it can become an effective communication medium, with feedback to the sender. The written word provides the widest coverage, but most rural communities are composed of a high proportion of illiterates and there is frequently a multiplicity of local languages.

There is another factor which must be taken into account. Studies of the perception and conceptual thinking of illiterate rural people indicate that they do not seem to have developed a series of fundamental logical concepts and symbol processes which might be deemed essential in recipients. It has been found that there is often little concept of conservation of quantity, mass, number, or area, or of the idea of horizontal and vertical, or even of a straight line. Yet such village people have experience and personalities; they are adult in attitude and like to be consulted; any attempt to approach them otherwise would be deeply and rightly resented. Coverage for such an audience presents another dimension to the challenge for social communication. Not enough is known. Skilled and penetrating research in this field by professional psychologists could provide valuable guidance to the communicator.

All materials produced require field testing with a sample of the target audience before they are produced in bulk. Only in this way can the communicator be reasonably assured that the message is being understood and interpreted as intended. The absence of this process of field testing has been a major criticism of the product of information services.

Instruction in the use, care, and maintenance of sophisticated equipment is obvious, but another factor is the need to train the contact personnel in the optimal use of materials produced, however simple they may be. Using teaching posters as wallpaper in clinics is all too common as is the misuse of flannelgraphs by instructors, whose aim seems to be to try to put up all the pieces in the shortest possible time. Such training is the responsibility of the communicator.

Social communication is not an end in itself, but a means to an end, meaningless unless the content is clearly defined. It should not be regarded as being solely aimed at those in need of assistance. In the preliminary stages of a program, it may be more important to influence the decisionmakers and ensure adequate mutual understanding among the divers professional personnel involved in the program.

CONCLUSION

The case studies considered by this conference should provide many guidelines regarding the way in which government might be activated to take effective action in tackling their nutritional problems. Based on practical experience, a few tentative suggestions are put forward for consideration.

For governments which have not formulated a national food and nutrition policy/program, the techniques of social communication should be applied to motivate the required changes in the attitudes of technical, administrative, and political groups. For governments which have demonstrated the will to accord priority and allocate resources for an effective, long term, nationwide policy/program on improved nutrition, technical assistance should be readily available. This technical assistance will involve teamwork by scientists, planners, and administrators, and it is unlikely that such teamwork will come about through spontaneous generation. Taking the magnitude of the problem into consideration, numerous teams would have to be created, but nutrition programmers and nutrition administrators are in very short supply. Through training workshops and courses it should be possible to overcome this shortage of expert personnel and the work of the teams might be regarded as operational research in applied nutrition, through which policy/program preparation and execution can be improved continuously. A major training effort should be aimed at the provision of local counterparts, who, in due course, will be responsible for the long term implementation of programs. If funding for food and nutrition programs could be coordinated, it would save much time and effort; if the format for project proposals could be simplified and their processing speeded up, it would help governments greatly. The length of the gestation period for a project proposal varies directly with the size of the funding organization, with no known means of inducing early delivery.

Each country is a sovereign state and technical assistance, from whatever source, is assistance to that country's policy/program. There should be no such thing as a World Bank program, a WHO project, an FAO survey, or a SIDA center. If governments would coordinate technical assistance so that all technical assistance is regarded as part of their own program, the degree of coordination at international headquarters would become comparatively irrelevant, but the desire for identified credit is strong and governments tend to play off one source of funding against another or one organization against another, because it has been profitable to do so.

The results of many years of work and effort to improve nutritional status, by many people in many countries, is reaching the stage when action can be considered in a new light. The era of prestige projects in development and the worship of economic growth is giving way to consideration of human welfare and the quality of life. The timing seems right to launch a major effort to apply available knowledge for the better nutrition of all mankind.

DISCUSSION (THE SYMBIOSIS OF SCIENTIST, PLANNER, AND ADMINISTRATOR)

Thomson

I have prepared this paper so that it will touch on points relevant to the objectives of the conference; but I hope also that it will provoke discussion, because I do not for a moment expect that everything that has been said will be accepted as valid. I'm sure that much is not generally applicable throughout all the countries where malnutrition is a problem, but I think this diversity is something that must be taken into careful account. The theme of the paper is the need for interdepartmental, interdisciplinary approaches to nutrition programs and the need for nutrition programs to be based on the best available scientific knowledge. The application of that knowledge depends on adequate planning, effective administration, and appropriate communication.

Perhaps lack of attention to the administrative machinery required for nutrition program implementation has given rise to the disappointingly meager results after years of effort. Effective action to combat malnutrition and to enhance the nutritional status of populations has been hampered by the rivalry and lack of accord which exists between international agencies and even between different departments of the same organization. At the national level this bureaucratic malady has been intensified. In the paper, illustrations are given of the ways in which the lack of accord has frustrated action, and I'm quite sure that those around this table can give many more examples.

Antrobus

I would like to give my vote of appreciation for Ewen Thomson's very sensitive overview of the nutrition scene. Nearly all of his comments are germane to our situation in the Caribbean. I do not know whether it is very reassuring or very depressing to find so many similarities already evident in all the parts of the world we have mentioned!

Solimano

Ewen has given us a framework from a technical point of view, demonstrating some weaknesses and limitations that I think we will have to look at carefully when we review the hypotheses based on experience. What I think we are going to see from the different case studies is that some problems can be solved and others cannot and that there are some very important forces outside of *any* scheme that really determine the achievement of success.

From this chance to share experience, we may demonstrate how things work in the real world and which factors are the most influential. Many times, from experience, you think you are accomplishing a lot, but when you stop and look, you find that things have not changed very much.

Soekirman

I would also like to congratulate Mr. Thomson on his paper and note that many of these problems really did arise in my country. I would like to speak to your comment on the need for policy and program planning to proceed in parallel. In my experience, it is sometimes difficult to write a program because there is no policy yet. In Indonesia, the president issues the policy, and then, starting with that policy, we work out the program. To work out the program, you need the money to invite people to work, and that in turn depends on policy.

After our principal policy was declared by the president, it was formulated in the resultant plan. From that we made a checklist of what should be developed further. After the nutrition section was written into the five-year development plan, we noticed a peculiar situation in which some important points were missing. We are not too upset, however, because we will have the opportunity to improve it later. The important thing for now is that nutrition has been written into the five-year development plan. We can start from that to develop a program.

Now, it seems that for the next policy plan there must be a program first. It will be difficult to persuade the high level policymaker to make a clear food and nutrition policy, for instance, before we have a clear program. They say: "After you have a coherent program, we will enact policy as a follow-up." So, first there was a policy, and then we tried to develop a more elaborate program, and then we realized that, to work out this program, you need more detailed policy. Now, the policymaker again asks for a good program in order to make policy. So the two are intertwined, but sometimes the policy must come first in order to start the program.

Thomson
It is merely a question of terminology, but I think that, possibly, what is described as the "nutrition policy" of Indonesia, I would rather call a presidential "statement of intent," with guidelines as to what should be done. From that, there will develop a national program and, when there are institutional bases and the manpower capability, the results of various intervention measures should give a guide to program policy for the next five-year development plan. But it does need time to build up.

A lot has already been done. A very great deal has been undertaken in Indonesia, but I think that, in the third five-year development plan, there will be opportunity for the development of a food and nutrition policy program.

Latham
When Ewen Thomson and I were recently in Indonesia, working with Soekirman and his colleagues, we met with representatives of the various ministries and were asked the question: what other country can we use as an example of an ideal national nutrition program that works? Ewen has spoken to us of the elements necessary for a rational and sound nutrition program. Yet, when we had to answer that question, we were at a loss to point to any such ideal nutrition program.

Perhaps one of the case studies presented here will illustrate an ideal situation, but I believe that each of them will show some measures of success and some measures of failure. By putting them all together and using Ewen Thomson's framework, we might be able to see which parts of each program are most likely to lead to success. One obviously can't have a blueprint that is suitable for Ghana, the Philippines, Indonesia, and Zambia. But I wonder if anybody knows of any program that we have missed, that does seem to have been a model of success?

Sai

I think, Michael, that if one narrowed the definition of program and didn't only look at "national" nutrition programs, it should be possible to identify individual programs or groups of projects that have succeeded. I think we owe it to ourselves to identify those because it may be that, from them, we can learn more general lessons.

What needs to be addressed explicitly is that we do not know the extent to which indirect factors affect nutrition as opposed to the effects of direct intervention activities. As a result of that particular lack of knowledge, it is difficult to get a proper mix of direct intervention activities and encouragement of indirect trends.

Barnes

Could you please give an example of what you mean by each, direct and indirect?

Sai

Let us call supplementary feeding of children a direct action. An indirect factor in that particular program would be the availability of potable water in the community. We know that there is a synergism between disease and malnutrition, but we don't know if, in fact, the provision of potable water *itself* and the education of the people in the utilization of that potable water, *without* the nutrition supplementation program, might not be able to influence nutrition more than supplementation alone.

I have given this example on a project scale. It could also be broadened to the national socioeconomic sphere. If we do have some examples that can be used as a testing model situation, we should try to study those to enlarge on the point.

Soekirman

This uncertainty represents a big probem in Indonesia because many people think that the program should be based on the importance of the determinants. The planning people say to the nutritionists: "You told us there are many important determinants: economic, public health, and cultural, among others, but which one is most important?" Our answer has to be that for a country like Indonesia, the most important is *all* at once. If you want to develop a nutrition program, all components should be there. Nutrition is a system, and every component is important. It is no use to give supplementary feeding for children if there is no water, no sanitation, no vaccination.

With Mr. Thomson and Dr. Latham, we are developing a program where nutrition is an input of the whole process: we do not have a "nutrition program" per se, but only a nutrition input into development. Nutritional status was written into the five-year plan in Indonesia as one of the indicators of successful development. The planners want to know how to measure nutritional status, and, of course, you cannot measure it if there is no nutritional input in the program. Therefore, the planners agree to incorporate nutrition. Now, it is important for the planners to get from the nutritionists a good program so that they can allocate budgets. For a developing country, there is little need to talk about what is written in academic papers looking for the relative importance of the determinants. All the determinants are involved.

Sai
I certainly did not mean that all the determinants are not important. You have to establish priorities, however: you have a certain allocation of funds, and you want to use that amount to carry you furthest. It may be that in the Indonesian situation, if I understand you correctly, the minimum package, with inputs from various sectors, must be spearheaded by the nutrition group. It may be that, in *another* situation, a minimum package to influence nutrition can be spearheaded, not by the nutrition group at all, but by an agriculture, health, or economics group. It is this kind of realistic orientation of programs that I was trying to bring up.

Montgomery
This question of distinguishing between direct and indirect intervention is one that I think is important for us to explore as we look at the country experiences. Can you use an analytical framework which says that a *direct* intervention is one which a government makes with the knowledge and purpose of affecting the problem and an *indirect* intervention is one which you *discover* is an *un*expected consequence of some other action that the government is taking? Then, an indirect intervention would become a direct intervention if the policymaker discovers that it has a bigger influence than the direct things being done all along.

So, instead of a school feeding program, the nutrition officer says, "Let's build reservoirs." Then the building of reservoirs becomes the concern of the nutrition group. In examining what works best and how it works, under what circumstances, it might be best to focus on direct interventions, meaning those which you intentionally undertake with the expectation of improving the condition that gives rise to the problem.

Winikoff
There seems to be a definitional problem here, resulting from the many uses of "direct" and "indirect" as descriptive terms. I believe Fred Sai described the possibility of a conscious "direct" decision to do something which will "indirectly" affect the malnutrition problem. In other words, he formulated a

distinction between dealing with nutrition problems by using *food* or by manipulating another aspect of health care or environmental sanitation. This second group of interventions might, via improvement in nutritional status, change the morbidity and mortality statistics *more* effectively than food distribution. Whether, in fact, we call that health/environmental intervention "direct" or "indirect" in an administrative sense is another question. Based on John Montgomery's framework, it would depend on whether policy-makers *understand* and *intend* to influence nutritional status with programs in other sectors.

Maletnlema

In fact, the idea of converting indirect into direct would appear to advocate putting everything under the nutrition program so that eventually nutrition would devour all other programs. This is obviously an unacceptable trend for many government officials, and, in the end, it might be that nutrition itself was devoured by other program interests! It is better to leave the indirect interventions to be carried out by nonnutrition people, with the knowledge that they are contributing a lot to the nutrition program.

Thomson

Without getting into the semantics of this, I *would* like to suggest that one of the great needs is studies of indirect action, in particular, of agricultural action in relation to nutrition. I suspect that there are many agricultural policies, budgets, and programs which are detrimental nutritionally and that studies of this nature can identify the indirect factors which are beneficial and/or detrimental to nutritional status.

Solon

I would like to add a comment on regional training. I have been part of and thankful for such training, although I was trained in London and sent to Africa for field experience. At the time, I said we ought to bring this training to Asia. The Asians are brought to London, which is very foreign to us, while we should be back in our own countries to do something more relevant. Changing the venue of training to Asian countries for the Asians would be more appropriate. Even if we do not find advisers right in Asia, we can invite experts to come to Asia and plan with Asian planners: not *advise* Asian planners, but *teach* Asians to be planners. Eventually we will be able to stand on our own.

Soekirman

I agree that *most* of the training in the countries in Asia should be regional, but it is not always necessary. It depends in part on the educational level. For instance, the national program director, a high level post, should be trained internationally.

We are now facing the problem of staffing a big program supported by the World Bank. We would like to train, in one year, about six national officers for this special program. These will be high-ranking officials, and we have no one to teach them nationally.

We propose to divide our training and send some people abroad, for a short time, for them to have an idea of how the international network operates and the experience of seeing what other people are doing. Then, for the second echelon, we agree that the training should be regional and national. In this case, we invite consultants or lecturers to come and give of their experience.

Maletnlema

I do like the idea of organizing courses locally, but in fact, you cannot have only one uniform type of training even on a national scale. In the Philippines, for instance, one area might be completely different from another, and to have all the training combined might prove impossible. Eventually, you come down to regional planning for areas which are similar, yet even this is difficult. International experts may help with training, but it would be extremely difficult to get people who know the local conditions sufficiently to do the organizing and training of regional planners.

Thomson

Obviously, if courses are local, any expatriate coming in must know a great deal about the background of the area. There are, however, certain principles which an expatriate can bring as a basis for consideration. As I tried to make clear in my presentation, however, I believe that one must make maximum use of the local teaching ability of the country. Whatever contribution there may be from outside is only a supplement to the basis which is already there.

Maletnlema

You tell us also that nutrition administration is a particular art which is, at the moment, not taught. I do not know whether you mean to introduce yet another school, but I do not welcome the idea of teaching administration of nutrition. We were told about training planners, so we spare a person to go and learn planning. Now, we would have to spare another person to go and train for administration!

This immediately brings up our very large problem of manpower resources. The few trained people that can be used on this program are also needed for many other programs. Currently, I think we are combining administration with planning. I am doing the administration and the planning: I have not been trained for either of these, but I find myself being almost everything at once!

Thomson

I would like to clear up one thing, if I may. In nutrition programs, it is not necessarily a separate administrator that is required. It is that whoever, at whatever level, is in charge of the programs must have knowledge of administrative processes. This should be part of the normal training of anyone who could be described as a nutrition program officer.

Wray

I think, especially out at the working level, we need to keep in mind that the apprenticeship is really much more important than any kind of formal training you could ever hope to provide. I am inclined, at this point, to think that *everybody*, right up to the minister, probably should have some kind of apprenticeship. Maybe that is going too far, but certainly the people working in the program can only learn, finally, to solve some of the problems by working in the field. If this is true, then in order to provide this kind of training, whether we are talking about the local level or the regional level or the national level or international level, we need some pilot projects or some models.

When you talk about a "model" program, people often think that you mean some kind of ideal, unrealistic, unachievable program. Obviously, that has to be avoided. Still, there is a need, at some reasonably local level, for some adequate examples of the kind of program that you want to establish. We have problems with demonstration projects and models only because we have not gotten *beyond that* level to the national level. There remains a very important place for such programs as centers for training, if nothing else. Such projects can also be a place where local people work out solutions for local problems before tackling things on too large a scale. But the question persists: Why have we failed to get beyond the demonstration level to the national level? Is there any place for "models" in your countries? How could they be used as a place to provide learning experiences?

Solon

Ewen hit the nail right on the head when he said that a series of pilot projects does not equal a nutrition program. I agree and have been saying that it is time to expand the "applied nutrition projects."

The Philippines have been hamstrung by so-called applied nutrition projects for ten years. In that time, the projects have only expanded to 600 schools, but we have about 36,000 schools in 42,000 villages! But, because the ANPs were introduced by international agencies, we were so contented that we did not try to make changes. The assistance itself became a restraint. In addition, many people, especially at the rural level, do not like to start a project unless assistance comes in the form of imported, nice-looking things. This, in fact, developed into a constraining situation where we could hardly move because our own projects were designed for the government by others and not by the government for itself.

How many children have already died because of lack of aggressive expansion of the programs? Now, in the Philippines, we speak bravely of expanding the program nationwide despite limited resources. The expansion itself stimulated the resources of the country. We even realigned the thinking of the many international agencies to look at the country's program the way *we* wanted it to operate.

Often, I think we limit ourselves to pilot and model projects because we are afraid to fail. We would like success to come first. Success is important, but there must also be a timetable to expand and cover the whole country. We can truly influence government by setting a large effort going throughout the country, showing that the problem is not a limited pocket problem but a nationwide problem that needs a nationwide effort.

Thomson
As a footnote to your point on the way in which applied nutrition projects were imposed by international agencies, I would like to mention the 1964-66 ANP program in Zambia, which Dr. Sai came out to evaluate. Later, I carried out an analysis of all that had led up to this program and found that there were 22 re. ons why it had failed, each one of which alone would have been sufficient to insure failure! This was the result of theory utterly irrelevant to the needs of the country!

It related back to the tendency of international agencies to define policy on the basis of wishful thinking, unrelated to attainable goals. Once idealistic policy has been formulated, it is presumed that programs will be planned to implement the policy so that planning for the unattainable is a mandatory exercise.

Maletnlema
The question of the placement of a nutrition program—be it a national program or a single small project—in the Ministry of Health, Ministry of Agriculture, or the president's office, creates enormous difficulties which are also related to the system of international aid.

If we look at the international system, we see, within the United Nations itself, in the WHO and the FAO, nutrition units in each of the organizations, which, believe it or not, are often in conflict. This is, perhaps, an outstanding example, but there are many others almost at the same level. Each group has its own ideas on what nutrition programs should do and how they should be carried out.

In our developing countries, whenever you want to start a program, whether you like it or not, whether you ask for international help or not, eventually it comes. Therefore, you get all the interagency conflicts reproduced within the recipient country.

Depending on which is the most powerful of the donor groups that come, you find your nutrition program placed in one ministry or another. We have had this very experience, and, for about six years, we have been battling. Meanwhile, nutrition keeps trotting from one place to another: from agriculture to the prime minister's office to health, and is not settled as yet.

Solimano
I think we need to look at the assumptions we start with in this area. Usually, we who are concerned with nutrition very quickly get into the nutrition questions and start talking about the different programs we want to implement. In

fact, I think this is not the heart of the problem. In institutions all around the world, there are programs and methodologies to deal with problems of implementation.

The basic difficulty is our underlying assumption that nutrition as a priority has been accepted by governments and that governments want to solve nutrition problems. From that assumption, we begin to talk about school feeding, education, health, and so on, but the situation is much more complex because *not* all governments want to or can solve the problem. Priorities set in the allocation of funds are closely related to the patterns of development and socioeconomic policies that a particular government is following. We may say that we have to distribute income better, but equality of income distribution is not necessarily the goal of the government. Yet, income distribution and employment policy, I am sure, are often more effective nutritionally than providing milk or new foods or proteins, especially for the groups that really are in need.

We will have to examine how we can go out and learn from the nutrition programs themselves what needs to be done next. Here we are, people from different governments, who have held or at present hold positions, so that at least part of the decisions are their own responsibility. How can food and nutrition become issues in different government policies? What does it mean to introduce food and nutrition in terms, not of a nutrition program, but of socioeconomic development? What is it going to mean for the overall policy of a government?

The failure of the nutrition sector is that, in some way, it has been too selective. It has failed to go deeply into the factors that influence a real solution to the nutrition problem. There are countries where the problem has been solved without a specific nutrition program because it is not needed, because part of the general government policy takes care of the situation. We can contribute something to knowledge if we are able to define approaches which will demonstrate the interaction between food and nutrition on one hand and government policies on the other.

Barnes
If I were forced into a corner to answer Michael's earlier question, to cite examples of national approaches that have been largely successful, I would, of course, choose China and Cuba. Ewen Thomson cites the food technology-profit motive conflict, and we also could note the breast feeding-artificial formula conflict. The power of the profit motive is always on the technology side. One really begins to wonder if it is going to be possible to solve these problems without a very imperious government and possibly without a more planned economy.

Adam Smith, in discussing economics, used a nutritional example when he said it is not for his love of humanity that we expect the baker to provide our daily bread, but rather from his own self-interest. I do wonder if we *can* have a free-floating economy and a free profit motive and simultaneously solve these nutrition problems.

This question may become more important as we face progressively greater shortages, not only on the food side, but on the fertilizer side, and the energy side, and the irrigation side as well. I simply raise that as one of the questions that we are going to have to face if we genuinely want to feed everyone.

Thomson

You raise an interesting point on the importance of government in a centrally directed economy. I would couple this with possibly the only successful nutrition program I know: the United Kingdom during wartime. People were nutritionally healthier than they have ever been before or since, and it was due to a centrally controlled economy. It would not have been possible otherwise.

14 NUTRITION AND CULTURE   Michael C. Latham

On a topic such as the one that's been assigned to me, the relationship between culture and nutrition with reference to government policy and planning, you might expect to hear a short anthropological treatise on the most bizarre food habits of some exotic people in some remote corner of the world and the difficulties in changing these practices.

Although it may be true that existing or traditional cultural practices constitute an important cause of malnutrition in some particular countries, or parts of countries, I really do not believe that these are the overriding and important detriments to nutrition that they have sometimes been made out to be. I would rather look at the obverse side of the coin because, in nutrition policy, I believe we should be much more concerned about the devastating effects of Western influence—of the introduction of inappropriate technologies and of the effect on nutrition of interference with traditional cultures—rather than the other way around.

There are other reasons for taking this perhaps contrary approach. One is because I think the anthropological literature is already very rich in observational studies of the food practices, traditional beliefs, and above all, food taboos of people who, in the eyes of Westerners and sometimes of their own national governments, are seen as "primitive" or "nonmodernized." Secondly, I think sociologists and nutritionists often have overstated the importance of traditional food beliefs as causes of prevalent nutritional problems.

Thirdly, there have been too many sweeping, yet unsubstantiated, statements concerning the rigidity of food habits and the impossibility of changing them. In fact, major changes *have* occurred, and continue to occur, in food habits and preferences, although some, unfortunately, are not desirable changes. The potato, for example, is not indigenous to Ireland but was transferred there from the New World. Yet the potato became the staple food of Ireland. As another instance, when one looks at Africa today, one sees many parts of the continent where maize or cassava form the staple. These are not crops indigenous to Africa. So there have been major innovations, and people *do* change their food habits.

A fourth reason for my emphasis is that I believe nutritionists have had it drummed into their heads that they must be aware of the culture of the people with whom they are working, but they have often failed to examine things that are wrong or undesirable in their own traditions and their own practices.

Let us face it, we all have our traditional beliefs about food, and there is no society that I know of where people, in general, eat all the foods that are available to them. Many Chinese, for example, believe that milk, that rather anemic white fluid that comes from the udder of a cow, is an undesirable or unpleasant thing to eat. But they eat bird's nests; they eat eggs that are many years old. Many Americans think that the French habit of eating snails or frogs' legs is revolting, but they themselves consume unlikely things such as spiny lobster or shrimp, and some even eat rattlesnakes. Englishmen are perhaps shocked that some people eat dogs, horses, and rats, yet *they* eat raw oysters and jellied eels. I dare say that the speaker from Scotland even eats haggis—and I won't tell you what that contains!

But, as I said before, I do not wish to dwell on these kinds of food habits because I do not believe that they are terribly important causes of malnutrition. There are many traditional food habits that are good; there are a few traditional food habits that perhaps are nutritionally bad. The majority of them fall somewhere in between.

Now, without being an amateur anthropologist, I want to turn the table and very briefly examine some of the bad effects that Western influence and certain inappropriate technologies may be having on nutrition in poor countries. I think these issues are of special relevance today and are of considerable importance for nutrition policy and planning. By raising them, I do not mean to be antitechnology, but I aim to draw attention to some existing or potential problems. I honestly believe that more government action needs to be taken to control the effects of these inappropriate technological influences than to change traditional cultural food habits.

The problem of Western technology raises many important political, economic, and social issues that may be of greater importance than some of the other strictly "nutritional" issues that we consider. What may be desirable is that a group of African and Asian anthropologists investigate some of the bizarre and undesirable practices of the West and determine the reasons that these practices are so pervasive when they move into other cultures. Investigations of this kind might be much more fruitful than research into the practice of eating slugs or snails or puppy dogs' tails.

After this preamble, let me illustrate my point by providing four related examples. These are: (1) the increasing use of the bottle, which is replacing breast feeding; (2) the introduction of commercially manufactured high protein weaning foods; (3) the spreading of the milling industry into remote areas; and (4) the widespread use of the birth control pill. I am not going to provide a case study on any one of these, but I believe that each one deserves such treatment. For the present, however, I will just say a few words about each to serve as examples.

First, let us look at bottle feedings. I am sure that, for at least 9 out of 10 of you, I'm preaching to the converted when I mention that the rapid spread of bottle feeding, replacing breast feeding, for young babies is having disastrous consequences, both in terms of health and also in terms of economics. The baby bottle has been termed "the baby killer" and that is just what it is in many places. The artificial formula or powdered milk is so expensive that the mixture gets overdiluted, leading to serious malnutrition in infants. Contamination of the water and inherent difficulties in preparing a relatively sterile mixture result in infection and diarrhea, major causes of morbidity and

death. Yet bottle feeding is spreading because of Western influence, because
of advertising, because of profits to be made by manufacturers, because of
unfortunate medical influence and for a host of other socioeconomic reasons.

In addition to affecting the health of babies and causing many deaths, reduction in breast feeding increases fertility leading to a narrower spacing
between children. It has recently been postulated that breast feeding may be
having more effect in many countries in controlling fertility than all the birth
control methods put together in those countries. Breast feeding definitely
delays ovulation.

Breast feeding clearly affects child development, but it also has very important economic consequences that are vital for planners to understand. Bottle
feeding is extremely expensive for the family. The cost is often half the minimum wage or more in countries where, often, more than 60% of the population earns less than the minimum wage. The economic implications for a
nation as a whole are also tremendous if one considers the amount of milk
that would have to be imported if all breast feeding were to cease.

The second example of technological influence is the introduction of what
Jelliffe has termed "commerciogenic" low cost protein-rich foods. In the last
twenty or thirty years, a huge effort has been made, with much UN agency
and bilateral aid financing, to promote the manufacture of protein-rich weaning foods. We are all familiar with products such as Incaparina, Pro-Nutro,
and so on. Additional efforts have also been supported by commercial firms,
and often they, too, have received subsidies and been provided special treatment by governments. These efforts have all been undertaken with the very
laudable aim of reducing protein calorie malnutrition among the poor in the
countries involved.

Barry Popkin and I, about three years ago, undertook a simulated study of
some of the so-called "low-cost" protein-rich foods available in India.[1] Taking existing incomes of the lowest 40% of the population and current figures
available for household purchasing, we determined what the effect would be
if poor Indian families diverted some of their income to purchase the recommended amounts of these commerciogenic foods. The assumption we made
was that a family already spending 70 or 80% of its income on food (which is
very common in many developing countries) could not increase the *total*
amount spent on food. If these families were to purchase commerciogenic
foods, therefore, they would have to divert some income from the purchase
of other foods. We found that in all cases, the reduction in the purchase of
rice, beans, or whatever they were buying and the purchase of the new commercial foods resulted in a reduction in total availability of both calories and
protein for these families. Therefore, the commercial foods, unless given away
free or highly subsidized, can have a negative nutritional effect on the poor
even though their aim is to improve nutrition.

Clearly the major beneficiaries, as in the case of bottle feeding, are the
manufacturers, often subsidiaries of large multinational corporations. These

foods may, of course, also benefit the middle class family. They may be benefiting the United States as well, because many of the new products are based
on soybeans, which are largely grown in the United States. But these foods
are harming the poor. The whole effort was part of a misguided attempt to
deal with the protein problem separately from the food problem.

The third example I will discuss is the milling industry. It has been well
documented that the spread of this industry across Asia brought with it increased risk of the scourge of beriberi because the mills produced highly refined rice, deficient in thiamine and other nutrients. Beriberi, in many parts
of the Far East, became the major killing disease. I don't think we yet know
the potential for harm, in terms of reduced nutrients, from highly milled
maize and other cereals in the developing countries.

Another aspect of this issue has recently been raised by Collier, working in
Indonesia, who showed a serious loss of income and of jobs for the very poor
in certain rural areas of Java caused by the introduction of small rice mills.
Many of the rural poor were dependent for their income on the provision of
labor for the hand-milling of rice. The introduction of small mills deprived
this large group of people of a means of support, and, through reduced income, the mills are having a negative effect on nutrition.

The fourth example I want to mention is the oral anovulants—the contraceptive pills. Though we all share a grave concern for the giddy spiraling of
population in many countries, particularly in Asia, and although the pill is
probably the most effective pregnancy preventive, nevertheless, the implications of the rapid increase in use of this new technology, especially in developing countries, has not been adequately investigated. These pills do not
consist of a simple chemical whose effects are well understood or which is
eliminated quickly from the body. They consist of very powerful hormones,
whose complete action is not understood and whose long term effects really
have never been fully investigated.

What lies down the road for women who take the pill beginning in late
adolescence and continuing almost through to the menopause, we really do
not know. We have, in recent years, learned that the related compound DES,
when taken to prevent miscarriage, can result, 15 or 20 years later, in vaginal
cancer in the daughters of mothers who took this drug.

We know that the pill has effects on carbohydrate metabolism. We know,
too, that these oral anovulants can result in increased requirements for certain
nutrients, such as folic acid and vitamin B6. Deficiency of folic acid is probably the second most common cause of nutritional anemia, after iron-deficiency anemia, in many of the developing countries. If the pill is causing folic acid
deficiency anemia in the United States or the United Kingdom, what is it
doing in India where this type of anemia is already fairly common? Despite
all these unanswered questions, no large scale monitoring of women taking
the pill in family planning programs in developing countries has been reported.

Another area which should be of even greater concern is the possible effect of these oral anovulants, particularly those high in estrogen, on the quantity of, or even the ability of women to produce, breast milk. In many poor communities, if sufficient breast milk is not available, the infant has little chance of survival, let alone of growing properly. Estrogen is the hormone drug that is commonly used to suppress lactation in those who do not intend to breast feed their infants or who wish to have the milk in their breasts dried up. In developing countries, many women are put on the pill very soon after delivery and at the beginning of lactation. No adequate study of the possible effects of this practice has been completed. There are definite benefits from the contraceptive pill, and there are risks involved in pregnancy and delivery. More study is needed of the relative risks and benefits, with specific reference to use in the developing world.

The foregoing are just four examples of the introduction to other cultures of new techniques from the industrialized countries, the consequences of which may sometimes be undesirable. All four cases have some things in common. First, each case results from a technological innovation. Ours is the world of technology, and the common attitude is that technology should provide all the solutions: if you have a problem, all you need is a technological fix.

Second, each case involves, in some way, our Western and particularly American practice of treating symptoms rather than causes. We have hungry Americans, as I am sure Ken Schlossberg will tell you, so we provide them, or at least some of them, with food stamps rather than with jobs. We have heroin addicts, so we replace the heroin with another drug, methadone. We are always looking for some kind of social aspirin.

Third, in each case, we have an industry ready to make a huge profit with little concern for the problems of the consumer. In some of the cases, the large multinational corporations are particularly involved.

Fourth, in three of the four cases, we have a medical profession, my profession, being a party to the introduction of undesirable changes. This is in part because of lack of appropriate training as well as conditioning to an assumption of the intrinsic superiority of technologic solutions.

Fifth, in all four cases, the new technology has come from the West, and is introduced in poor countries with little study of or concern for its potential consequences there.

Sixth, and last, in all four cases the affluent in the nonindustrialized countries either benefit from the technology, or at least are not harmed by it, whereas the poor, the underprivileged, the deprived suffer the most from its ill effects.

In conclusion, by raising these examples and by discussing these issues, I am not suggesting that these, or all technological innovations, are bad or should not be introduced. I am not opposed to the pill. I am not opposed to milling of cereals. I am not even totally opposed to high-protein weaning foods. I am certainly not opposed to technology. But I am recommending that, in government policy planning, the consequences of the introduction of alien technologies and foreign ideas and practices be carefully studied and that appropriate action be taken to minimize the ill effects of their introduction. I will conclude by suggesting that, in sum, alien cultural influences may already be having a much more serious effect on the nutrition of the poor in nonindustrialized countries than are their present food habits or current rigid food taboos.

DISCUSSION (NUTRITION AND CULTURE)

Schlossberg

Can I ask you, Michael, as one of my American colleagues who has appeared many times as an eloquent witness before Senate committees, if you have a choice, in approaching the problem, between dealing with the fundamental social conditions—a very difficult, perhaps impossible task—and alternatively, an available technological avenue, how you can avoid taking the technological avenue? If for instance, what you want to do socially requires fundamental, revolutionary, political change, which does not seem to be at hand and which to you, as a planner, may be totally unavailable, while you do have available a variety of technological tools, are you not in an almost impossible position? Do you not have to take those technological tools and use them as best you can?

Latham

I'm trying to suggest that you can use those technological tools, but that first you must be honest about who is going to benefit, and that second, you must consider who is going to be harmed by them. At any rate, you should evaluate the potential risks of adopting the technology. I think the issue of protein-rich weaning food is an example. In introducing these programs and subsidizing them, the United States, AID, and others should have realized and admitted that these were going to have very little positive impact on the poor in developing countries but were going to have some good effect on the middle class. They would also be of benefit to the United States by enabling it to get rid of surplus foods. I think the problem has been that we have been inclined to camouflage the situation and to delude ourselves and others that the benefits were going to be widespread to those most in need.

I am not opposed to the introduction of new technologies, but the question is whether the technology is appropriate and whether it will benefit the most needy. Therefore we must look at the objectives of our programs and then determine whether a new technology will help achieve these objectives and not do harm. In the case of the high protein foods, if these were desirable and necessary, then they should have been subsidized or given away free to those most in need, as they were in some countries. In the case of the pill, which in my view is a very important birth control device, we need to look at its drawbacks as well as its benefits. One might add a new corrective technology by providing, for example, folic acid in the pills for the six days of the month when one does not take the anovulent, in order to alleviate the folic acid problem. One should consider the problem of the pills' effect on breast feeding and perhaps decide not to introduce them to women who are breast feeding, or at any rate not early in the breast-feeding cycle.

I think one can use appropriate technologies after examining the potential problems. I am suggesting that in the past we have often used the technology, but we have not first examined the problems. I think we have ignored the consumer in favor of the producer, and we have ignored the very poor in the introduction of many of these technologies which are, in fact, designed to benefit the not so poor.

Technology is not bad in itself, and I agree with Ken that often, when stymied, one has to go along with some form of new technology. I think, however, that we need to examine each approach and consider its impact on the existing culture and its appropriateness rather than, as in the past, to believe that Western change is desirable, that it is "modernization," and "this is good." Often, what was done before we came along, was, in fact, not so bad after all.

Sai

Michael, you took a lot of my argument away with the very last words of your presentation. Originally it appeared as if you questioned the use of technology without first understanding *all* of its implications. I would put on the table that this is an impossible task and is not a very useful way of going about things.

I will use your own analogy of treating symptoms rather than causes. You and I, as practitioners of medicine, know that, if you have a patient with a bad headache, and you must go to the laboratory to decide whether it is malaria or typhoid, there is still the aspirin that you will prescribe for the pain, no matter which is the underlying disease. The mistake is if, after that prescription for headache in general, you stop there and do not find out the basic cause so that you can deal with it rationally. I do think we have life situations where we have such pressing problems that, if a technology comes in which looks as if it will work, the only way you can test it fully is to put it into programs and study it.

I agree entirely that the mistake has been to generalize the application of certain technologies without building locality-specific or culture-specific studies into their use. You will be happy to learn that, with regard to the pill in Africa, serious attempts are being made to understand and correct this error.

When you have a situation with rapid, dynamic change in a community, it is an oversimplification to want to address technology to the general mass of the community. There is a very great difference between the developed and the developing world in this respect: the first countries to develop did so reasonably slowly, without too many of these shortcut technologies. By the time the shortcut technologies became available, a large proportion of the population was able to benefit from them. In the developing world, you have a situation where the development is not as widespread throughout the population. Therefore, by withholding certain technologies, you may be withholding help for a marginal group that needs it.

When I evaluated the FAFFA weaning-food program in Ethiopia, we had to make this clear immediately. This program was targeted at perhaps 25% of the under-5's population. It was not a particularly useful exercise to keep

weaning food production outside of industrial processes, however, because
this 25% of the population is also from the group that uses industrially produced pasta a great deal. By creating a polyvalent industry which made
FAFFA *and* wheat products, one would be able to utilize the overhead of the
very high demand bread and pasta industry to maintain the baby food enterprise, literally, for free. I think, therefore, that there are choices. I would like
to temper your very excellent analysis of the situation by noting also some of
the ways in which technology can be harnessed.

Barnes

I would add that the pill has a much lower mortality than does pregnancy
itself and certainly a much lower morbidity. To be specific, a million 35- to
45-year-old sexually active women, practicing no contraception, will have a
death rate of 500 per year, and those taking the pill will have a death rate in
the neighborhood of fifteen. Now that is a differential that makes the technology really valid. This is a US statistic, but the benefit is higher in Africa
because pill users' death rate is lower, and pregnancy death rate is higher!

Sandoval

I agree with most of what Dr. Latham said also, yet I am going to play devil's
advocate. A lot of people in this room, at present, have children. How many
of your children were breast fed? There are numerous reasons, which we are
not going to discuss, why women might desire to avoid breast feeding although it may be hard to understand from the point of view of a pediatrician.
Nevertheless, in any social condition, there is a desire for what is perceived as
self-improvement and this leads to a demand for artificial feeding. Of course,
the desire can be stimulated by commercials and other advertising, but that is
part of what people perceive as social progress. It is hard to stop. I am not
saying it is correct; I am just saying we have to deal with it.

What we consider "adequate living standards" implies, in a way, certain
expenses. It is, therefore, bound to produce a reduction of disposable income
unless total income rises. For instance, the use of shoes implies some cost.
Now, we do not examine whether shoes are good or bad. But it is an expense
and produces a reduction in available cash. The money that goes for shoes,
theoretically, could be used for other expenses, but we do not tell people not
to buy shoes.

I do not think it is moral to say to someone, "Breast feeding is good for
you, but not for me because my wife is a doctor and she has to work." This is
the other side of the coin that should be taken into account. Of course, we
are not talking about a program here; we are talking about everyday life.
There is a desire in populations to use modern technology. They want better
living conditions and may have standards totally beyond the reach of their
capabilities or their education. Nevertheless, there is a pattern of desire, and
we must take this into account.

Solon

My own attitude to technology is both yes and no. Yes, because I am for
technology, as long as it is local technology, well-controlled technology, well-
administered technology, and technology that does not import things. I was
in China last June, and I think the secret of their advancement is that they
use local technology: their equipment is made within the commune, and they
do not have to import spare parts from all over the world.

This came up in our country, about a year ago, when I was forced to decide
on a technology to use for a low cost weaning food. After the declaration of a
nationwide approach in nutrition, commercial firms came to my office in
droves, offering low cost weaning food and wanting new plants simply for
grinding fish and shrimp and drying them. They came up with a multimillion
dollar plan on the theory that a multimillion dollar proposal would come out
less costly eventually by serving large numbers of people.

In fact, I finally decided to support the village Nutri-Pak which is built on a
very simple technology. It is still a technology, of course. It moves from
pounding to grinding. A grinder costs less than US$50 in our country, and the
sun is there free for drying. High level technology for drying costs more than
₱30,000 with the added assurance that it really kills bacterial organisms. Our
people have always eaten dried fish with high counts of bacteria, however,
but they are not harmed because all dried fish is cured in fire. Fire is still the
best treatment!

We use a sealer as well in our production. It costs about US$50 and is a low
level technology which packages in plastic on a very simple machine that can
be brought into the village. My caution is that technology is inherent in progress, and we have to move forward. We need technology, but it has to be
toned down to the local operating capability and local maintenance capability. It must be for the greater good of the greater number of people, well-
administered, and at low cost.

Thomson

I agree entirely that the appropriate standard of technology varies in each
culture and from village level to provincial level to national level. Indeed, it is
what is truly appropriate that is wanted.

Vamoer

Certainly, it is really criminal if a technology is imported into a country and
adopted despite known detrimental effects on the poor. But you may have a
situation where inappropriate technology has been established previously
with the nutritional aspects completely ignored, either purposely or because
there was nobody to point them out. The question then becomes: what do
you do with it? The problem is reversing a decision.

For example, in Zambia, we are faced with a problem of technology—milling the maize. Previously, we all ate roller meal, 86% extraction, and, by
analysis, 9.5% protein. Now that we have a milling industry, we have a highly

refined flour called breakfast meal, which is 50% extraction, and this is in the region 5-6% protein. This is the meal that has become popular with the high income bracket. Because of its status and social copying, it is also the flour now bought by the ones who really need the less refined, 86% extraction. Now, how do we reverse the process? How do we go back to eating something which is nutritionally better than what is eaten by habit?

We considered fortifying the meal with amino acids. Recently, we were advised by political experts that the best way to control consumption of the refined meal would be to increase the price and thus reduce the demand. Our previous experience with this type of advice was with beer, which used to be 15 ngwe. Experts said, "Increase the price and reduce the drunkenness." We increased the price to 18; the demand went up. We increased it to 25 ngwe; the demand went even higher. Now, we are at almost 50 ngwe per bottle and demand is still higher!

In any event, the price policy itself did not stop drinking. We still do not know what to do about maize. We have investigated why people prefer the more highly refined meal and find that:

• They like the whiteness of the refined flour.
• They prefer its packaging: an attractive polyethylene bag with artistic printing and flowers, as opposed to the paper of the roller meal, which looks like a bag of cement.
• They like the fact that the highly refined flour is packaged in bags from 2.5 to 25 kg, while the smallest package of roller meal is 25 kg.

We went to the millers and said, "Why don't you change your milling since this refined maize is nutritionally bad for the people?" And they answered, "We are a profit-making organization, and this *is* the demand of the population. In fact, the demand for the breakfast meal is 25% higher than for the roller meal." So we said, "Why not make the roller meal package as attractive and as small as the one for the breakfast meal?" They reply with cost figures: "If we put the roller meal in the same packaging as the breakfast meal, then the cost will go up and we will have to increase the price."

Sai
No. Add the extra cost to the refined meal! Instead of thinking of beer, think of the two specific things that you have. Put the price of the new package on the breakfast meal, irrespective of the cost of production. Make it three or four times the price of the roller meal. This has been done before: when the Yugoslavs wanted to change from maize to wheat, they slapped a huge tax on maize.

Schlossberg
Price is very interesting. There are certain levels at which price makes no difference, and there are levels at which price suddenly makes a great difference. For instance, in the United States in the last several years, the price of meat went up quite a bit. It had been taken as gospel that Americans would

never stop eating meat, no matter what the price. Yet, when the price did go up 100 to 200%, they did stop. There *was a point* at which Americans reduced meat consumption and traded down to lower-priced food items. I think you can play around with price, and it might well work.

Solimano

We all agree on the importance of technology, but I think what Michael has said is very important in terms of what the cultural background means and how technology should be applied. It is important to develop criteria to evaluate when and how to use technology.

I think the developing countries have the responsibility—not the US Congress—to decide what type of help they are going to accept. Many times, in developing countries, we just accept what comes. We have to consider if that approach is reasonable. We are not against technology, but we have to see how the technology applies to our development and national trends. We need very sober and objective evaluations because there is a strong tendency to communicate successes and not failures with regard to technological innovations. We learn of the product that has been successful but not much else; even researchers do not often relate their failures.

Antrobus

I think that one can add to this consideration of cultural factors and nutrition what one might call the dependency syndrome of the developing countries, which has existed for centuries. Now, several countries are making a conscious effort to shed the syndrome, not knowing whether it is possible. This attitude is linked to the need for aid and, therefore, the automatic recourse to solutions from outside of the country itself. It may extend to a whole cultural outlook which encourages receptivity to the entry of many undesirable and perhaps inadequately resolved solutions into the country.

15 NUTRITION AND HEALTH POLICY   Joe D. Wray

One of the first things that comes to mind in thinking about the relationship between nutrition and health policy is that much of what is said and done in the name of health policy is, in fact, very little related to health and much more closely related to sickness. Much of what we do as physicians, much of what goes on in administrative health, is concerned with sickness and coping with sickness. Yet, if our concern is with health, then surely nutrition should be a central issue, especially in the early years of life. No environmental factor is more important than good nutrition if we are concerned about good health.

My own perspective on the relationship between nutrition and health has been profoundly affected by my experience in a number of countries, where I have seen the devastating effect of malnutrition on young children. These consequences are well known to many people in this room. My appreciation of the importance of nutrition has been heightened by some of the historical evidence from more affluent countries, and it seems worthwhile to review some of that evidence here.

Just about a hundred years ago, Louis Pasteur, Robert Koch, and some of the other pioneer medical scientists were laying the groundwork for the medical-technologic approach that still dominates our medical thinking. The germ theory came into being approximately a century ago, and we have yet to escape from it. At that same time, however, in the continent of Europe, death rates were already falling and in some countries had begun to fall a good many decades before. It is interesting for pediatricians to contemplate that while overall mortality was declining, infant mortality rates held steady through the nineteenth century and then, around the turn of the century, began to fall precipitously in Europe and in the United States.

Among the best data available are those from New York City.[1] There we know that infant mortality fell from around 140 per thousand at the turn of the century, to well below 60 per thousand in the space of about 30 years. And yet, at *no* time in those 30 years did the medical profession have any specific, effective, preventive or curative measures that were capable of bringing about that change. The fall in mortality occurred, primarily, because fewer and fewer children were dying from diarrheal diseases and respiratory infections, as is clearly apparent in figure 1. As we look back, the only way we can account for this is to assume that there must have been changes in exposure to and in resistance to infection, and it seems likely that these changes were related, above all else, to nutrition.

Thomas McKeown and his colleagues, who reviewed general mortality changes in several European countries for which adequate data are available, came to this same conclusion.[2] They found evidence, first of all, that most of the decline came about because of a decrease in deaths from infectious diseases. They then reviewed the state of medical science and public health at that time as well as the many changes accompanying industrial development.

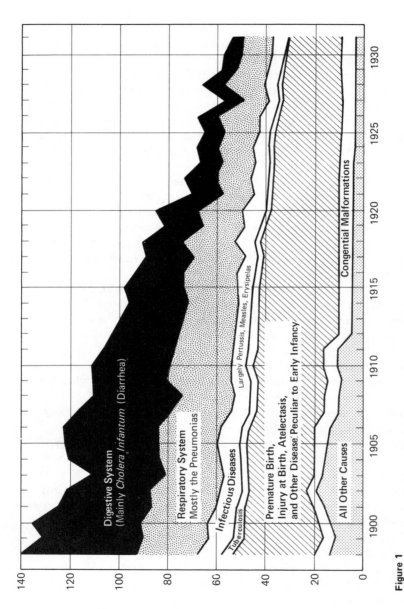

Figure 1
Infant mortality, New York City, 1898-1931. Source: See ref. 1

None of these changes, in their opinion, were sufficient to account for the
decreased mortality. They could, however, be accounted for by increased
resistance to infection because of better nutrition. There is evidence that
gradual changes in European agricultural practices during that period produced both qualitative and quantitative improvements in the food supply!
There were also improvements in marketing and distribution which made
food more readily accessible and the supply more dependable. Thus, their
hypothesis that better nutrition was responsible seems tenable.

McKeown had, in fact, carried out an analysis of similar data from England
and Wales many years ago (1942). Figure 2 shows clearly that decade by
decade, in the late nineteenth century, mortality from infectious diseases
decreased both relatively and absolutely. With specific regard to infant mortality, Titmuss[3] also showed that a decrease in deaths from infectious diseases
accounted for two-thirds of the fall in mortality between 1900 and 1925,
when, as was the case in New York City, there were no effective curative or
specific preventive measures that could account for such a decrease.

Where this has led me, in thinking about nutrition and health, is to doubt
that the Western, scientific, hospital-oriented medical tradition is the powerful panacea that I had thought it was when I finished medical school. When I
first went abroad to work, my assumption was that if we wanted for mothers
and children in poor countries the same levels of health that women and
children in the West were enjoying, then we needed better hospitals. It took
me about five years to get over that. Finally, before I left Turkey, I realized

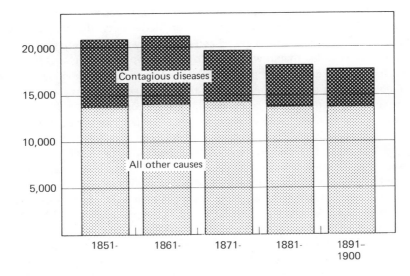

Figure 2
Mean annual death rates from contagious diseases and all other causes, England and
Wales, by decade, 1851-1900. Source: See ref. 2

that many of the children we were treating as well as possible in the hospital in Ankara should never have been there, and would never have been there if they had had an adequate diet and decent, simple primary care in the villages where they lived.

As my thinking has evolved over the years since then, I have realized that, as a product of Western medicoscientific culture, I had, in fact, attributed the health status of mothers and children in rich countries to the health care that they received. I had assumed, therefore, that what women and children in poor countries needed was the same kind of health care. As I learned a little bit more about the history of the decline of mortality rates, I came to appreciate the fact that the improvement in the health status of mothers and children in the United States, in the United Kingdom, and in other rich countries may very well have had much more to do with some indirect factors, specifically with nutrition, and little to do with health care per se.

We might do well to remind ourselves that these changes came about altogether independently of national policies and national planning. No one in New York City, in 1900, sat down and thought, "Well, the way to improve the health of mothers and children is to improve their nutrition; therefore, we must have a policy and make some plans." Instead, improvements came about as a consequence of changes in the overall standard of living produced by many factors operating in ways that were not fully understood then, or now. But the result of these complex changes was that mothers and children were better fed, birth weights improved, and fewer babies died of diarrheal diseases and respiratory infections.

As a physician, I am, of course, committed to the proposition that health care *can* make a difference, although as Walsh McDermott[1] has pointed out our position with regard to diarrheal and respiratory deaths in infants is only slightly better today than it was in 1930. If we accept, however, that better health care is needed, how should we relate nutrition to health policy? Surely the policymakers should be more aware than they seem to be of the relation between good nutrition and good health. Thus we could, in all good conscience, urge the health policymakers to give equal priority to nutrition. This is not a completely satisfactory conclusion, however. It seems to me that as we look at the difference between rich countries and poor countries today, we see that the countries with the resources—human, physical, fiscal, etc.—to mount effective nutrition policies and programs at the national level or to mount effective health care programs at the national level, are the ones that need them least. And, as we heard earlier, the countries that *need* either effective, broad, national nutrition programs or effective, broad, national health care programs, or both, are the ones that are lacking in the manpower and other resources that would make these things possible. I have been driven to the position endorsed by others earlier: that the focus of both nutrition policy and health policy has to be out at the community level, built around technology that is applicable, whenever possible, at that level.

Realistically, however, we must be careful not to go too far. With regard to health technology, there are some necessary things that really cannot be done at the village level. We are not at the point where intermediate technology in villages can produce polio vaccine, for example, or "the pill." But the list of essential things that cannot be done at the village level is short.

A related issue troubles me in regard to weaning foods. There *are* many cultures, many people, living in situations where, at the village level, there exists a combination of foods which could be mixed to provide a nutritionally adequate diet for weaning children. On the other hand, there are large numbers of people who live in situations where there is no way they can grow their own food and where the right combinations are difficult to obtain. The millions of rural-urban migrants comprising the un- or under-employed populations of mushrooming squatter-slum settlements in most large cities in the developing world are obvious examples. Thus, there are situations where the only solution, it seems to me, is to provide some sort of premixed nutritionally adequate weaning food at a price that poor people can afford.

To be sure, there have been careful and reasonably sustained attempts to develop such foods. "Incaparina" in Central America and "Balahar" in India are but two of many examples, and the results with all of them have been less than spectacular. So unspectacular, in fact, that in the minds of some the basic concept has been discredited. I think this is tragic. Rather than blaming the concept, we should reexamine our attempts to apply it—and continue until we succeed or find a more effective alternative.

The need of the urban poor is desperate. In cities where 20% of the population struggle to survive on 1% of the income, or where 20 or 25% of the heads of households are unemployed, there is no feasible alternative. If people are to be left to their own economic devices, they must have an adequate affordable food for weaning children. If the government is planning subsidized programs, the need is the same: a nutritionally adequate product that can be produced cheaply for mass distribution. Thus, I am prepared to argue that the development of such food products, and of effective methods for persuading people to use them ought to be a cornerstone of nutrition *and* health policies.

Aside from a short list of needs that can be met by technology, I believe that we must think in terms of both nutrition and health policies that are based on the resources, wherever possible, of the local community. Given the interaction between nutrition and disease, and given the importance of nutrition to the health of individuals, nutrition and health policies need to be intimately interrelated. I believe that many of the problems that confront the health planners and the nutrition planners should be dealt with through the same infrastructure. Unfortunately, it is precisely the infrastructure that is lacking in most poor countries, as we are all well aware. The superstructure at central levels tends to be overblown, while it dwindles away to little or nothing at the periphery—where the people are. Yet if we wish to do anything about health *or* nutrition, there must be a connection between the center and the periphery. Another cornerstone, then, of any nutrition *or* health policy must be the extension and improvement of the infrastructure.

Whether this infrastructure is to be the responsibility of the health sector, a rural development program, or some other agency, the need is essentially the same. Furthermore, those administrative skills that are called for in managing nutrition programs out at the village level and in managing the necessary support system are essentially the same for health care or family planning programs as they are for nutrition, whatever the sponsoring agency. And I think, finally, that sometimes in trying to separate out health and nutrition and deal with them differently, we may be creating or aggravating problems that could be better handled if we used a more integrated approach.

DISCUSSION (NUTRITION AND HEALTH POLICY)

Barnes

One thing puzzles me: why explain the drop in childhood death rate by a change in immunity? Haven't you failed to mention sanitation: the introduction of flushing toilets and the spread of pure water through those decades? I have always felt that it's more important to have a plumber on your city block than a doctor, and I wonder why articles speak of the ratio of doctors to population instead of the ratio of plumbers to population!

Mellor

Because the doctors write articles!

Wray

McDermott is the person who has looked at that New York data most carefully. He points out that you can pinpoint on the mortality-rate-by-year curve, the dates at which various "public health" events occurred. For example, in 1907, the Croton water supply began to be chlorinated, and then, a few years later, laws were passed requiring pasteurization of milk. You can look at those specific events, and others like them, and find that there is no discernible effect on the slope of the declining curve.

The issues here were well covered by Dr. Edward Kass, in his presidential address to the American Society of Infectious Diseases.[4] He presented the curves of mortality from tuberculosis, diphtheria, measles, whooping cough and scarlet fever shown in figure 3. The graphs indicate, for each disease, the points in time at which the causative organism was identified, antitoxins or vaccines were developed, or specific therapeutic measures became available. Figure 4 shows tuberculosis death rates in the United States from 1900 to 1960. In all cases, death rates from all these diseases had begun to fall before modern medical science had any impact and by the time specific therapy became available were but a fraction of their initial levels.

This is the reason that I incline to attribute the changes more to changes in resistance than to environmental sanitation. I do not deny the importance of environmental sanitation at all. On the other hand, environmental sanitation per se, plumbing on your block, surely has nothing to do with rates of diphtheria, scarlet fever, or tuberculosis, although crowding in homes might. Actually, there is a whole package of changes involved in improved standards of living. Among other things, in New York City, between 1900 and 1930, refrigeration became more easily available, along with better plumbing. I am sure that was an important factor in reducing diarrheal disease. But that alone cannot account for the total change.

Sai

I think that the antibiotic example that you mentioned is important. The TB curve was falling, but, at any rate in Scotland, where the incidence was very much higher and where the local sanitation and general environmental

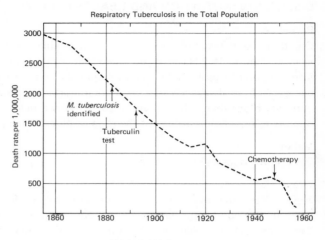

Respiratory Tuberculosis in the Total Population

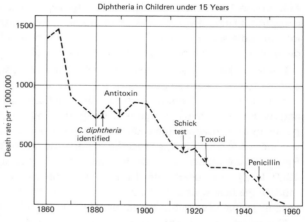

Diphtheria in Children under 15 Years

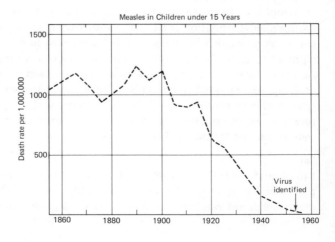

Measles in Children under 15 Years

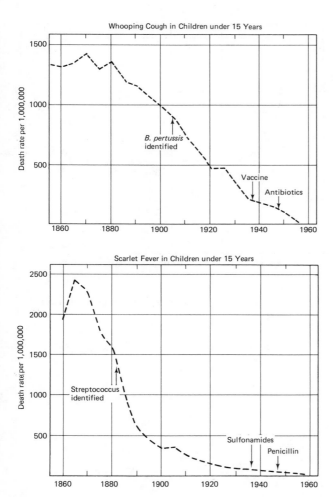

Figure 3
Mean annual death rates from various diseases, England and Wales, 1860-1960.
Source: See ref. 4

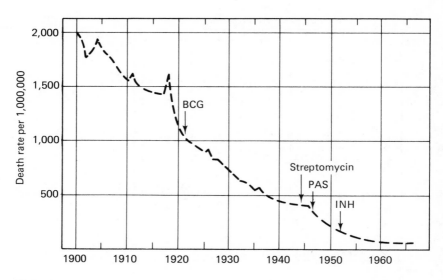

Figure 4
Mean annual death rate from tuberculosis, all forms, all races, total population, United States, 1900-1966.

background was not as good as in the London area, the change in the curve, when streptomycin was introduced, was really much more dramatic. I use this as an example because it shows that, given a lower developmental level, the impact of the technology may be greater.

You might not, however, be able to *maintain* that impact unless you change the total environment, too. I will give you an example. Yaws had almost completely disappeared from Accra in Ghana before penicillin became widely available, but there was a very large incidence of yaws in the rest of the country. A massive campaign, using penicillin, wiped out yaws from the rest of the country, but, on resurveillance in recent years, we find that it keeps creeping back into various sections of the country, while it has not been able to creep back into Accra. So the logical conclusion is that these environmental changes have helped; the general upgrading of living standard helps solve the problem if it operates over a long enough time scale. But given appropriate technologies *now*, you can make the change very much faster. A caveat is that unless, pari passu, you also try to take care of other environmental problems, you cannot maintain your advance. I think, as an old health planner, that this is the way I would like to rephrase your statement.

Latham

I think what Joe Wray has said is terribly important, but I also share Allan Barnes' views that some of the other changes were also important. It was during the terms of three particularly strong mayors in New York City that all this occurred. A lot of other things were happening at the same time, some of which were directly nutritional, for example, the introduction of milk stations for children.

Joe's comment on the need to integrate health and nutrition policy is very important and very relevant, and we need to do this. But there is a problem, I think, with nutrition which differentiates it from some other aspects of health policy. One controls smallpox almost entirely by a health activity; one controls polio by a health activity. On the other hand, to improve nutrition we need very much the contribution of agriculture, of education of social development, etc. So, though, within the health policy, nutrition needs to be a significant component, "nutrition policy" goes far beyond a "health policy" per se. The complexity of the picture increases because we have to involve several other disciplines and many ministries.

Schlossberg

I want to emphasize that the thing to do is to keep in mind the long term objective and, perhaps, not worry so much about the steps by which that objective is achieved. More specifically, the objective is to improve the standard of living. As someone who has worked in politics, I am fascinated with the way certain problems seem to be more attractive to governments than other problems, regardless of the scientific or statistical case for the importance of one problem as opposed to another.

For instance, in the United States, we had a serious problem of malnutrition in the low income population. We have an equally serious and, perhaps, a more severe problem of poor housing in that same population. If I could somehow make the case that bad housing causes disease, I think I might be able to get something done about housing. But that is a very difficult case to make. For whatever reason, nutrition, as an issue, was the easier case to make and, therefore, attained support that the housing issue did not. I think that may have been a function of the fact that food is readily available, or at least appeared to be so, whereas housing, materials, labor, etc., were not so readily available. Now, in fact, I really cannot tell you what effect the approximately $8 billion invested annually in nutrition has had in eliminating the respiratory diseases that occur in the bad housing.

If, in a less developed country, it is easy to make a case for dealing with environmental health problems as an attractive and feasible route to improve the standard of living, it might well be in the interest of nutrition advocates to arrange with health planners and/or physicians that both groups forego their most immediate interest (providing food to improve nutritional standards or medical services to cure the sick) and agree on something that would be desirable from both of their standpoints, although not a prime concern of either: the improvement of basic public health standards. By doing this, they might build a coalition between two groups that have different interests, but somehow find a common concern. And in fostering that common concern, they then might begin to deal with each other's specific interest.

Wray
Coming out of the medical tradition and looking at these problems, I have been shocked and distressed at the lack of hard data that would help one make the kind of choice you are proposing. The trouble here is that the data that are avilable do not help us build a very strong case for environmental sanitation. It is really a very confusing set of situations, the result of different blends of causes and effects.

Schlossberg
I think the problem is relying on data. Why do you have to rely on data to make a case that environmental sanitation is a public good?

Sai
Actually, there *are* statistics. When you look at the PAHO study of mortality in infants and children, you see that 5% of mortality is directly attributable to malnutrition alone. In 55%, poor nutrition is an associated cause of death. Among that 55%, diarrheal diseases are the major cause of mortality and diarrheal diseases are largely related to water and other environmental conditions.

Wray
That is the assumption that many people make, and it is widely and frequent-

ly repeated that diarrheal disease in infants is "largely related to water and other environmental conditions." But it hasn't been very well substantiated. Nor, indeed, was that the conclusion of Puffer and Serrano, who carried out the PAHO study you cited.[5] Look at the specific field studies: in Guatemala, for example, an attempt was made to compare the impact of nutrition, per se, versus health care, including improved water supply. The health services, water supply, latrines, etc., that were provided, were, according to the authors, far more extensive, comprehensive, and costly than is likely to be available in most countries. Yet, they had relatively little impact, and nutrition alone had *more* impact in improving health indicators, both morbidity and mortality, in preschool children. That was also my experience in Candelaria, Colombia.

Soekirman

To expand on your point, Joe, we are convinced in Indonesia by hard data that nutrition should be an important component of health policy. In a suburb of Jakarta there was a study on health care in which all health services were maximized: nurses were supplied, primary care was given, all vaccinations were complete, but without any educational input on health and nutrition. Within five years, infant mortality dropped from 110 per thousand to 60, but childhood mortality remained the same. The prevalence of PCM, grades one and two, remained the same, at about 30%, and vitamin A deficiency remained the same. Here are facts with which to convince the policymakers: here, for example, we have health services minus nutrition and do *not* solve the nutrition problem.

Wray

Environmental sanitation, apart from medical services, surely affects the health of adults, but if you focus on infants, the connection is not that clear. There is no doubt that household and maternal hygiene have an impact, but, on the basis of the evidence available, I think diarrheal diseases are tied in more closely to nutrition.

Ken, you asked why we have to have data. If we are going to have to assign priorities, if, as is sometimes the case, because of limited resources, you have to choose between putting your money into nutrition versus putting it into water supply, you would like to have some hard data. You would like to make the most rational choice. On the basis of data that I know, if I had to make that choice, I would choose nutrition. But I would do it while telling you that I am not happy with the quality of the data.

Schlossberg

Let me respond to that. I am trying to say that *if* it is believed that sanitation is the problem, and if *that* is what you can get the government to spend its money on, then take it and run with it. And then, after you have done that, if you still have problems, you can say, "All right, now we have to take step two." Obviously, nutrition is an important component here, and you can make a case for it. But why undermine something that is good by trying to nail the data down to such a fine point that you confuse the politicians?

Wray

I appreciate the point you want to make: if you can "sell" only one of two more or less equally useful issues to the decisionmakers then do what you can. My difficulty with the case in point, however, is that I simply do not believe that the two—environmental sanitation and nutrition—are equal. As I have tried to make clear, there is *very* little evidence that environmental sanitation per se has any effect on infant mortality, in spite of constantly reiterated slogans about its importance. There *is* some evidence that nutrition makes a difference. Thus, if you care about children, you push nutrition, no matter what the decisionmakers are willing to "buy."

16 NUTRITION AND POLITICAL PROCESS   John D. Montgomery

Many factors influence the nutritional state of a population. Government policies are only one factor, but they cannot be ignored in our discussions or our research because there are many situations in which their influence is decisive.

The task of the nutrition planner is to discover, promote, and manage public interventions that are scientifically practical, politically feasible, and economically viable. Moreover, his success depends upon what he can do to improve the performance of other actors in the policy arena, including the Ministry of Agriculture, the Ministry of Education, the Ministry of Community Development, the Ministry of Commerce and Industry, the economic planners, and the importers. These agencies are performing functions they may not consider relevant to the function of nutrition planner. When he decides to make them relevant, he is trying to link "indirect" effects into "direct" nutrition interventions. Most of the work of nutrition planners working on a national scale involves mobilizing and joining with resources assigned for other purposes. Converting "indirect" effects to "direct" policies is the central task of nutrition planners.

One of the most interesting stories I have heard is the Indonesian case in which, as I interpret the history, three different policies were adopted in succession. In each instance, an activity "external" to nutrition became the direct responsibility of the nutritionists. In all countries with which I am familiar, nutrition policy came about through such transitions or accretions, producing incremental growth. Nutrition programs do not spring full-blown; they are pragmatically and incrementally adjusted by finding one thing that works and moving into other things that might work to reinforce the desired effect.

The student of nutrition policies is concerned with the processes by which programs move from indirect to direct interventions. I believe that more knowledge of these processes, drawn from comparative experiences, can be of great value in developing strategies for improving nutritional standards. I take this issue to be the peculiar concern of policy analysts.

Since most countries do not start with a comprehensive nutrition program, it becomes all the more important for the policymaker to discover the interests of different participants in formation and execution of policies that are to become elements in a coherent national strategy. These interests are not identical. The politician likes a child feeding program in the school system because it affects so many schools, so many children, and so many parents. He is not necessarily concerned to discover that that is not the best way to get at the most vulnerable segment of population. The nutrition planner has to consider such divergent interests; he has to add different goals together, to consider different sets of interests, and to find out ways of bringing them into some kind of compatible relationship (figure 1).

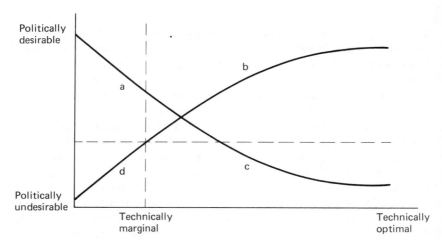

Figure 1
A conceptual model of political decisionmaking.

Consider the case of the US Department of Agriculture, which, for many years, wanted to send surplus grains abroad simply because they were surplus, regardless of the priority needs of countries on the receiving end. Or consider whether people getting food stamps in the United States are necessarily getting the foods they need most. The challenge in both cases is to make the most of resources that are made available. Even physicians have their own special interests, and they are not necessarily identical with those of the most disadvantaged elements of the population. In short, nutrition policies can be conceived of as a play in which everybody has a role, but the actors are not all saying the same lines. The person who is planning nutrition policies must understand the roles of all the players, or at least the ones he wants to have on his side. He must understand something about the process of coalition building in developing a satisfactory, sustained program.

Our ultimate need as planners is to discover *how* to learn what works and what does not. My approach to this may be a little different from the focus of others. I am certainly not trying to substitute it for the biomedical sciences, but to plead for professional nutritionists to learn how *to treat policy and policy decisions as data.* Making policy the object of study is not the same as examining interactions between food and health or the incidence and medical consequences of malnutrition. It is now quite feasible to make use of current operating experience as a basis for improving government performance.

In order to use policy as data, that is, in order to form hypotheses about government interventions and subsequently test them, we have to perform two tasks. First, we have to have a taxonomy, classifying the content or substance of decisions, which is sufficiently standard to permit others to observe practices and detect patterns in different situations. When one has only unique country experience to work with, there is little prospect of transferring the knowledge thus developed.

The second task is equally important: to look at the processes or sequences of events that occur as policies unfold in order to identify patterns of experience. There are regular sequences in which decisions are made in each area of public policy. But these sequences are not apparent unless there is also a taxonomy of the processes of decisionmaking.

The taxonomy I propose to use in approaching the first task takes the form of a matrix (table 1).

There is no field of government action which embraces as many different kinds of policies as does nutrition. One must begin to disaggregate the concept of "nutrition policy" into its basic elements so that it can be examined in three major dimensions: technological, institutional, and motivational elements.

The most obvious, or "first order" decisions, involve technological choices. The choice of technology can be characterized by the point in human activity at which the government intervenes. Such points in the case of nutrition are listed on the top line: the farm, the mill, the market, the home, the soup kitchen. One can go on indefinitely, but I picked these because they all have very distinctive characteristics from the point of view of the policy analyst.

Second order decisions address the question: who is going to carry out the changes required at these points? What administrative organization is required? At farm level interventions, one probably has to work through the Ministry of Agriculture. At the mill, one probably is going to have to work through a millers' association, the Ministry of Commerce and Industry, and so forth. In dealing with the market, there is the Ministry of Economic Planning, the import control devices, the tax people, the shopkeepers, and the regulatory agencies. As we heard in the case of Zambian flour milling, one cannot pull just one of these levers without setting into motion a complicated set of interactions.

If governments choose to intervene at the home level, they usually work through mothers' and women's clubs, through the Ministry of Community Development, perhaps also a Ministry of Agriculture and, if there is one, a Ministry of Communications. They may also work through the media. An intervention through the school system means working through the Ministry of Education. A soup kitchen scheme requires some kind of welfare agency, perhaps including the private sector. Nutrition planners decide on the mobilization of different administrative resources in terms of the technology or entry point through which they plan to intervene.

In many, perhaps most, cases, governments make this decision first. First order decisions tell you which choices to make in the second order. Conversely, if you start with second order decisions, you limit your access or entry points. If you make decisions in both categories at once, it is difficult to

Table 1
A matrix showing the interaction of decisions regarding technological, institutional, and motivational choices that are associated with different "entry points" for nutrition programs

Point of Entry (Decision Options)	1 Farm	2 Mill	3 Market	4 Home	5 School	6 Soup Kitchen
First order decisions (technology)	Agricultural innovations	Food enrichment	Food products	Food preparation	"Hot lunches"	Prepared food distribution
Second order decisions (organization)	Farmers; Ministry of Agriculture, Research, and Extension	Millers; Ministry of Commerce, Industry	Commercial sector; multi-nationals	Wives; home extension services; mass media	Teachers, administrators; Ministry of Education	Volunteer workers, welfare agencies
Third-order decisions (motivation)	Price supports, subsidies	Regulation, price supports, taxes	Taxes, import policies	Education, health concerns	Regulations as discipline	Risk of starvation or malnutrition
Primary beneficiaries	Entire population	Entire population	Middle classes	Lower classes	Children	Very poor, urban classes

calculate how to gain affirmative interaction, reinforcement, and mutuality among the participants.

Third order decisions have to do with the clients or the supposed or intended beneficiaries of policy. These decisions depend on what clients have to do and why they will want to do it. Once these facts are known, nutrition planners can mobilize various resources at the government's command to gain popular support and participation. If nutrition planners forget the beneficiaries, it does not matter how good their technology is or how beautiful their administrative organization. Third order decisions are the ones that count. That is where the payoff is if you are really talking about *nourishing people* and not simply designing a nice-looking program or using appropriate technology. This is a truism, but knowing it is not the same as acting on it.

If the farmer is supposed to plant an improved seed, planners should ask themselves, why should he? Will he get seed at a bargain? Will he get a price support or subsidy? Will he have to pay a tax on purchases of unimproved seeds? Such policies are adopted in order to make clients' participation worth their while. These decisions are usually made independently of the first and second order decisions; governments rarely start with a third order decision, although maybe sometimes they should.

In the case of the mill, the question is how to persuade consumers to pay the extra cost of the iodized salt or enriched grain. Even if the cost is the same, there sometimes have to be policies to persuade people to depart from traditional preferences. Governments have to create motivation to change if they expect their citizens to respond.

In the case of the home, ways have to be found to persuade the mothers to try something different. Getting people to eat new foods is often not easy. Sometimes nutrition policies require members of the family who have traditionally had the first choice of food—the elders, for example—to sit back and let expectant mothers or infants have the first choice. These kinds of behavioral changes involve the cultural patterns that we talked about before.

In dealing with motivation through schools, one begins with the ministry in order to reach teachers. They, in turn, will have to become concerned with school lunches, and more than that, with seeing that they are mixed properly and consumed by those for whom they are intended. Even the soup kitchen approach is difficult in many countries because the very poorest people in society often hesitate to come to a soup kitchen, even when they receive food free. Often the people you are trying hardest to reach are just below the margin of being reachable. The very poorest people do not read the newspapers or use the streetcars because they do not have small change. They bear hidden costs in gaining access to public services. To them, transportation is a problem. So is pride: they are ashamed to come to a soup kitchen.

Third order decisions are the critical policy instrument in reaching the people who need help the most, as contrasted with people who are just above the economic line of marginality.

My own interest is in identifying answers to these questions as they appear in the country programs. In applying these three orders of decisionmaking, I hope to gain some insights that will permit me to compare the experiences of countries that are carrying out similar programs.

In the interest of time, I have confined my discussion to the first of the two tasks I mentioned at the outset: developing a taxonomy of nutrition decisions that will permit us to compare them in terms of content. The process variable, the second analytical task, represents an even more complex range of issues.

DISCUSSION (NUTRITION AND POLITICAL PROCESS)

Thomson

You advocate taking policy as data. In this exercise, what would be the definition of policy?

Montgomery

I regard a policy as an intentional intervention by the government with the expectation of improving an identified problem or condition.

Sai

I would like you to elaborate on that area of your presentation dealing with deriving a program to maximize the efficiency of an indirect approach when you discover that it has an effect. It appeared to me as if you were giving indirect approaches some kind of priority in the situation and that you might almost ignore the direct approaches.

Montgomery

No. What I was referring to was the incremental process by which you start out knowing that you are going to do something, and then you discover that somebody else is doing something that is even more important, so you redirect your efforts in order to take advantage of his. If, on the other hand, you discover that somebody else is doing something that is undermining your efforts, you begin to negotiate with him. That means that you have taken what was an indirect effect and converted it into a direct effect, and this process by which you consciously address yourself to an enlarging scope of intervention, is, to me, the way in which policy is made in the real world.

Sai

Now you have just made one other point that I want to emphasize: in the context of accretion of efforts, minimizing a retardation might be as important as anything else.

Montgomery

Exactly.

Schlossberg

I really do not understand what you mean by "minimize a retardation."

Sai

When you are pursuing a policy, there may be activities which will increase the effectiveness of your program; other things will tend to diminish the effectiveness of the program. I am saying that in mounting an ever increasing quantity of programs, anticipating and preventing those situations which might hold you back could be as important as identifying those activities which, added together, will make you move forward.

Montgomery

Under nutrition programs, you might, for example, intervene to reduce the importation of Coca-Cola because that is taking place at the cost of better nutrition for a certain part of the population.

Sai
That's right.

Montgomery
Now that becomes a nutrition policy as well as an import policy or licensing policy.

Antrobus
Jack, does your model accommodate the possibility of decision order one and two as being more or less simultaneous?

Montgomery
That is a very good observation because I do talk about these decision orders as if they were made separately, as if somebody sat in a dark room and said, "Now, let's see. Here it is two o'clock, and it's time to make a decision." The world is not like that. What I am trying to do is use these decision orders as analytical tools for examining experience and structuring it.

Some decisions may never be made explicitly, but something happens anyway. Decisions may be made in very different sequences, for different reasons, affecting different kinds of programs. We need to know what that order is, because the sequence affects the substance. Some decisions perhaps preclude other actions in the future. If you make two decisions simultaneously, or if you make none, some kind of program will unfold, but its course is hard to predict and harder to control.

Antrobus
But once you put down the orders of decisions, you suggest a priority rating for them.

Montgomery
Priority in sequence is not necessarily the same as priority in importance. The first order decisions, technology, are in some ways less important than either the second or third order decisions, but they are the ones that tend to interest professional nutritionists.

Maletnlema
In your very first statement, you said that the government makes a decision in one area or another which eventually will influence nutrition and that very often this area is either only remotely related to the cause of the nutritionist or sometimes not at all. There may even be entirely political decisions which may be detrimental to nutrition. Then you go on to say that the nutrition planner should discover which interventions are most effective and probably try to utilize this.

Montgomery
And which interventions are most practical.

Maletnlema
Yes, and which ones are the most practical. Now, how do we marry the two? Because here is someone making a decision using very different inputs from those of the nutritionist. Very often, this decisionmaking person is quite unrelated to the nutritionist.

Montgomery
That is a very profound question. I think there is a trade-off. You can refer to the table showing the optimum choices from the point of view of the nutritionist and the optimum choices from the point of view of the politician. Where these intersect, you could say, "Well that's what I can get away with." In reality, such choices represent very complicated political processes with trade-offs and bargaining. You are going to lose a few, and you are going to win a few.

López
And you have to assume that you don't have all the answers.

Barnes
As a matter of interest, how similar is this to the paradigm you constructed for education? In other words, how related are the solutions to different problems?

Montgomery
Nutrition policies are not very similar to those in education. On the other hand, the optimum way to carry out land reform seems to have many lessons for nutrition policies. Some of the things we find by comparing different policies are essentially common sense, like the necessity for decentralization, community involvement, and appropriate technology. It is noteworthy that these issues touch mostly on second and third order decisions. Occasionally, an educationist comes in and says, "What I need is a satellite; then I can reach everybody and give them a standard education. In four years, everybody in this country is going to come out with a Harvard Ph.D." This is obviously an inappropriate technology. But it is not really surprising that there are people who think that way about education. And there are people who think that way about nutrition.

The place where specialists most often get in trouble is in second and third order decisions. But there is a different weight to each of the three decision orders for each one of these policies, which you will note if you look closely at them. For example, take the mill case. There, technology is quite important, but if you get it so that it works, then the consumer may not have as much importance because he buys what exists on the market. Note here that I tried to arrange the decisions in order of ascendancy as social interventions. If you arrange them in order of the relative *importance* of first, second, and third order decisions, you would come up with an entirely different way of looking at the problem.

If you happen to be in a situation where there is a very strong government, then decisionmakers can adopt policies in accordance with the capacity of the government to make first and second order decisions, and everybody else has to go along. If you happen to be in a situation where there is not strong central focus on the nutrition problem, then you had better start with the third order decision and try to find ways to get people to change their habits. The decision order analysis is a kind of diagnostic tool as well as an instrument for making historical comparisons.

To make this analysis work, we would probably have to go into each country. At a conference such as this, we can examine country studies in a preliminary way, but in order to find out who decided what and how they went about it and what sort of levers they had to pull, one would have to develop special techniques and special access. In the end, that is what I think we will need to do.

Policy sciences are somewhat like the science of economics as it was 50 years ago. It was just beginning to think of asking questions, testing some very general assumptions, and figuring out ways of compiling data. Now, for the first time, after thousands of years of human experience with agriculture, we are beginning to look at compiling some data about nutrition. Next, we are going to have to learn something about nutrition policies.

17 NUTRITION AND AGRICULTURAL POLICY
John W. Mellor

I would like to approach the topic of agricultural policy from the perspective of development policy and nutrition. The differences in title are modest, but they should be made explicit. I am going to talk substantially about agriculture and agricultural policy, but I want to emphasize that just as most nutrition programs fail because the general economic strategy is not conducive to their success, so most agricultural development programs fail, because the general strategy is not conducive to their success.

Thus, I want to take a little broader approach and talk about development policy, not just agricultural policy. I also want to note that nutrition is subsidiary to development policy, because no country starts with nutrition policy and then wraps development policy around it. One starts with a development policy, and that policy may be conducive to desirable nutrition policy, or it may not. If it is not, you will still have programs for nutrition, but they will not work.

I think there are really three basic reasons why specific programs in nutrition, or agriculture, or in other areas fail. First of all, they may be poorly conceived as programs. The second reason why programs may fail, even though they may be well conceived, basically logical, and founded on correct scientific premises (in the case of nutrition, human biology), is that they may be poorly executed or administered. This is involved in part of what John Montgomery discussed. In the third case, the one that I want to deal with, you may have well-conceived programs which have good administrators in charge, but the programs may still fail. And that is because the economic environment or the development environment more broadly is unsuitable to success.

I might say, incidentally, far too often we blame poor implementation when really the problem is that the general environment is wrong. For example, it is generally said that Indians are good planners but poor administrators. Now that seems like a very strange view when we look at the quality of the administrative services in India and their reputation in the colonial period for administering particular types of programs. One recognizes that it should not be all that difficult to move from law and order to true development. A lot of the specific programs in India fail, in fact, because of a very inhospitable economic environment for those programs and not because the administrators are poor implementors.

I would like to leap from that background to a few comments about what I see as some crucial environmental needs for effective nutrition programs. I use the term "program" to mean something fairly specific, such as the direct delivery of certain nutrients to expectant mothers or to infant children, or to adolescents. I will deal with the question of the general economic environmental needs for success of specific programs. I can list three requirements, and, as we always say, "I'm sure there are more of them."

The first of these environmental needs is sufficient food production, given the distribution of income in society, to ensure an adequate caloric supply for the mass of people through the market mechanisms. I am making an assumption that nutrition programs are not appropriate tools for providing a basic caloric supply for the mass of the population and that market mechanisms are the efficient way of doing that. Perhaps one should include protein along with calories in that statement, but I feel a little uneasy about that because protein may be a bit more complex.

In my view, one of the most serious problems of nutrition programs in low income countries has been the fact that the development strategies in those countries did not have a place for major expansion of agricultural production or for massive imports of food. Therefore, the caloric supply has been deficient, given the distribution of income, to provide adequate calories for lower income people.

There is an important problem of distribution of income, which needs to be commented on specifically. I think we all recognize that India, when we adjust for body size, climate, and so on, may not be much worse off than mainland China in caloric supply per capita. However, as long as India maintains a distribution of income which is essentially the same as that of the United States, it will not be able to provide adequate calories for the lower income people without a massive increase in the total supply of calories. If, on the other hand, they had a distribution of income unlike the United States and very much like that of China, then their existing supply of calories might be adequate to provide a basis for effective nutrition programs. So we cannot divorce the question of distribution from that of total supply.

The second environmental need is sufficiently productive employment to insure the requisite purchasing power which, in turn, assures adequate caloric intake by the mass of people. Furthermore, that productive employment, which insures purchasing power, has to be in a context which does not significantly impair health in other ways. There is a very complicated set of problems here, so let me give some examples. One of Michael Latham's students has some absolutely fascinating data, still fairly preliminary. Looking at data from Kerala, in southern India, this student has found that, first of all, increased income earned by the female member of the family has a much larger effect in improving the health of children than does increased income on the part of the male member of the family. She also finds that, while there exists a direct relationship in which increased income earned by the female member of the family improves the health of the children, there is also a relationship in which, as the number of hours per year worked by the female member of the family *outside* of the household goes up, the health of the children goes down. Actually, it is rather obvious: you would expect that with mother absent and not looking after the children, they would suffer.

You have a dilemma here in that, if you attempt to improve the health of the children by having the mother earn more money, she is likely to augment that by working even more hours. Yet, that is actually going to hurt the health of the children. There are obviously some interesting trade-offs and calculations which you can make as to at just what point the health of the children is optimum. Actually, the lesson that I want to draw is a very different one: not the idea of working around the margin so that these poor women toil maximally and cause minimum damage to their children's health, but the point that raising the productivity of the labor of poor people is very important in the strategy of improving their condition.

I would like to cite one other bit of evidence. There is a very careful study by Abdullah Farook of how people in Bangladesh use their time. He entitled the study "The Hard-Working Poor," which may seem very peculiar because the upper-income classes, if not we, individually, share the view that the poor sit around idle most of the time. Farook's study shows that among the lower income classes in Bangladesh, male workers average something over 3,000 hours a year of what he calls productive employment. Productive employment includes both working for cash income as well as doing all those things necessary to the welfare and survival of the family, like cooking food and scratching up some vegetables or wheat fallen on the side of the road.

While the male members thus work a little over 3,000 hours per year, female members of the family, as studies in the United States also show, work significantly more hours. Females are working 10 to 15% more hours than the male members. Not much of that is done for cash wages outside of the household, but their total productive work is quite high. So, although I will talk quite a lot about the importance of employment-oriented strategies and increased employment in raising the funds of the poor, we must always keep in mind that, in general, the poor are not idle. When you stop to think about it, the rich people in the world would never be so foolish as to have the poor sitting around idle and the rich working! It is much more likely, with the rich running things, to be the other way around.

So, we must keep in mind that we do have to have more purchasing power in the hands of the poor in order to purchase enough food, but we also have to be concerned with the level of productivity, as well as the total amount of employment. I would add that we should be, in this context, particularly concerned about the use of women's time and look at it very much as an interaction with the use of male time. If I can be pardoned for digression, I think we need to be very careful not to impose Western middle class answers to the problems of lower class women in low income countries. My impression is that lower class women in low income countries desperately want to get *out* of the paid labor force so that they can do the things which reduce the death rates of their children. Of course, this is a radically different problem from the one facing middle class women in high income societies or, probably, middle class women in low income societies.

The third environmental need may seem peculiar at first, but I do believe one needs a rural environment adequately attractive to the educated people necessary for program success. What do I mean by attractive rural environment? I would prefer to define that entirely in pragmatic terms: a rural environment providing whatever is necessary to get those people who can implement programs in rural areas actually out into the rural areas. Now, the specifics will obviously depend on the specific requirements of those people. If you are able to use mostly people from the local rural environment, then it may not have to be quite as fancy an environment as if you are drawing people from an urban environment to go out there. So again, we have very complex trade-offs between the type of people who will staff an institutional framework and the nature of the environment needed.

The basic point I want to make is that any kind of program dealing with rural people has to be highly decentralized and locally oriented. Since the environment itself is highly variable, the solutions have to be highly variable, and that takes a good deal of delegation of authority and responsibility. To achieve that goal, one has to have some really good people in the rural areas. I simply do not believe one is going to get competent people to go to rural areas by having ministers of agriculture and commerce go to agricultural colleges and give lectures exhorting students to go back to the villages. I think something has to be done to make those places genuinely more attractive.

Let me say in passing that probably the most delightful experience I have had was the two years that I spent living in a village in India, but I would want to make a very clear distinction between spending two years in such a village and in spending a lifetime there. I would not have considered it such a delightful experience if I thought I was going to spend my whole life in that village, and I think a lot of people in low income countries take the same position.

I would like to say just a word or two about the kind of development strategy which does *not* meet the above conditions. I am going to put this in very brief terms and, therefore, grossly oversimplify, but it is the kind of development strategy which explains a great deal of the failure in nutrition programs in the world. I use a shorthand terminology for this strategy. I call it "capital-oriented strategy."

This is a development plan which, in essence, says that capital is the source of growth and maintains that, even in countries which are labor surplus and have a lot of idle or underemployed labor, you cannot mobilize that labor unless you create capital to combine with the labor. That is not such an implausible view. In putting this simply, I want to be very cautious not to give the impression that I think that this theory is a theory of idiots. It is a well thought out, internally consistent view of economic development.

Now, if you see capital as a basic source of growth and see it as necessary to mobilize labor, a number of very important implications for the economic environment follow from that. First of all, if you are going to maximize growth in your capital stock and, therefore, in the long run, maximize growth of employment, you want to maximize savings. This is because savings lie behind investment. Therefore, you want to be very careful that income does *not* get into the hands of people who will spend most of it on consumption. You want to keep the income, in the capitalist version of this strategy, in the hands of rich people who are said to save a high proportion (most of Latin America to the contrary, incidentally). In the socialist version of this strategy, you want to keep money in the hands of the government, and the government then should put it entirely into the capital goods industry: the heavy industries, machine building, and to a certain extent, steel.

Now, if you do not want to put income into the hands of the poor, you must be very careful not to employ them because we find, virtually universally, that if you employ the poor, you have to pay them wages. If you pay them wages, you are putting more income into their hands, and they spend that income. Then the demand for the consumer goods goes up, and that tends to suck resources out of capital goods production. That is effectively, I think, why we have low employment growth in most economic development strategies in the world; because most of them are the capital-oriented, capital-intensive kind of strategy.

You will notice, however, that this strategy immediately defeats the second crucial environmental factor for successful nutrition programs: provision of adequate purchasing power. Notice something else: if you are not going to emphasize consumer goods, and, if indeed you are going to keep resources *away* from consumer goods, you are not going to emphasize agriculture. If you have this capital-oriented view of economic growth, you should not put resources into the agricultural sector because agriculture is a consumer goods producing sector. All increased agricultural production will do is provide more consumer goods for the labor force. It will not contribute to capital formation. You will not have growth, capital-style, and the argument runs, you will, therefore, not be able to create employment in the long run.

Incidentally, with this view of growth, in both the capitalist and the socialist version you are supposed to check every once in a while to see if the time has come to start consuming. But what you always find out is that the time has not come yet. If you just wait five more years, if it is a socialist economy, or, since capitalist economies do not plan in five-year segments, in "some more years," you will have even more capital and then an even greater capacity to increase consumption. That, of course, has been the basis of a big debate in the Soviet Union and is what much of the criticism of Khrushchev was about: he was for beginning to switch towards consumption. So my point is that, in the capital-intensive strategy, you not only should not create employment, but you also should not do anything in the agricultural sector.

Let me now switch into what is involved in an employment-oriented strategy of growth and point out what is perhaps the crucial problem here. The alternative view of economic growth is that growth is a function, not just of one factor of production: capital, but of two factors of production: capital and labor. To increase the utilization of capital, you have to do what the capital-oriented strategy says: abstain from consumption, put resources into producing capital goods. However, in order to increase utilization of labor, even though there may be unemployed, relatively idle labor of low productivity, you do have to increase the supply of consumer goods. You have to increase the supply of agricultural commodities and other consumer goods to back up the wages which you pay. Even mainland China found, in the Great Leap Forward, that they could not employ vast quantities of labor without paying a wage, without increasing the supply of consumer goods. Of course, one crucial difference between China now and the Great Leap Forward period is that they now emphasize the production of consumer goods in order to mobilize labor for productive purposes.

Let me give you a figure at this point. In India, we find that, if you increase incomes by $1.00 in the lower 20% of the income distribution, that is the labor class, you will increase expenditure on grain alone by about 60 cents: or 60% of incremental income goes to grain. A total of about 85% goes to purchases of all agricultural commodities for consumption, including grain, and then when you put in the agricultural component of textile purchases, you are up to about 90%. So, if you believe that labor can be used productively, but that to mobilize it you have to pay a wage which will be spent, a heavy burden falls on the agricultural sector. Therefore, the crucial element of the employment-oriented strategy, which is needed to fulfill the second condition for effective nutrition programs, also requires that you fulfill the first condition, mainly enlarged supplies of food.

Two very able economists, Maurice Dobb, from England, and A. K. Sen, from India, thought about growth in similar terms, but instead of coming out with the strategic position which I am suggesting to you, they came out with exactly the same position as the capital-intensive strategy. They saw growth as requiring two factors of production: capital and labor. They saw labor expending its income largely on agricultural commodities, but they saw agricultural production as being very much subject to diminishing returns, increasing costs, and hence, very capital-intensive. They said, following a long history of economic thought, that agricultural production is limited by land area, and, therefore, faced with limited land area, increased agricultural production depends for any given increment in production, on larger and larger inputs of labor and other resources into the land. That means that the costs of increments to production are constantly going higher, and will very soon price labor out of the market in the competition with capital. Therefore, they claim, agriculture will have to switch to using more and more capital-intensive production processes.

Now, of course, in practice that never happens. We never see labor in a low income country getting priced out of the market relative to capital because of the simple fact of rising food prices. The reason for that is perfectly obvious: long before labor costs get up to a very high level, middle class people are rioting in the streets about increasing food prices. This will bring the government down unless the government does something to stop those rising prices.

What the government does in order to stop rising food prices, though it never admits what it is doing, is the only thing that can be done: *cut down the demand for food.* The way you cut down the demand for food is to reduce the incomes of the people who spend the bulk of their income on food. So, you have to cut back on your employment program. You do that through fiscal and monetary policy, and you end up back in the same boat as the capital-intensive strategy.

This explains why what is usually referred to as the Green Revolution is so crucial to the employment-oriented strategy of growth and so crucial to creating a favorable environment for nutrition programs. What the Green Revolution provides is new agricultural production technologies which, yes, do increase the cost of production per acre, but where they work—and, of course, they don't work in very many places at the moment—they increase yields per acre much more than commensurately. Thus, the cost of production per unit of output declines. This is what is crucial: how much does it cost to produce a ton of wheat, not how much does it cost to produce an acre of wheat.

A lot of people say, "If that is your definition of the Green Revolution, there hasn't been much," and that, of course, is correct. I think, however, what the Green Revolution is all about is not a few varieties of wheat and rice sprinkled here and there in the world. The Green Revolution is a revolution in our approach to biological sciences which offers us considerable promise of bringing down costs of production of grain over very large areas and bringing very large increases of production while the cost is coming down. It is not going to give us those results, however, unless we make the effort to develop the right institutional framework. In this context of technological change with sharply increased supplies of agricultural commodities, the incomes of rural people will increase very sharply providing the price of the commodities does not decline. And that can have some very salutary effects.

If the incomes of rural people are at the outset fairly broadly distributed, as they are in the peasant agricultures of essentially all of Asia and most of Africa, one tends to have a consumption pattern in which very little of the increased income—about 10%—is spent on the basic grain which has produced the incremental income. Rather, the income is spent on consumption of a fairly large range of labor-intensively produced commodities, in turn creating a substantial increase in employment. Because we are all somewhat antiagriculture—viscerally, if not intellectually—we usually think first of all of producing textiles, transistor radios, bicycles, and so on. We find, however, in consumer budget data for peasant farmers in India falling largely in the 5th, 6th, and 7th deciles of income distribution that they spend about 35% of increments to their income on agricultural commodities: not grain, but livestock commodities, vegetables, and so forth. In India, this is substantially milk, but in Thailand, it would be heavily pork, in Indonesia, I suppose, mostly chicken. These livestock products, as well as vegetables and fruits, tend to be produced labor-intensively; thus quite a lot of employment is generated, both on the agricultural side and the industrial side.

Increased employment transfers incomes to even lower income people who then, of course, use those incomes in large part to purchase the grain, which generates the rural income in the first place. I want to make it clear that, although I can describe a rather neat, closed circle of relationships here, it takes a very astute governmental policy to see that it all continues to work nicely. I do not want to suggest at all that it works naturally all by itself.

Finally, once one has a substantial increase in agricultural production and larger rural incomes, then there are secondary effects from that increased rural income. With further increases in employment and income in rural areas, there arises a very substantial demand for rural infrastructure and services: roads, other types of communication, rural electrification. Now, one also has the means to pay for it, shared between consumption expenditure by agriculturists, production expenditure by agriculturists, and the small and medium scale industries which begin to find a favorable environment under those circumstances. That contributes, again, to meeting the third condition for effective nutrition programs: an attractive living environment for the educated people necessary to staff the program institutions. With higher rural incomes, the consumer goods of the urban society presumably become more widely available. Similarly, better medical services and better education may further make the rural environment a less unattractive place in which to live.

The point I want to emphasize is that I think the basic infrastructure is important to success of any kind of program, including nutrition programs. In order to get the right people out there, you need a very expensive infrastructure. You cannot support that infrastructure unless you have a rather broad-based development effort in the rural area. To put it at its simplest, you cannot run roads and electrification out just to service an applied nutrition program. It has to be paid for by a much broader range of activities.

DISCUSSION (NUTRITION AND AGRICULTURAL POLICY)

Wray

As a pediatrician, my exposure to the economic literature is limited, in addition to which a large portion of what I have seen is difficult for a nonspecialist to comprehend. However, from the things that I have read in recent months, it seems that economists are attempting to evaluate the results of the so-called first development decade, particularly in terms of income distribution in the early '60s versus the early '70s, and have found little improvement; in fact, many of the poor are worse off. It may be that I am reading a biased segment of the literature, but I get the impression that some of the fundamental economic assumptions about development that we attempted to apply in the '50s and '60s have been fairly thoroughly discredited.

Mellor

Unfortunately, that is not quite true, although some of us are working very hard to make it true.

I think I was reasonably even-handed in my presentation of the two points of view on economic growth by grossly oversimplifying both, so that one can pick holes in whichever one chooses from the way I presented it. What I described as a capital-intensive approach was the ascendant way of looking at economic development from the middle 1950s up until, more or less, the present. I think it is fair to say the whole epoch is epitomized by the Indian second five-year plan of 1956 to 1961. This period is very well documented, partly because a lot of very bright Indian economists have gone around the world talking at conferences, and also because the bulk of the first-rate development economists of the West were in India at about that time because it was a big, interesting case in point. Several things were learned as the Indian second and third plans went on.

First of all it was discovered that the specific form which investment took, in these capital-intensive approaches, ended up giving us awfully slow growth. There is a lot of damage done by putting so much emphasis on growth *versus* distribution. One of the really crucial criticisms of the developing programs of the late '50s and '60s is they gave us awfully *slow growth as well as poor distribution.* If they had given us the growth rate which had been promised, the poor would have gotten (at least by the standards of the rich) some decent amount of trickle-down. But with the very slow growth rate and then a structure which also trickled rather slowly, even by the standards of the rich people, the trickle-down was not decent. This must be emphasized.

Secondly, it turns out that, with this strategy, it was not really possible to contain fully the leakages into greater consumption and greater pressure on agriculture. So that, sooner or later, agriculture appeared to fail. Now that need not have happened. What could have happened, in theory, is that you kept the incomes of the poor down and, therefore, you didn't get much demand for agricultural commodities. After all, it is much more the growth in per capita income than growth in population that gives us food crises. The two are somewhat related, of course, but per capita income growth is the real moving force in the food-crisis piece. It turns out that those incomes just could not be contained as much as had been thought was possible. So you had pressure on agriculture and rising food prices, even without having gone the employment-consumption route.

One reason why I put so much emphasis on this problem of diminishing returns in agriculture is that I find it a rather useless exercise to look back at the Indian second plan and debate whether they made a mistake or not. There were a lot of political factors which pushed them in the direction they took. It was very important to Nehru to get some centralization of the very large and at the same time divided country, and the capital-intensive plan did tend to encourage centralization of authority. Nehru needed a plan which would bring large quantities of foreign aid into the hands of the *central* government which it could then distribute out to consolidate its power. It is very well for us to say that it does not matter whether India is one big country or lots of small ones. Yet, while it might suit Americans better if India had become lots of small countries, I do not think it would have suited Mr. Nehru to have lots of small ones. And it probably did not suit Indians in general to have lots of small ones.

Perhaps more important, it is by no means clear that the foreign experts, to say nothing about the Indian experts, knew how in the world to increase agricultural production at that point in time. I think it is quite obvious that if the second plan had emphasized agriculture more, what one would have had was more of an ineffectual community development program and more investment in massive, large scale irrigation schemes, which also may have provided very low rates of return. We really have had a substantial increase in knowledge about how to develop agriculture in the last decade and a half. In fact, it is that which, in my view, puts a new complexion on the game, whether we look at it broadly in terms of development strategy, or whether we look at it narrowly in terms of the environment for nutritional programs.

I think there *is* a Green Revolution despite the fact that most people do not like the term. There really is a revolution involved, but not in the sense that we can suddenly move to 20% growth rates in agriculture. What we are hoping for is to go from a 2% growth rate to a 3½% growth rate in agriculture. The implications involved in that and the way it is being approached are revolutionary, and we should recognize that.

I think one wants to be careful about saying that the old views are discredited. I think that there were some unrealistic elements in the old view which call for some reexamination. Also, I think we have learned something very new, and that is how to move on the agricultural side. It is that which gives us the new ball game, which, as I say, has tremendous implications for human welfare in general and for nutrition in particular.

Montgomery
It seems to me that this kind of macro view, which you are criticizing, has a counterpart in the field of technology. The notion that it is more efficient to undertake massive, technologically rich, and capital-intensive investment programs cuts across all of the sectors of development. This includes a preference for big dams as against small ones, big machines against small ones, satellites against community programs for education; and I suspect one would find the same sort of thing in nutrition. The expectation is that you can find a couple of things that will be easy and quick and take a fairly small amount of intensive managerial or technical expertise at the beginning and then be self-enforcing. Now, I think this, which I call a second order dimension of these choices, is also being attacked because people are finding the small dams more cost-effective than big ones in many cases. In fact, they are finding that we are getting the real growth from what we ought to call the "appropriate" or "intermediate" technologies, after the British terminology. I think, therefore, that this is an ideal time for us to be looking at the interventions which require more intensive and thorough social permeation and more types of involvement by more people in the decisionmaking.

Mellor
On this matter of constantly looking for the inexpensive—let us call it "the cheap"—program which would solve all your problems: I think the reason we have such tremendous drive to do that is that we basically, as societies, do not want to do the big programs because these *do* involve major changes for the society.

Let me make several points in a very simple way. First of all, if you are going to do something on nutrition, there have to be some fairly basic changes in quite a few societies. I might say, these are changes to which American policies, in general, are quite opposed, even though we are very much in favor of the objectives of the little programs. On the other hand, at the same time that agriculture is so basic in all of this, I want to emphasize that, particularly in agricultural development, you have to have a decentralization of responsibility so that programs can be tuned to highly variable conditions.

What we must remember is that in many low-income countries, and quite possibly all, simply because they are new countries, there are tremendous divisive forces, particularly regional divisive forces. Central governments have a desire, with which I am very sympathetic, to hold the countries together. Yet, it seems to me that they very often face a conflict between the measures which appear to them to hold the country together by centralizing a number of activities and the decentralized approach I recommend for rural development and effective nutrition programs. I hinted at this in regard to India. I also think it would be true in Ethiopia, at the present time. So, there may be tremendous conflicts here which push the national strategy in a way which is simply inconsistent with success of the specific programs we are talking about.

Maletnlema

In talking about why programs fail, you listed three points, the first one being how the program is conceived. The way I look at this, one must combine it with your number two and three. In other words, if your program is poorly conceived, it means that the execution and the administration will be poor. Also, in conceiving your program you *must* look at the economic and social environment and whether they are going to be conducive to success or not. So really, it boils down to only one reason: that is, programs fail because of being poorly conceived.

You then went further and described the requirements for effective programs and, in your number three, said there should be an attractive rural environment for the people needed to make the project a success. Are you thinking of the staff who are going to run the program, or are you thinking of the people who are going to be affected by the program? If you are thinking of the staff who are going to run the program, and of providing them with an attractive environment so that they stay, then this is only a short-term effect. Eventually, that environment will change, as the program nears its objective. One should, I think, look at it from the point of view of the people who are served by the program: that their environment should change in such a way that the project staff will want to live there and that the local people will want to continue the program in their own area and not simply depend on the people from outside. The moment you create an attractive staff environment, different from that of the people being served by the program, then certainly you have created a tension which will not be very conducive to the success of the program.

A fourth point which you did not mention, and which is important, but probably not subject to analysis by economists, is local interest. For a program to be effective, it must interest the people. In other words, if you take your program to the people, and they are not interested, then it does not matter what calculations you have carried out, you will fail in the end. If the populace sees its own needs very differently, they will do everything to make your program fail.

Montgomery

When dealing with this issue of poor conception, I think we must not overlook the importance of the hidden hand: poorly conceived programs sometimes are very successful. It is a mistake to insist upon purity of conception. You may have resources that are made available to you simply because of impure conception. Sometimes the bastards are the most productive elements in society. I think what we need to do is to take something which is certainly conceived in sin, like some international food aid program—bad first order decisions—and look at the conditions under which the second and third order decisions are made. That is, we must examine the administrative arrangements and means by which the people who need the program the most are motivated to use it.

Thomson

In reference to the environmental needs of the program, the second requirement was sufficient paid employment, but many parts of East and Central
Africa with which I am familiar are only marginally on the money economy.
In these areas, there is no likelihood, in the foreseeable future, of coming
sufficiently into the money economy to achieve that environmental condition
required for a program. The indications are that, in these parts, about 20-40%
of the children under five suffer from protein calorie malnutrition, roughly
the same percentage as one sees in the employed communities.

To identify what needs to be done, I feel one must study the way in which
the 60% succeed in raising their families successfully, even though they are
not on the money economy. Once this is known, then there is a way of getting out an effective program in areas such as these.

Mellor

I tried to use very general terms because I believe so much that conditions
vary, and one must mold programs to the conditions. By the term "income,"
I did not mean just money income. I think very often we monetize more as
we raise incomes in a real sense, but that may not necessarily be the case. In
fact, I wouldn't disagree with what Ewen has said.

Soekirman

First of all, I would like to comment on agricultural development strategy. I
may be biased, but I feel that we are practicing in Indonesia what Dr. Mellor
advocates. Agricultural development is the backbone of our development
plans at the moment. Any capital-intensive programs are meant to support
agricultural development. For instance, the revenue from oil is used to build
fertilizer factories to stimulate agricultural development.

Our nutrition group in Indonesia tries to demonstrate to policymakers that
this is already a nutrition-oriented policy; that a development strategy with
concentrated priority on agricultural development means that the government
is doing something for the nutrition of the people: providing enough food.
That is, in fact, the first objective of development in Indonesia. It seems successful, and this year will probably be the first year with no imports of rice, a
milestone in the history of Indonesia.

Income redistribution in Indonesia is done, first of all, through local development. It is a "package" that we call BIMAS and IMAS: the farmers get a
subsidy for fertilizer, all agricultural inputs, credit, even money for the management of the farms. Then, once the farmers get results, there is a second
phase in which they do not get cash for the management of farms, but only
the other agricultural inputs. This is one means of the distribution of income,
practiced throughout the country.

Second, beginning last year, there are a lot of rural development programs
which allocate much money to rural areas. The central government provides,
in each village, money for health centers, for roads, for irrigation (interacting

with agricultural development), and for schools. The government even gives money outright to the village community as an incentive to develop their village. The government is trying to develop the "underdeveloped villages" into "advanced villages." The "advanced village" is one that can move ahead on its own, without government influence.

We feel that the total environment is the critical factor in development: for example, in one interesting study, more than three thousand medical doctors throughout Indonesia were asked about morbidity and mortality in their families. It was found that their infant mortality is very low, 15 per thousand—as low as a developed country. Most of these people have very good environmental, socioeconomic, and educational conditions. Attention to individual components of development is not enough, so we try to convince the planners that *every* component should be in rural development. Health services have priority, now, and sanitation is second. We maintain, however, that sanitation and health services are not complete because there is no nutrition component. Therefore, we are trying to convince the planners, step-wise, that development occurs only when all components are there.

We nutrition people try to join in these overall development approaches because the government already had a plan for other components of development. They had sanitation programs, providing latrines and water supply and, in rural areas, agriculture and labor-intensive work, but no nutrition at all. Thus, we tried to fit the nutrition input in the second part of the development plan. Yet, the question the planners always ask is, "Okay, if I let you come in with this nutrition component, how will it relate to the rest of the plan?" This remains an important question: how to relate the impact of agricultural development to nutrition, labor-intensive work to nutrition, home economics education to nutrition, rural extension education to nutrition, and so forth, and how to demonstrate to the government how our programs and plans are interrelated. Actually, we believe that nutrition programs will only be effective if there is a basis for them in rural development.

Solon

John, how do you develop a loan system where a small farm holder can get a loan without collateral? We can do some of this now with jeeps and helicopters, bringing the bank right to the farm, and farmers can get loans without collateral for fertilizer and for equipment that is supposed to increase the income of small farmers. Yet, we continue to have a problem with other people buying their fertilizer from the small farm holder so that it becomes cheaper for them as well. Although we have increased production, there is still this problem of misuse of the program by big land holders who like to get the fertilizer at low cost.

Your discussion of broader development policy brings to mind my experience at the time I was appointed director of the nutrition council. Six government members were sitting there when I said that one of the policy directions should be to improve the economic condition of the family. The chairman looked at me and said, "What are you now? Are you the National Economic Development Authority?" That really put me in my place.

It is seen as impertinent when a nutrition body tries to influence economic development authorities by saying, "Change your approach to economic conditions in the country." Who are we in nutrition to use nutrition and health as a lever to change economic conditions? In the end, I simply fell back and said, "Well, I just want to increase the income generating activities in the home." Maybe that is the only way we can make progress.

Later, when I was designing the Philippine Nutrition Program, I asked myself, "What am I trying to do?" I was designing for the whole country as if I were going to do it all by myself. Then I realized that everything has to be done by all the ministries, and if every ministry did do its job and fulfilled its objectives, we would not need a "nutrition program." This was apparent when I visited China. I asked, "Do you have a nutrition program?" They said, "No." But as far as my eyes could see, there were no malnourished children. Why? Health services were very good; agricultural production was tops; economic conditions were within reason.

Wray
Food is rationed, prices controlled.

Solon
I realize the Chinese model entails a lot of modification of government structure, but, even within the present structure of income distribution, improvement would occur if each ministry did its job. Nutrition, whether the ministries like it or not, is a part of every structure of government.

I do not think you need a separate council to run a nutrition program. I realized that when I started to design what each department should do. In health, one does not have to go outside the basic health services. It is simply intensifying environmental sanitation, intensifying medical care, intensifying education. With the agriculture ministry, it is the same thing: intensify appropriate production. So what I am really trying to do is simple: coordinate the ministries so that they carry out their responsibilities pertinent to nutrition. This is exactly what we did: we asked them to agree that they have to carry out their functions at a different level.

Winikoff
This is precisely the paradox we are here to explore. We look at the situation worldwide and find that often countries *without* nutrition policies or nutrition councils *do* solve their problem, and countries *with* nutrition policies often do not. What is happening?

Barnes
Well, if all people did their jobs, we would have utopia. Not only would malnutrition disappear, but a lot of other problems as well!

Wray

What amazed me in China, to expand on Florentino's comments, was how little thought they give to nutrition education. I asked over and over again: "What do you teach mothers about nutrition?" And they said over and over again: "We don't have to teach people to eat the right foods; we just have to make the foods available."

Montgomery

And there are no rival attractions for consumption.

Solon

And the services are available in both health and food.

Latham

I think many of us would share John's hopes that governments are moving in the direction of his "school" of philosophy of economics. One of the things he did not discuss is the possibility of looking at measurements of development in different terms. Previously, one looked at per capita incomes and gross national product rather than some of the things that nutritionists would be interested in, such as infant mortality rates and rates of malnutrition, which, in my view, are better measures of development.

Secondly, John talked about increasing the attractiveness of the rural areas in order that people who are needed to work stay out there. The other side of the coin is in stopping migration to the cities, or encouraging return to rural areas.

López

I have been surprised to discover, in all these comments, a parallel to the common wisdom about population policies: the conclusion is always that you need better living standards, better education, better health, and then maybe you will have a reduction in birth rates. And the same thing appears to be true about nutrition. If you could only raise peoples' standards of living, if only they could have better health services, better educational services, you would find that children would not die of malnutrition. This leads me to underscore Soekirman's earlier comment, which is that what you really need is the political will to introduce nutrition into government policies. Better still, not nutrition into the overall policies, but a redirection of the overall policies of governments in order to be able to bring better nutritional standards to the population.

This leads me to the question of whether you need directed economics in order to improve peoples' nutrition. From my own personal experience, I am beginning to discover that the crucial factor is really a process of introducing income redistributive goals to overall government policies. Which kind of system you use to carry that out is not necessarily important. But you must have more than just an intention. You must back that intention with actual steps, mechanisms, programs, and policies. Unfortunately, it is a long term process, and we are all thinking of the problems here and now and looking for immediate solutions.

Latham
Yes, and I think we should come back to Beverly's very important comment at the beginning, noting the tendency to label economic development and improvement in economic output as the answer to all our problems. She gave a very striking example from Mexico demonstrating how various economic indices had improved while the rate of malnutrition did not improve. I think we need to continue to come back to this. We can have all kinds of so-called improvement taking place and nutrition not changing. We must not forget that.

18 NUTRITION AND ECONOMIC POLICY F. James Levinson

My task of discussing "economic policy" has been made easier by John Mellor's presentation, because the most important economic policies affecting nutrition are the very ones he just mentioned. I think that is so probably by a wide margin.

There are a whole range of decisions that face planning commissions and finance ministries encompassing monetary and fiscal issues and industrial policies. I think, on the whole, it is unlikely that decisions in these areas will be made on the basis of their effects on nutrition or, in most countries, in fact, on the basis of their effects on the welfare of the poor in general. This has more to do with the political basis for such decision making, which I will deal with later.

For the moment, I would like to reflect on imports and exports. Those of us who have studied India do not give much attention to this area, yet there are countries for which import and export policies are critically important to nutrition. I think, for example, of the Caribbean countries and in particular of Jamaica which, as I recall, imports about 60% of its calories, as well as Chile, which continues to import a substantial amount of its food.

I have been impressed with some of the thinking on the nutritional implications of import policies, particularly at the Caribbean Food and Nutrition Institute. They are trying to decide just what are the best things to import when a country must bring from the outside such a large portion of its food requirements. We have seen some very sensible policies, and we have seen others that maybe are a little less sensible. I remember, for example, looking over some of the import and export figures for Ghana some years back and finding funds earmarked for imported infant milk formulas or what we might call breast milk substitutes.

Clearly, this is an area that has important implications for nutrition in those countries that are importing and even exporting a good deal of food. It may, in fact, make eminent good sense for certain countries in Central America to export their meat if they take the earned foreign exchange and import less expensive commodities. In addition, these less costly commodities usually have higher income elasticities of demand among the poor and would thus have a more significant nutritional impact on this group.

As I mentioned at the outset, however, I think the most important set of policies for nutrition are those that John Mellor discussed. It is well to emphasize the critical importance of food-grain production coupled with employment as a means of improving nutrition, health and well-being. As Joe Wray points out so often, this improved health is also an essential precondition for successful population and family planning programs.

You cannot pursue effective employment policies unless you have your food grain situation in relatively good shape. Furthermore, you are unlikely to have an ongoing, effective agricultural production system unless you are able to reinforce that system with significant effective demand, which is in turn generated by increased employment of the poor. Now, the question that arises is whether, in fact, this kind of a system alone will be adequate to deal with the health and malnutrition problems that we see in the world. Most probably, there is a need for explicit attention to these problems and a need for the kinds of direct nutrition and health programs we will be discussing during the week. I am continually struck, for example, by the fact that there still exist desperately poor landless agricultural laborers in the Indian Punjab which, by any measure, is a beehive of both employment and production activity. It seems, then, that significant nutrition improvement requires some more direct means of increasing the real income or real resources of the poor.

Unemployment in the Punjab is certainly lower than in other parts of India and lower than before this production spurt took place. One can still find, however, large numbers of simply desperately poor employed landless laborers, their poverty reflected in remarkably high levels of malnutrition. We found, in one district of Punjab, the staggering figure of just under 50% of the children aged 6 to 24 months suffering from second or third degree malnutrition. So, realistically, there clearly is need for more explicit attention to the problems facing this group.

One could argue, in fact, that the primary determinant of a country's success in its public health and nutrition activities and its effectiveness in reaching the poor, is the political orientation of the government. With all too few exceptions, most low income countries simply have no real political mandate to redistribute resources. Even where there is some receptivity, land reform policies and actual income transfers usually are too overt a means of redistribution.

There are lots of less overt means, in theory, of redistributing income. This calls to mind some interesting deliberations associated with the Woodrow Wilson-Brookings project on income distribution, where the economy was examined sector by sector in an attempt to figure out which instruments were likely to have an effect on the distribution of income. One after another, it was found that the theoretically effective means of redistribution were, in reality, usually circumvented by those who preferred to leave things as they were. In terms of distributing income to the poor, then, the macroeconomic approaches, while they are appealing in theory, sometimes have not proved to be very effective means of redistributing income in practice. Some of our colleagues from the LDCs challenge us on this topic, saying, "Income redistribution is one of those things which we can say very easily and is all very well on paper, but how do you do it? How do you really distribute income to the poor? Is there a formula to do this?"

The question is really whether there are any other means that might be possible. One of these that comes to mind, with respect to nutrition, is what some of us have come to refer to as "consumption planning," taking a term that originated in Pakistan. This is the notion that planning consumption is, in fact, as important as planning production. Pakistan, in fact, adopted as its policy the provision of "adequate" (or defined) amounts of seven or eight "essential" commodities to all income groups through combinations of production, price, and distribution policies. I found some other countries using rather similar language: for example, Jamaica in its recent planning work. One important implication of this trend is that countries such as Pakistan are beginning to think through agricultural land use policies, not only in terms of production per se, the conventional purpose of land use exercises, but for purposes of understanding the implications for distribution and consumption.

In addition, Pakistan has paid more explicit attention to subsidized consumption. Here, we get into an area that is traditionally controversial and frequently receives bad press: Bruce Johnston basically dismissed it out of hand, Leonard Joy joyfully embraced it, and, as I recall, John Mellor waffled on it. The last time I heard him talk about it, John said that subsidized consumption, ration-type systems, because of their very high administrative opportunity costs, are the kinds of programs that one wants to employ on a short term basis only, but not for longer term nutrition improvements. Yet, these subsidized food consumption programs do provide the poor an opportunity to buy below the market price at least limited amounts of those commodities which they are most likely to purchase. Since they cannot afford to pay the market price, such a scheme is, in fact, a transfer of income, with an increase of real income for the poor.

If, in fact, there is a need for a redistribution of resources in order to do something about the problems of the poor, then perhaps we should begin reconsidering the subsidized consumption concept. Since it is already being pursued in a number of countries, this does represent a type of indirect redistribution which has proven possible. Sri Lanka and Egypt spend roughly 20% of their budgets subsidizing the price of rice and bread, respectively, to assure that the poor are able to consume at least minimal amounts at prices they can afford. Similarly, Pakistan, India, Bangladesh, and Peru, along with a few towns in Guatemala, have pursued such policies. The United States' food stamp program is another example, in fact one of a very few which employs a means test in this kind of subsidized distribution. In the other countries, ration cards are distributed, and anyone can stand in line although the programs are, I think, effectively biased toward the poor.

Child feeding programs also transfer resources to the poor, assuming that the poor children are the consumers of the food. One can say in fact, that, on the whole, because ill health and malnutrition are concentrated among the poor, even if health and nutrition programs were evenly distributed across the whole population, they would inherently be biased toward and would favor the poor. The poor would benefit more because they are more in need.

Experience has shown that we have not been too much more successful in reaching the poor with our nutrition interventions than we have been with development programs as a whole. The direct nutrition interventions seem to fall into two categories: those which do transfer some resources to the poor and those which do not. Child feeding would fall into the first category, while nutrition education would fall into the second. At some stage in the process of nutrition planning, one tries to determine which groups in the population can benefit from relatively easy, inexpensive interventions that do not involve real income transfers, such as nutrition education. There are cases where benefits can be derived from such an approach, but one needs to distinguish those from cases where the *only* effective interventions are those which involve a resource transfer.

There is a group studying the subsidized consumption approach to resource transfer in order to see whether there are specific sets of preconditions under which such systems might be effective in low income countries. We have not yet completed the study, but I can venture a guess at two of those preconditions (beyond the basic one of having the kind of government that would even consider such a program in the first place).

One is a coupling of such policies with the kind of employment patterns and employment emphasis that John Mellor spoke about. This is critically necessary to boost income and effective demand and put continued pressure on the agricultural production sector. The second precondition, for many countries, is a certain level of food aid, per se. This aid can serve to make employment-oriented policies possible in the short run and also provide governments with the means of initiating such subsidized consumption systems.

I find myself an advocate, on the whole, with respect to food aid, despite all of the problems we have associated with it. Food aid seems critically important as a means of permitting the kinds of participatory employment and production-oriented agricultural development patterns that John Mellor was talking about. Food aid, as John also points out in one of his papers, can help a country pursue these policies in spite of major reverses in agricultural production caused by weather and natural disasters. In some sense, food aid provides insurance.

There has been some evidence that food aid will have the effect of depressing agricultural production domestically. There is some evidence from Colombia, but most comes from India where perhaps it *has* had that depressing effect. If, however, a country can pursue high employment policies at the same time as it receives food aid, it probably can offset the depressing effect of the aid on agricultural production.

I should mention here the initial returns of some research into the question of food aid which seem to indicate that in some countries—not India, not Bangladesh, but in countries which are somewhat better off and which trade in food grains—there has been remarkable success in "untying" the food aid that is provided, and transforming it from "food aid" into foreign exchange earnings. The United States provides the aid as food, sends it overseas, and expects the food to be used to feed people who were not being fed before. In fact, based on data up to approximately 1972, what we find in many countries, again not in the poorest countries and not in times of serious food scarcity, is that this objective is circumvented. What these countries do, quite simply, is to reduce the food that they would otherwise import by roughly the same amount as the donated food and/or increase by roughly that amount their exports of other foods. So, the net amount of food in the country, the net food availability, remains the same. Presumably, nutritional well-being in the country remains the same, while the country's foreign exchange position improves.

Now, this process is not necessarily a bad thing for development. If you think foreign exchange earnings are beneficial for development, then this utilization of food aid is beneficial. But we should not delude ourselves into thinking that such utilization improves nutritional well-being. Depending on the utilization of the foreign exchange, we may not even be able to claim that food aid used in this fashion has any positive effect on the poor.

DISCUSSION (NUTRITION AND ECONOMIC POLICY)

Sai

May I add a specific example of how I think, in the agricultural sector, income distribution to the poor can take place? It is too early to state its full impact in Ghana yet, but "Operation Feed Yourself" has as one of its major ingredients the free or near-free provision of good cereal grain seeds, fertilizer, extension service, and crop protection service, coupled with harvest collection and an immediate guaranteed payment for surplus commodity produced. I think this is classically the way of getting income to the poor.

Mellor

One small simplistic comment on this delivery question: it seems to me that it is absolute nonsense to think that you can have a society in which very rich people are servants to very poor people. And that is what we are setting up when we have complex institutional structures, manned by high income people, rendering services to very poor people with extremely low incomes.

There is just no way that society will pay for that. You might say, it *can* pay for it, but it will not. You see this in the United States: it does not make any sense to think that you can provide first-class medical services to people with $5,000 a year income and have those services rendered by people who are making $60,000 a year. It just takes too much income redistribution through that particular process itself, and it is not going to be done.

Thus, you have to have some kind of "reasonable" degree of equity if you are going to provide services to low income people. Coming in on the back door of what Jim was saying, I would note that for the basic services, you have to get income to low income people, and let them provide for themselves. But then I go a step further and say that, even with the supplementary services, you are not going to get very far as long as you have any major income disparities. I do not know how to define a major income disparity exactly. It is something greater than what exists in the United States, I guess, if you are an American, but if you are not an American, maybe you define some other guideline.

Maletnlema

I would like to hear some comments on food aid and food aid policy. I find this has sometimes, in some countries, a strong negative impact on local production. You find UNICEF, the World Food Program, Catholic Relief Service, CARE, all pouring food into countries with the very good intention of helping people, but often with no coordination or relation to needs. I would like to hear the economists speak on the effect of this kind of aid on local efforts.

Mellor

Food aid certainly is going to form a very major portion of total American aid over the next several years, so, while I do not disagree at all that food aid may be used in a very counterproductive way, I think it is very important to search for a positive way of using it.

Probably, the best way to put it is: if someone from Mars came down to earth and heard that in a lot of countries a lot of people were very hungry, and then heard that it was proposed to move food from a place that had surplus food to the people in the place where there was hunger, he would say, "My goodness, that's a very sensible program." Then, if he were told, "No, no, that's not; that's very bad for the place receiving the food," he would say, "My goodness, you're a terribly ingenious people if somehow you can make it bad to get more food for people who are hungry."

The fact of the matter is that we are very ingenious people, and we have discovered how to make getting more food into places where people are hungry a bad thing. But I would say that we should stop being so ingenious. Food aid legislation should be designed to increase the possibility that food aid will be useful rather than harmful. I do not disagree with your position on this; I just hope we can improve the situation somewhat.

Sai

I think that food aid, if properly monitored, can be of real assistance. In the sub-Sahara zone, all across West Africa, there are preharvest food shortages. In this circumstance, aid is helpful, but it does not have to come from outside of the shores of the country. This is where we get confused: some countries in West Africa ought to be able now to make aid move from their own southern areas to the north. The north is often so depressed that there is no entrepreneurial pool for bringing foodstuffs in. Yet, if the northern people are to be able to do a good agricultural job for the next season, they must have food. That is one place where aid can be useful.

In addition, when you have a large scale project, as we have in the Volta River project, which displaced 70,000 people, and you have built housing for them, but you have not been able to set up agricultural activities for them, you need at least one or two seasons in which they are given food while their land is opened up. This is a classic example of a type of successful food aid program, carried out by the World Food Program.

There are other basic ingredients in the World Food Program which are also good, and I think those should be identified. One of the things that I consider important is the fact that some of the foods were brought in, not to feed the people being rehabilitated, but to sell in the commercial sector. This eliminated the need to spend foreign exchange for some imported goods, such as soya oil and butter. These very high value commodities were actually sold, and the money was used to pay people being resettled to build their own roads and to make their own farms.

While the basic staple was being distributed to the adults, a milk scheme was going on for their children. This kind of a mixture tests the market and identifies what needs food aid can supply without interfering with the production of the country. Using the food in that particular way is a good aspect of the food aid program.

Antrobus

On the other hand, in these young child supplementary feeding programs, to what extent do the administrative costs offset some of the other advantages? There is often an illusion that these foods are entirely free, whereas, in fact, the mere cost of administration and distribution is of a large order. Perhaps a resourceful and imaginative government could do something much more efficient on its own. Some preliminary data in the Caribbean suggest that the administration and distribution is done in a very uneconomic way.

Levinson

One response is that any country that has the same kind of consumption behavior that John Mellor described for India would do much better to give that aid dollar to the poor directly. If the poor person spends 85% of the dollar on agricultural commodities, that is going to be a lot more efficient than putting the food aid dollar through a bureaucracy. On the other hand, there are countries where one simply cannot take that dollar and give it to the poor. There are countries where, for one reason or another, unless one addresses the vulnerable groups explicitly, the market system, which includes family behavior, will not take care of the problem. In such a case, government intervention is necessary.

Solon

I would like to add some further statements of caution. First, in a lot of countries, these food commodities are affected by weevils. Often, we do not have good control of food storage, especially when it gets down to the village level. I notice that the local government is then blamed by the people for giving foods unfit for human consumption. The government can be seriously affected here because it usually will not say that the food comes from another country, and it is the government that is simply delivering these foods.

Second, this donated food interferes with what we are trying to do with the educational approach, making people realize that rice, fish, and vegetables are the mainstay of the child's diet. Donated foods often replace local staples with something absolutely foreign, such as bulgur wheat, rolled oats and CSB (corn-soy blend), a name which does not mean anything at all in the village. If only they called it "Corn and Beans," that would be a lot better. In fact, why can't it be donated as corn and as beans separately? We are already eating corn; we are eating beans—when you blend it, it becomes something altogether foreign. We need to make changes so that food aid is coupled with education on consumption of indigenous food. Third, we thought of selling this food, and we are still considering it. It might be sold in a cooperative facility or variety store in the village. We think some people in the village would buy it for animal feed and the profit would go for the benefit of the poor. Or else, we could sell the baby foods. Never mind if it is fed to the rich babies, as long as we can get money to subsidize the poor babies' nutritious indigenous food they like to eat.

I hope this idea will be reexamined carefully because it would be more useful if we could buy subsidized, locally acceptable foods already eaten by the people with money that we could gain from selling food commodities.

Latham

I usually agree with Jim Levinson, but with regard to food aid I do think that if a country is getting foreign shipments free and, at the same moment, in the same harbor, corn is being sent out of that country, then that is immoral both for the donor country and the recipient country. It is very expensive to move donated grain a thousand miles inland in Tanzania or Kenya, and it is an undesirable thing to do from the point of view of local agriculture. We should not be party to it. Obviously, foreign aid for the small, hungry countries is very important, but so often it is used for political purposes on the part of the donor. 85% of US PL 480 in Latin America went to Chile in the last two years and that may not be entirely based on nutritional considerations or nutritional needs. I think this kind of food aid is highly undesirable.

Levinson

Which says something, in turn, about the criteria that ought to be established for the recipient of food aid.

Montgomery

I would like to suggest that such criteria really ought to be based on experience. So far, nobody has discussed the food for work programs, which, in fact, were used in several countries, with reasonably good payoffs. In several countries, follow-up studies showed that they did succeed in using food to pay people to build local infrastructure. Therefore, I would suggest that the standard not be the "perfectly conceived" program or the "perfectly delivered" program, but that we find the criteria from experience.

Barnes

Was the overhead on the food for work program excessive?

Montgomery

I do not think so. The follow-up studies that I have seen suggested that some were pretty prudent. The overhead may have been more than you would like to have, but the programs did get the food to people who were not going to get it otherwise. It was a case of feeding the rich kids as well as the poor, but at least the poor got something.

Maletnlema

If the food aid is tied to a specific program with a goal, then certainly I accept it entirely. Its administration is then a bit easier in that it is handled within a certain group. In the case of the refugees that Fred cited, people were being shifted from one place to another, and they were helped to reestablish themselves. We have a refugee group in Tanzania that has come in from another country, and they have to reestablish themselves. Here, it is perfectly acceptable, in fact essential, to give aid in the form of food.

There is, however, another aspect. When this food, donated with good intention, comes to a country, it lands in the entry port. From there on, the government has to take care of it, and the donor is not really concerned about what will happen after it reaches the port. The moment the food lands, an announcement is made to the press everywhere that such and such a country has donated so much to such a country.

Yet, from experience, about 50%, if not more, of this food is wasted—just as good as throwing it into the sea. It does not go anywhere, but rots at the port. Then, the distribution upcountry is done in such a way that a lot of it will end up in the hands, or in the stomachs, of children who do not really need it. The distribution to the people who require it is not easy. Very often the government cannot afford to do it, as there is no existing system for this kind of distribution.

In Tanzania, for example, milk has been used as a means of attracting mothers and children to child welfare clinics. This may seem to be very good because mothers will come in large numbers and bring their children. But what about the day the milk stops? One day it certainly will stop, as the supply is never regular. Will that be the end of the MCH clinic? Since the MCH clinic is really supposed to cover so many other things that are more important than the food itself, the distribution may be doing harm. The donor should have looked into the other effects of bringing in food.

I should add that in most cases it is not the recipient country which is asking for this food. It often comes as an offer that is put to you, and if you refuse—and I have had the guts to refuse—you may get in trouble with the politicians because the aid is thought to be good and looks good on the surface.

On the other hand, if you do manage to get the food over a period of time, and this was the case with UNICEF dry skim milk in Tanzania, people get accustomed to it. It is good if you get the mothers and children used to having better foods, provided you can maintain the supply of the food. But if it stops, there may be no alternative but to change to something quite different, or import. For example, now we have had to change to CSM mix and CSB, which are quite different from dry skim milk.

Vamoer

Laymen, like myself, do not really understand what is involved in the political decisions behind food aid. We think it is being given free when, in actual fact, it is used as a foreign policy tool to implement the foreign policy of the donor country. If in the final analysis, the improvement of nutritional status in developing countries depends on increased food production, the donor countries should really think in terms of aiding countries in food *production*.

In addition, the people themselves should be involved in decisionmaking and in carrying out the projects. Many millions of dollars are poured into aid programs in the Sahel region. Why can't the countries that donate foodstuffs identify areas in the region, say Nigeria or Ghana, which are capable of producing food in excess and aid *those* countries as a whole, or on a regional basis, to produce more? Is it not better for those who really want to help developing countries to implement projects to produce more, rather than wait for a disaster and then pour in food aid?

Schlossberg

By way of clarification, although everybody may know this: the food aid program in the United States, popularly called Food for Peace, doesn't exist as "Food for Peace." The name of the law is the Agricultural Trade and Development Act; that's the Food for Peace program law. The first purpose of the Agricultural Trade and Development Act is to develop markets for US products, and one of the prime purposes of donating food to a country, as conceived by the United States, was to develop a commercial market for those products. This is the true fact of the matter.

In 1961, when President Kennedy was elected, he wanted to do something dramatic in terms of overseas aid. At the same time, George McGovern had been defeated for the Senate and was without a job for a year before he could run again, so they created an office of Food for Peace. This was just an invented office that had no legislative standing whatsoever. Soon, people began to believe that there was a greater humanitarian aspect to this program, but the primary purpose was to dispose of surpluses and to develop markets and, incidentally, to use the aid in a way that would serve the national interest of the United States. The momentum of that effort did create a program and, in a sense, an obligation on the part of the United States which is being redefined in the foreign aid debate and in legislation.

Throughout the whole world food conference year, there was a debate in the United States and in the Congress over the use of American food aid for anything but strictly humanitarian purposes. Previously, there had been no restriction on its use. For the first time, in 1975, the foreign aid legislation of the United States was divided into two very distinct kinds of foreign aid. One is strictly economic, and the other is the so-called military defense aid. In the past, they were tied together for domestic political purposes. The new foreign aid bill for economic purposes provides somewhere between $200 and 250 million more for nutrition and, specifically, for agricultural development. It also provides greater incentive for the sale of commodities tied to nutrition and agricultural development projects.

In a sense, you had something that started out as a very self-interested program but appears to be turning into a program that is more useful to other countries. Incidentally, this is in spite of the fact that there are no more surpluses; there is no longer the need, at the moment at least, to develop markets. Yet, at the same time, the humanitarian demands on the United States became embarrassing. Hard choices had to be made between selling and donating. To the extent that our aid program now is used to develop internal agricultural productivity in other countries, it releases us from a difficult problem: do we have enough food to do everything that we want to do?

Sandoval

I have sat and listened to comments about moral food distribution and about food policy versus food programs, but nobody has mentioned the end result of the whole effort in terms of health. How long are we going to pursue a given program and to what end? Nobody mentions what, if anything, we expect from these food recipients, although we know that, in certain cases, food can be put to work, as in the "food for work" projects. Incidentally, I do not think that after the donated milk runs out, MCH clinics will necessarily shut down in Tanzania. We have been through a similar experience. In Panama, we stopped giving milk many years ago, yet there is the same attendance at the clinics.

Wray

Because you are giving something else though. This is important.

Sandoval

Yes, we are giving medical care. The point is, I think, that a very important aspect of food programs is the goal, which cannot be simply giving food. That is meaningless by itself. We must continue to examine our basic goals.

Wray

This issue of food aid is an immensely complex one, but very interesting and very relevant. I still cannot comprehend how anyone can object to trying to find ways to get food from where it sits to the children who need it. From the comments that have come from Tanzania, the Philippines, and Zambia, it seems to me that what is hopeful about this whole issue of food aid is the fact that there is now, clearly, the competence within these countries and the will on the part of responsible people to set their own conditions and to avoid having the food crammed down their throats, if you will pardon a figure of speech. Rather, the recipients will define conditions and adapt the food aid to their own needs. So many millions of tons of food have rotted at the ports, so many millions of tons of food have gone into the wrong channels, that we ought now to be able to learn from these experiences and use the food creatively. I do not see how we can deny the need of people, especially the malnourished children, or how we can escape the obligation to find ways of getting this food to those people who need it. We certainly must have the know-how to tackle this problem.

Maletnlema

If it were just a question of food going to poor people, people who need it, there would be no trouble. It is the things that are tied to the food that cause trouble. If these could be stripped off, and one could simply bring the food in and donate it to the people who need it without the "political strings," we would have an ideal situation.

Latham
Just as we criticize inappropriate technologies, I think we can criticize inappropriate use of food aid. I do not think anyone in this room is against food aid as such, but there are facets which are bad. I have, indeed, been in the harbor in Mombasa and seen Kenyan corn going out on one ship and US corn coming in on another. I think this is inappropriate food aid, and a man from Mars would think it ridiculous as well.

I think, however, that the World Food Program, which has been very selective in its aid, has often been very helpful. For example, as Maletnlema mentioned, helping refugees during the years while both agriculture and industry were developed. There *are* appropriate, well-defined uses for food aid, but much of the food aid that is being given is inappropriate.

Food for work is sometimes good; for example, if the work builds a school or a dispensary. I think, however, that there is a tendency in some famine areas to use food for work inappropriately. For instance, there are programs which build roads from "nowhere in particular to nowhere in general," as Jean Mayer points out. Some of these projects are designed for the sake of the Protestant ethic: work before you get food. Yet the food has often gone to able-bodied men, while the women, children, and old people remain deprived. That is inappropriate.

This whole question of US food aid is being reexamined, and many in the Senate are very concerned. Senators Kennedy and Humphrey have been working on this, and they have enough clout to make changes. I think there is in the works a new food aid bill which has a very good chance of passing. If it does become law, I think it will change the whole complexion of US food aid and make it much more acceptable. We hear comments from people like Dr. Maletnlema who is very much involved in this problem on a day-to-day basis. These workers often feel innately hostile to food aid for what are, I think, very good reasons.

Levinson
It is ironic that the first people to challenge the general and indiscriminate use of food aid were the proponents of a food aid philosophy which most of us would find immoral: the triage argument. The argument often concludes that we should channel our aid only to those countries which are pursuing effective population programs. These arguments may be faulty as well as immoral, but they have triggered the notion of utilizing our food aid more selectively and establishing certain kinds of criteria. The question of which standards to use is interesting.

John Mellor, in one of his papers, suggested a few possible criteria. He talked about aiding countries that are pursuing rural development, developing small and medium scale industry, and are employment oriented. Also, he mentioned countries which are taking long range steps to pursue agricultural development. These tend, on the whole, to be countries with basically decentralized political systems.

Some of the Senatorial groups working on this issue are thinking of restricting most or all of our food aid to countries either on the International Development Association (IDA) list, or the UN's Most Seriously Affected (MSA) list. I think such a decision would bring us closer to the necessary criteria. Certainly if we use need as a standard, we would have less cases of the food coming in on one ship and going out on another.

Mellor

I think the food aid question is important, and, therefore, I would like to comment briefly. Food aid can be used to support any number of different development strategies in a low income country. In the late 1950s and early 1960s, it was very effective in India in supporting the capital-intensive strategy. What food aid did in India was to displace commercial imports and release the foreign exchange necessary for importing capital-intensive capital goods.

It should be clear that this strategy was the one which the government of India had chosen and was the one which the American "Indianists" were supporting. It was the generally supported Western view of how to do economic development at that point in time, though we are all playing Monday morning quarterback on it now. Food aid could also, of course, support a strategy in which one tries to increase *total* consumption of food in a country and, in that case, would be very much consistent with a vigorous push in the agricultural sector.

I hope one thing is very clear from my earlier comments. That is, an increase, even a large increase in supply of food, whether it is from domestic production or whether it is from imports, in low income countries, need not be depressing of food prices and, therefore, discouraging to production. It need not be depressing of food prices if one follows a strategy of getting additional income and purchasing power into the hands of low income people. This is so because demand will rise more or less proportionately with supply in that case, something that would not happen in a rich country.

There are very few people in rich countries who will buy more grain if their incomes increase, but there are plenty of people in India and Tanzania and Ethiopia and Costa Rica who will push up their consumption of grain if their incomes are pushed up. So, food imports need not be depressing of prices any more than increased domestic production need be. It all depends on the combining strategy.

In this context, and putting it fairly brutally, I don't think low income countries are ever going to get foreign aid in a context which meets their needs if they wait for Western liberals to figure out how to do it. The poor will have to organize and figure out what they want and then put on the heat themselves. I think we are beginning to see some of that. The unity of low income countries and the Committee of 77 has had a very major impact.

Certainly, there is a problem figuring out how to use this food aid. What is the most effective way? Low income countries have to get together on that. Currently, the environment in the United States to respond to such pressure has improved considerably. We see the seeds of some pretty good legislation. The current foreign assistance act, for instance, was passed by the largest majority which has ever supported foreign aid legislation in the House. This represents a real change, in some respects.

In essence, the current food aid innovation is to stiffen the terms for the old-style PL 480 so that you pay higher interest rates on the loans and have to repay, in dollars, much sooner than was the case in the past. There is very little "concessionary" element in it, but there is the option of, in effect, converting this rather hard loan into a grant by putting the proceeds into agricultural development programs. The motivating concern was to meet the argument that PL 480 served the purpose of reducing domestic production by an amount equivalent to the increase in imports. Now, the United States would say, "All right, if you're going to get this food on concessionary terms, you have to spend the proceeds to increase your own agricultural production."

Obviously this thrust is never going to work unless there is a real desire to move in that direction in the recipient country. The recipient country has to have accepted what I am terming a new strategy of economic growth. My own personal view is that the United States should really believe in the position which it is espousing here and should try, as difficult as it may be, to administer the aid that way. In that event, recipient countries will not be able to convert loans to concessionary terms unless they have a program which will raise incomes of the poor and, therefore, provide demand. We ought always to think about demand and supply shifting together.

Probably the most worrisome feature is that just at the time when food aid may be very effective because attitudes both in the United States and in recipient countries are changing, the supply in the United States is drying up. As a result, it is going to be increasingly difficult to allocate significant quantities of grain from the United States, because there will be a measurable impact on domestic US prices. Thus, there is going to be a conflict on a front from which we never had it before. The prospects for substantial food aid had, in fact, looked quite good until the latest Russian wheat deal. If I can size up the political situation without being a politician, this grain sale has made aid a more difficult problem for some congressmen and senators. It may well be, and is perhaps likely, that in a few years US food production will be up enough to put on pressure for expansion of food aid, and hopefully in a productive context.

There has been some inclination within the United States to take a position of encouragement for a low level guarantee of a minimum food supply for everybody in the world. We ran through some calculations on this, and, in fact, it is not an unreasonable prospect in terms of the total food supply available in the world, particularly in the rich countries of the world. Now, there would be tremendous problems figuring out how to implement something like this in the recipient countries, but again, I think it shows some switch in interest within part of the community in the United States towards a humanitarian concern and a development concern and in trying to use our food supply in that direction.

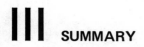

SUMMARY

19 POLITICAL COMMITMENT AND NUTRITION POLICY   Beverly Winikoff

This chapter is derived from the rather free flowing discussions which took place after presentation of the country studies. The discussions took place over eight hours, so that what follows is necessarily a synopsis of the conversation. Ideas attributed to particular participants were voiced by those persons during discussion. Use of a participant's name does not refer to any particular published work of that person. The editor assumes responsibility for any distortions which have occurred as a result of the condensation. It should be noted here that these sections are not intended as comprehensive presentations of each topic but represent the opinions of the participants as they surfaced at the conference.

The subject of politics has perhaps few equals in its potential for creating dissension and disruption in an otherwise orderly discussion. In this case, the subject commanded the most intense yet amiable interchanges on the role of national policy in dealing with nutrition problems. The word "ideology" was used frequently in the discussions, but not in its technical, political science meaning. It did not refer to any particular well-established set of ideas embraced and promulgated by any particular political party, world leader, or social scientist.

The aspect of ideology which the participants saw as crucial is the ability of political doctrine to produce the "commitment" or "political will" to deal with nutrition. This encompasses a general attitude of government in reordering priorities, so that solving nutritional problems through direct nutrition programs or by indirect government activities ranks high on the government's list of national goals. There was a conscious, if intuitive, acceptance of the proposition reached by Reutlinger and Selowsky after more systematic economic analysis: "Malnutrition is unlikely to disappear in the normal course of development: that is, in the course of normal per capita income growth even with greater emphasis on expansion of food production. Only policies deliberately designed to reallocate food or income can eliminate malnutrition."[1]

Real doubts remained, in fact, as to whether direct but isolated policy interventions designed to reallocate food and/or income will solve the basic problems of malnutrition among the very poor if there is not also an underlying prior commitment to social equity. The Chile case specifically addresses the proposition that government may tinker with systems for redistributing one or another resource in an effort to deal with a particular problem such as health, and yet, without a basic reordering of national social and economic priorities, never really reach the most needy. The possibility that a similar dynamic will haunt all "nutrition programs," and maybe all specifically oriented health and income programs as well, remains one of the large unexplained, and perhaps unprovable, hypotheses.

In this context, socialist countries and countries with directed economies can be seen to deal explicitly with food and nutrition problems. They deal with it, and quite effectively, but through different mechanisms than "nutrition programs"—because food needs and thus nutrition are at the very base of the system, not an addendum or an appendix to it. It would be a large error to conceive of these societies as ones which do not pay specific heed to the nutritional well-being of their populations.

Nutritionists and nutrition planners, on the other hand, have often accepted the proposition that small programs may be able to improve the situation without the need to tackle basic issues. Solimano, for one, feels that these "nutrition programs" and "nutrition interventions" usually only marginally affect the problem, however. The paradox, he points out, is that analyses of the situation generally reach the conclusion that very deep structural changes are needed in societies. Yet, when solutions are offered, in fact, they virtually always deal with special cases: the family, the vulnerable, the poorest, the malnourished, the first, second, or the third degree cases. One of Solimano and Hakim's basic propositions is that nutritionists have failed to make the case for inclusion of food and nutrition into the overall strategies, policies, and patterns of development in most countries.

In part because of these observations, Solimano and Hakim, in a recent paper,[2] stress that in any discussion of nutrition goals on an international level, the very deep ideological content of even the verbal formulations of the problem must be clearly recognized. This is true down to the individual level, for ideology often informs the actions that people pursue. Nutrition workers themselves are all influenced by the experiences they have had in the different political systems in which they have operated. Individual action, government programs, and even the different patterns and policies of development are influenced by ideology. The problem of food and nutrition is not a distinct case. Both empirical research and theoretical development in the field of nutrition must take into account the ideological factors involved, they reiterate.

At the same time as the influence of ideology must be understood, there is need to develop new approaches to the practical elements of nutrition programs. Attempted solutions to food and nutrition problems may continue to be marginal and static unless concern with the issue of nutrition reaches the key decisionmakers and influences the mechanism of policy formulation. Great weight should also be given to the planning and implementation of government activities.

Finally, Solimano and Hakim emphasize a need to tackle not only the nutrition problem itself, but ways to improve analysis of the whole area of nutrition and government policy. Up to the present, there has been little country-based data to work from, yet approaches being tried around the world are advertised as potential solutions. Are the approaches really solving any part of the general problem? Are they solving some specific problem? Are they solving

problems for the vulnerable or the group at risk? What are the implications—
political, social, and economic—of the proposed solutions?

As intelligent observers of government procedures and participants in political processes, the Bellagio participants understood quite clearly some inherent
limitations of nutrition advocacy. It was obvious, for example, that political
commitment is important precisely because governments function as political
entities. But from this very same fact flowed the realization that governments
act and react on many levels at once. Nutrition, health, and the well-being of
the population may often be subordinate to defense considerations, attempts
to deal with inflation and unemployment, and even projects undertaken largely to increase the popularity of the government itself: roads, dams, housing
projects. How far nutrition advocacy can proceed by riding the horse of "political commitment" as against "traditional" economic development is a difficult question. The stumbling blocks of hard political realities are likely to be
strewn across that path.

In defining the importance of ideology these workers were seeking a definition of their own role. At what point is concern with nutrition per se socially
useful? Which kinds of programs are best, given different circumstances of
government concern and general government policy? Are there circumstances
in which there is no role for a nutritionist, either because the environment is
so conducive to good nutrition or because the environment is so productive
of poor nutrition? In trying to disentangle the role of ideology and the underlying assumptions of an entire social system, two distinct though related
questions were discussed:

• Are there preconditions for success in solving the problem of malnutrition
in any given country?
• Is there such a thing—or should there be such a thing—as a nutrition policy
or program within a country?

THE CONCEPT OF PRECONDITIONS

General development, in terms of economic growth alone, and the distribution of that growth along already existing lines, seems to be inadequate or at
least unacceptably slow to eliminate malnutrition on a national basis. Indeed,
even increasing yield per hectare of cereal grains and increasing the income of
the farmers, while these may be necessary to solve the problem, do not seem
to guarantee the disappearance of malnutrition. Other elements necessary to
mounting a successful national effort may include political will of the government, effective health and education infrastructure, adequate employment
policies, and meaningful involvement of people themselves in planning and
implementing measures for their own nutritional improvement. Does this
mean, then, that there are countries where nothing can be done because political and economic conditions predetermine what will happen with any specific nutrition program? Or can nutrition advocates still work effectively where

the so-called preconditions remain unfulfilled?

To illustrate the notion of preconditions, Levinson suggests examining country experiences in light of the following question: if a nutrition advocate in some country received a telephone call from his president and was asked to take on responsibility for nutrition (a mandate similar to Dr. Solon's in the Philippines), in the context of that country would it be possible to launch a major, overall nutrition effort? Or, are there other basic preconditions missing?

To be explicit about the meaning of "preconditions," it should be stressed that there may be two separate sets of preconditions, one specifically for *program success* and another for *elimination of malnutrition*, which *may or may not* come about through successful programs.

This postulate is based on a concept of national functioning even wider than programs. It implies that there may be certain combinations of inputs which allow solution of the problem *without* a program and other combinations which allow the problem to be addressed only *with* a specific program. Preconditions, then, are not discussed merely as a means to mounting an effective program. The idea of a program is, after all, just one approach to solving the problem. The question remains: are there specific preconditions that can be examined and labeled as essential, in some proportion or another, to solving the problem?

Models of Preconditions

John Field[3] and F. James Levinson (chapter 18, this volume) note that significant nutrition improvement, where it has taken place among low income countries, has fallen basically into one of two patterns. The first is the pattern of countries that have achieved quite rapid rates of economic growth coupled with a reasonably participatory and equitable pattern of development, such as South Korea and Taiwan. The countries with both rapid growth and significant nutrition improvement have not, on the whole, addressed nutrition problems explicitly but have benefited from the spin-offs of their rapid and equitable growth. Other countries have achieved fairly rapid rates of growth but without this sense of equity, for example Brazil. The evidence of malnutrition in the northeast of Brazil speaks to the inadequacy of rapid growth alone as a solution to the problem.

The second successful pattern is exemplified by those countries that have opted for very major social changes: China, North Vietnam, and Cuba. These countries, on the whole, also did not address nutrition explicitly, but there has been fairly significant nutritional improvement as a result of the distributional reforms that have been undertaken. (Many social interventions in these nations have clear nutritional implications, moreover: food rationing, agricultural reform, and advice on infant care and family planning, to name a few.) The results, according to many observers, have apparently been astonishingly successful.

Most countries fall into neither of those categories, however, and it becomes much more difficult to see the appropriate path to nutritional improvement. Levinson points out that, in some sense, the whole concept of "international nutrition planning" makes the assumption that, even without very rapid and equitable growth, and even without very rapid major social changes, it is still possible to have a significant effect on malnutrition problems through more rational planning and more effective programs. With a few notable exceptions, such as fortification of foods with specific nutrients, this hypothesis probably has not been proven or disproven; the evidence is not in.

One might visualize national nutritional status more schematically as the result of a complex system in which certain key inputs have to be available in one of a number of minimum combinations. Just which combinations of inputs can produce the result of adequate nutrition for the entire population are as yet unknown, but may be discoverable by future research. In economic terminology, this is a multidimensional production function. The various dimensions might be

- level of agricultural production
- level of overall resources (affluence)
- nature of resource (income) distribution
- level of commitment to the poor
- nature of child care

Each variable would be represented by an axis. The task then would be to pick out the points of minimal combinations of inputs which permit achievement of the desired result: adequate nutrition. In reality, one might need either fewer or more variables (axes) than those proposed above to explain success when the exercises of plotting out points is actually attempted. The amount of time allocated to achieve goals might be stipulated as an overall constraint of the system.

A situation can be postulated, then, in which effective provision for nutrition would be possible if there were very great commitment, even if there were very little affluence. On the other hand, in a situation such as in the United States, there might be less on the commitment axis, but much on the affluence axis, with moderately effective programs. Presumably there would also be some points in between representing other combinations. Ultimately, one might be able to derive a surface, any point on or outside of which would give an effective solution of the problem.

Antrobus proposes a simpler two-dimensional model with each perpendicular coordinate representing a goal of development: affluence and social justice. Activity in developing countries, it seemed to many, often is directed towards increasing affluence. This thrust, in itself, may have a depressing effect on the other dimension, political will for social equity. Several years into this process, an overview of the situation may still find many people impoverished and unemployed in the face of impressive development figures.

This has already occurred in some developing countries. Nutrition advocates feel strongly that a political ideology of equitable distribution of the new affluence must be wedded to movement along the road to affluence.

In elaboration of this model, an optimistic prediction is that, once committed to social justice and having established a somewhat equitable distribution of resources, countries would not slip backwards in this regard. It was noted, however, that Chile is an example of a country that was rather violently wrenched downward along the equity axis. In addition, some African countries, which, at the time of independence were moving rapidly towards social justice suddenly, as affluence hit the ruling classes, seemed to move backwards.

Uses of Models in Advocacy and Policymaking

Joe Wray has noted that models of preconditions might be made more useful by identifying threshold values for prosperity, for commitment, and so forth. This would describe a minimum essential level which could then become a target in attempts to change each particular variable.

Of course, depending on the variable, there might or might not be a measurable minimum essential level. Beyond that, the threshold for one variable may shift as different levels of the others are attained.

Such a formulation of minimal levels should in no way be confused with "triage" or some other attempt to define a certain number of societies into a "hopeless" category for lack of minimal criteria. It would be a grave error for either national or international planning or aid organizations to attempt to use a model in this way. In fact, a dynamic model of the interrelationships of nutrition systems is useful in counteracting such thinking. If one can identify threshold level(s) for the crucial input(s) to make the system work, all resources and energy can be devoted to getting over that threshold.

For example, if one could, in fact, define an overall "prosperity" threshold, one might come to rather optimistic conclusions: it might well be the case that with a very equal distribution of resources, the necessary prosperity level is much lower than had been thought. According to most observers, the threshold value of prosperity is really intimately related to political commitment: a country need not necessarily be extremely rich to achieve nutritional goals. If China, with an extremely low per capita prosperity index, can eliminate the most blatant nutritional problems, other relatively poor societies can do it by pushing up the "social equity" variable. Triage then becomes irrelevant. The path to social equity may not have to follow the Chinese map, but at least the analysis can point out the choices available to decisionmakers.

One might choose to define threshold target levels for several quite specific variables, such as crop production. Yet at the same time, it must be borne in mind that different elements in the nutrition system do not often occur in isolation, so that where there is a food shortage, there may be other shortages, such as in the administrative or transportation infrastructure. A model similar to those described above might clarify the issues for policymakers, help them identify different potential strategies for dealing with the problem, and locate the most efficient combination of efforts.

These models demonstrate that there are many interlocking categories of action which might be studied in different types of countries. There does not exist one standard ideal program output, but a goal of "effectiveness in provision of adequate nutrition." "Effective nutrition" itself has many dimensions. Montgomery suggests an attempt to list the desired outcomes in order of their importance. The highest priority might be to deal with the most serious cases. The next problem might be to deal with cases early enough to have maximal impact on the creation of human potential for the country. The dynamics of the system might be studied by measuring the stages through which it deals with each task.

Typing countries into large, general categories gives only sketchy guidelines as to what is likely to be a tremendous success, what is likely to be a modest success, and so on. National experiences, in fact, tend to be on a continuum, rather than falling neatly into "types." It would be most useful, therefore, in future work, not only to identify prerequisites but to disentangle separate elements within the experiences in order to be able to transfer their lessons across situations.

Conceptualizations of the National Nutrition Problem and its Solution

Over time, it has become apparent that the most difficult nutrition problem to tackle, both conceptually and in practical terms, is that of protein calorie malnutrition, or undernutrition in general. Very successful, well-defined nutrition policies are possible to eliminate goiter, xerophthalmia, anemia, and so on, because the problems themselves are so specifically defined. The importance of dealing with these problems should not be underestimated simply because technological approaches have already been developed. There may still be significant political, economic, and administrative difficulties in mounting such programs. In fact, there is danger that the specific deficiency problems are inadvertently ignored during discussions of nutrition planning which emphasize changing political priorities and grander national designs. Special nutrient deficiencies represent subsystems within the total nutrition system, and, while they may be separable, many of these problems are often closely linked to other serious nutrition and health problems. Protein calorie malnutrition, on the other hand, represents the functioning of the entire nutrition system. It seems to have more complex roots and is more difficult to define, even schematically. The causal relationships involved have been diagramed in at least three different ways.

Thomson suggests a map of malnutrition "pathways" analogous to a metabolic pathways chart. His construct contains 128 interlocking factors and would be far too complex to use without the aid of a computer. For simplicity, Wray suggests that this complex "web of causation" involving production, transport, commerce, income, and health delivery, in the end comes down to the final common pathway of the mother providing nourishment to the baby. Thus, the very last link in the chain is the only constant. Nutritional effectiveness, it is clear, must always be measured by a function of actual intake by the child. According to Wray, working backwards through the model may allow one to identify first those problems which, when solved, would have the greatest "payoffs" or effectiveness/cost ratio.

A construct simpler than that of biochemical pathways might be made using the ecologic model of disease causation. Since 'malnutrition' is often treated as a disease, this concept may be quite appropriate, according to Solon. It emphasizes the importance of a proper balance between man (host) and food (agent) in which environmental changes influence the balance between the two. Solon constructs a model for malnutrition analogous to the well-known public-health "seesaw" and fulcrum model of disease:

food   man
_____
         ▲
    environment

Food factors would include both quality and quantity, and factors affecting man include age, knowledge, health practices, and so forth. Environmental forces include the political, economic, agricultural, and social factors.

Sandoval suggests a more "economic" model of causation, labeling the immediate problem as one of "low family-food availability": an imbalance between food offered (a result of production, storage, industrial, and distribution processes) and food required (a composite of physiologic "demand," education, food practices, income, etc.). In any one given political setting, there is room for improvement in each variable, he feels, but, as yet, hard data are not available to indicate how much increased production, for example, or improvement in storage or improvement in commerce will reduce malnutrition in every political context.

In all these schematic systems, however, response of the people is fundamental to any action in nutrition. This is encompassed within the food "demand" criterion and might be a dimension of the societal "prerequisite model" as well. Appropriate responses can be generated, according to Thomson, using the tool of "adequate social communication" to influence both societal change and programmatic efficiency.

An experimental approach to improved understanding of the causality of malnutrition has been proposed by Thomson. He suggests that one disaggregate the problem by studying how people *are* able to feed themselves adequately, as most do, even when they live under the most difficult conditions. This proposal takes cognizance of the fact that, even in groups where malnutrition is a common and serious problem, some mothers succeed in raising healthy children. How they accomplish this would have more relevance to appropriate interventions within that same socioeconomic context than sophisticated data showing that affluent people raise bigger and fatter children by feeding them milk, eggs, meat, etc.

An elaboration of this approach suggests that endemic problems are extensions of normal conditions: the end results of the functioning of the social system. According to Montgomery, this presents societies with a choice of dealing generally with the "normal" or specifically with the endemic "disasters" that result from "normal" functioning. The path chosen by both of the two types of countries which can claim nutrition success stories in the Field/ Levinson typology (i.e., (1) rapid, fairly equitably distributed economic development or (2) major social change) seems to be to direct most policy towards changing the "normal" (i.e., the functioning of the whole system) so that the number of "disasters" are reduced. The "middle" countries (those without either rapid, equitable growth *or* rapid major social change), on the other hand, seem to try to deal with the disasters, hoping to get them cleaned up. The "normal" continues to generate problems which are dealt with as they occur. According to an optimistic scenario, the entire system, with its packages of interventions, may eventually reach a point where its functioning changes qualitatively and improvement in the "normal" occurs. This highlights the importance of incremental approaches, and points to a strategy in which nutrition advocates in "middle" countries make an emotion-laden "emergency" the focal point for broader action which, in time, will begin to ameliorate the "normal."

The idea of addressing nutrition as part of an overall development approach has been stressed recently. Previously, the goal of nutritional improvement rode the crest either of a research thrust or a humanitarian effort. Neither of these tracks has yet produced an example of overwhelming success. Those committed to the nutrition planning approach, emphasizing integrated development, contend that this is because there have not yet been sufficient commitment or resources allocated. Most countries, however, do not have the institutional bases or the trained capacity to implement an overall program once it has been proposed. It should be remembered, too, that societies *never* have "enough" resources or administrative capacity to do everything that program advocates desire. Waiting for the "commitment and allocation" millenium may prove to be the same mistake as waiting for overall development to catch up with the needs of the poor, given present patterns of distribution.

It has been stated explicitly and by implication in the country "typology" approach, that the experiences of Cuba, China, and North Vietnam and perhaps Taiwan and South Korea as well, are nutrition success stories in which there was no nutrition policy nor any specific nutrition planning. Further consideration makes it clear, however, that, in all these cases, there was, in fact, a *food* policy. It was a much more directed food policy, moreover, than that of many other countries. It often included rationing food, price control, import control, and so on. Explicit health, housing, and sanitation policies were formulated in order to reach the rural people. These often emphasized use of *small* systems, the lowest levels of manpower in health delivery, immunization programs, and control of the important infectious diseases that relate to malnutrition. There are also income policies, as well as both rural and urban employment policies, to eliminate poverty. Agricultural policies have favored the small farmer and involved cooperatives and community participation.

In fact, these successful countries really may have had what is currently labeled a "development/nutrition policy" even though *they* haven't labeled it as such. In this light, they have already done what most nutrition planners are, at present, advocating as the path for the future. All of their strategies are included under the rubric of "nutrition policies" when that topic is elaborated. Many of the so-called successful countries may simply, because of their politics and ideology, choose not to label their overall policies as "nutrition." In any political context, however, some attention to all of the aspects of policy outlined above appears essential to successful attacks on the complexity of protein calorie malnutrition and undernutrition in general.

NUTRITION POLICY

The Nature of Nutrition Policy

This brings us to the second question: can there be, or should there be, such a thing as a "nutrition policy" as a separate national goal? This question took on special meaning in the context of the gathering at Bellagio: a collection of serious-minded people from all corners of the globe, committed to solving nutrition problems, asked themselves if, as nutrition planners, nutrition program officers, nutrition administrators, and nutrition advisers, they had, in fact, anything relevant to offer.

While all agreed that "development" would not alone take care of the problem of malnutrition—or at least not fast enough to avoid millions of excess deaths—there remained considerable uncertainty as to whether a new approach involving nutrition programs and nutrition planning could address the problem adequately either.

The discussion arose partly from the despair of frustration and partly from a curious kind of hope: frustration, obviously, at the many false starts, political reversals, and partial successes; frustration at the frequent demand that programs for the poor, in fact the poor themselves, display no inefficiencies of purchase or storage or use, while the inefficiencies of the middle classes and the rich are tolerated cheerfully; frustration because no human system yet devised is frictionless, with energy, time, and resources all used with complete efficiency. Yet, nutrition advocates may be called upon to devise programs of incredible complexity, dealing with the fundamental processes of production and distribution in society, touching on deeply ingrained habits of community preference and practice and, at the same time, to show quick and/or large-scale results. But there was optimism because, in some places, at least, nutrition problems have been addressed. Where governments have been willing to place food availability high on a list of priorities, the adequate feeding of all the people does not seem so very difficult.

Since in the real world of social functioning "everything is connected to everything else and vice versa," it might make sense to conceive of overall government policy as a "nutrition policy" because it has a nutrition *output.* On the other hand, it might be equally valid to contend that general nutrition policy *cannot exist* because it would encompass everything else as well. This argument perhaps emphasizes the importance of nutrition together with its many connections to other aspects of government activity. It is a naive perception, however, because the same analysis might be made of "employment policy," "education policy," "energy policy," etc. Yet, governments do, in fact, devote attention and resources to these other areas of national concern. This attention, in turn, creates and reinforces a constituency of advocates and beneficiaries of specialized programs and policies. As a result, few governments can ignore employment or education, for example, in planning for national goals.

Both the optimistic "development" school of nutrition policy theory (which maintains that overall increases in affluence will overtake nutrition problems without a specific nutrition policy) and the more pessimistic view (that *no* adequate solution to nutrition problems will be possible, either through development generally *or* through specific programs, without certain prerequisite government commitments to equity) share the same basic belief in an intrinsic relationship between nutrition and development patterns. On both sides of this coin, stress is laid on the importance of general government policy in creating an environment which bounds and constrains all nutritional outputs—whether through policy *or* program.

The question, therefore, might be rephrased to ask: are there circumstances when a separate food and/or nutrition policy is especially appropriate? This defines the issue more clearly, and leaves the key unresolved question one of emphasis: what are the ratios of specific "program" to overall "policy" that are likely to work? Which circumstances of general policy call for attention to special nutrition policies in order to achieve a substantial impact?

Students of the problem, such as Sai, have proposed that where a government's comprehensive development policy focuses on the quality of life of its citizens rather than abstract numerical indices, such as GNP, many of the most critical nutrition issues may take care of themselves. There are special circumstances, however, when even with a favorable policy environment, the desired result may not be achievable without specific attention to nutrition.

First, if the agricultural situation is very poor, due to the type of land in the country or the weather, then enough food cannot be produced. In this case, the basic policy, even if it is "people-oriented," must also spell out quite clearly the way in which adequate food is to be obtained for the population. Once there is enough food, a separate food and nutrition policy may not be necessary. Occasionally, however, even in those cases where socioeconomic *goals* are quite broad *and* adequate food supply is available, unexpected effects, deleterious to nutrition, may occur during the *implementation* of general government policy. Food and nutrition policy issues may thus need to be discussed so that overall policy, as it is implemented, can be made congruent with nutrition goals.

When state policy is tied to general economic growth rather than distribution of the increased income, a nutrition program or policy will be needed in order to avoid at least some of the adverse consequences of this approach to national development. In Ghana, for example, the cash-crop cocoa-producing belt is constantly encouraged to produce more cocoa. Achievement of this goal will enrich the national coffers; new cars and other luxury items will come into the country; the cocoa farmers themselves will have more money in hand. Yet, unless there is a deliberate effort to help them divert some of that cash into food and nutrition for their own people, these farmers may not be able to meet their nutrition needs. Costa Rica is another classic example of a similar situation, this time with a cash crop of coffee.

In Nigeria, currently, much wealth is being generated at the national level through production of oil, yet food and nutrition problems are not abating. In such a case, a specific food and nutrition policy is necessary because, apparently, national socioeconomic policy proceeds partly in conflict with individual family food and nutrition goals.

The review of national experiences which concludes that increased productivity *and* more equitable income distribution together will improve nutritional status with or without something called a "nutrition program" is, in fact, cause for optimism. This is so because it is seriously open to question whether, even in the most favorable government environment, nutrition advocates could ever have enough power to direct all the other sectors as needed for a successful interdisciplinary nutrition enterprise. Many important factors influencing nutrition are not part of the health system and are totally out of the control of both nutritionists and health personnel: production and agriculture, for example. Efforts motivated by nutrition considerations may well come up against a brick wall if the aim is to readjust overall government policies, even in small ways, simply for nutritional reasons.

Chile, as studied by Solimano and Hakim, is an example of a country which did not succeed even within a "progressive" development environment. There, a capitalist pattern of growth spurred both economic and social development but was not able to eliminate nutritional problems. Although the Chilean development system, and some of the factors influencing the nutrition problem, have changed more than once, the basic nutrition difficulties are still very much in evidence. This represents, perhaps, one of the clearest demonstrations of the ingrained and deep-seated nature of societal nutritional problems: changing policies, changing systems, or changing both systems *and* policies are all, at best, slow roads to solving a difficult problem.

Conceptually, Levinson proposes that the most logical approach to the policy issue would be *not* to have a nutrition policy per se, but rather to have a policy aimed at decreasing the overall deprivation of the poor. This would have the advantage of being heavily weighted, in any case, towards food, nutrition, and health because these are the most important ways to improve the welfare of the poor. It might, in fact, assure better priorities, on the whole, in health and nutrition. Decisionmakers might not be tempted as much by the programs one sees in many countries: catering colleges or food processing activities that are called "nutrition," which, in fact, have nothing to do with the welfare of the poor.

Such a policy would also mean that, as one looked at policies in other sectors, one would be able to have a better understanding of what they really meant for the poor. Levinson cites what might result from a nutritional evaluation of an agricultural production pattern. A nutritionist might note, "They are producing a little bit too much corn and not quite enough of other crops with higher niacin or tryptophan content. Therefore, they really ought to shift their cropping patterns." Yet, if one were concerned with the deprivation of the poor, one might ask, first of all, "What is the employment being generated by this particular pattern of production?" And, "Should we perhaps have another pattern that would be more income- and employment-generating in order that the poor can purchase the nutritious foods that they need?" There would be less emphasis on milligrams of amino acids, and such an overall policy aimed at decreasing deprivation of the poor would thus assure better integration with the other sectors of development. This approach appears sensible, even at the risk that it might end by putting a number of "nutrition policy" people out of business! This poverty-oriented tactic may be appropriate for addressing the most critical, widespread, and devastating problem of undernutrition but, on the other hand, it does not provide for efficient monitoring of special, local, or specific-nutrient nutritional problems. Nor, in fact, does it address nutrition-related problems, more and more apparent in all societies, which are not the results of poverty: obesity, diabetes, heart disease, to name a few.

Alan Berg[4] and others have developed hypotheses linking nutritional improvement and national development. Interestingly, and despite the fact that there is no hard evidence to support the optimism of many of these works, policymakers are often eager to believe the postulated connection whereby improved national nutrition status also improves the prospects for successful socioeconomic development. Reliance on policymakers' belief in this link seems to be part of the tactic of making nutritional priorities politically viable. The conduct of obsessive and extensive debates within governments on the necessity for "nutritional" policies can thus be seen as a political retreat. Nutrition advocates might reinforce their cause—and their potential political allies—by producing more hard data on the hypothesized importance of good nutrition to national well-being.

Politics and Nutrition Planners

Action in the Political Arena: Incrementalism One is led from an examination of overall government goals to an examination of *nutrition* policy in particular. This is an area more specifically defined than general state policy but more overarching than individual nutrition programs. Those who have worked within the political context often suggest, from the pragmatic point of view, that there should not be a hierarchical ranking of, first, policy and, then, a derivative program. Rather, it is claimed, if either must come first, it should be program—and then policy. This emphasis derives from the fear that if advocates forcefully push the formulation of a grandiose nutrition "policy," the actual "program" may get left out. Activity, for example, might be sidetracked by endless technical discussions. Furthermore, enunciation of policy tends to generate responses within the political system, and these may be unfavorable: some groups may become frightened and organize resistance to implementation. Planners may go from meeting to meeting without actually doing anything: without some program one obviously achieves nothing, whether there is a stated "policy" or not. Schlossberg advocates an incremental approach in which "program" comes first, generating a set of activities from which policy can be extrapolated. Other, expanded, programs may then be justified.

The model of "minimal prerequisites" proposed earlier could be very helpful from the point of view of the person who has to try to "get something done," according to those who have labored in the political arena. If the model included all of the relevant variables, the person with responsibility for developing an effective approach to the malnutrition problem could quickly look at each as it applied to his/her particular situation, and see whether it could be modified. One might conclude, after a look at all the variables, that the task was hopeless, or that there were only one or two which could be changed, or that all the things were present to allow a good program to be put together.

Schlossberg feels that perhaps the most important variable with which to work is extensive executive authority, as in the Philippine program. In that situation, the road to action is fairly clear, although implementation may pose unexpected difficulties. On the other hand, where government has a complex system for making decisions, one must look at many factors in order to decide how to develop the kind of support required to put together an effective program.

The concept of a nutrition model thus helps the political planner to identify important components and to identify the environment—particularly the government environment—in which those variables operate. The next step would be to outline different approaches that might be taken.

In the United States, Schlossberg recounted, those with a political role to play soon concluded that, although it seemed preferable, a straight "income" program to deal with the malnutrition problem could not be implemented. A conscious decision was made, as a result, to construct an argument and political support for *specific* intervention programs. As a result of the fact that it was not possible to launch a sustained and successful overall campaign against all aspects of poverty at once, there is not a sensible, cohesive attack on the problem. Instead, there is a Food Stamp Program, an attack on disease, a special program on rats, a special program on sewage: individual and continually changing attacks on individual pieces. Although conceptually this may represent a flawed approach, realistically and politically such a tactic may be necessary. At the same time, advocates felt that these were only intermediate measures to what should be some more fruitful reform.

In other circumstances, a nutrition planner might think it a waste of time to develop a food distribution or food stamp program because of the magnitude of the problem and the limited resources available. In such a situation, the planner might feel it more effective to spend time developing political support either to make basic changes or to launch a greatly expanded program. The planner might also perceive that the only way to develop political support would be to take whatever small program is available and use that little program as a basis for building support and turning it into a bigger program.

Students of nutrition policy are keenly aware of the context of political reality in which nutrition goals must be achieved and of the necessity for political allies. Levinson points out that, in many of the countries whose experiences were discussed, it is simply unrealistic to expect governments to launch major programs based on a policy of decreasing the overall deprivation of the poor. Very frankly, he notes, "it is not their mission and, right now, it is not their political mandate." The nutrition community can, however, marshal its considerable evidence on the magnitude and severity of the problem as a demonstration of the results of inequitable, nonparticipatory patterns of development. This may strengthen the hands of those within low income countries who would like to see these patterns change. There is strong sentiment that nutrition cannot wait forever: many nutrition advocates want to do something now. Using small gains as building blocks towards a larger structure of nutrition programs is one way to begin.

This approach has been used in the Philippines where the short term limited interventions are seen as only the first steps toward a long term goal. Massive community weighing of children is viewed as a vehicle for creating awareness in the community. The final measure of accomplishment of this program will be a demand from the community for continued action beyond weighing.

From the start, in the Philippines, food giveaways were rejected in favor of weighing and educating, because these activities were felt to have greater potential for stimulating long term activity.

Using the Language of Politics   At base, then, is political reality. Nutrition advocates can help to force the pace of political decisions by framing nutritional issues in political language, even setting up conditions for "rhetorical blackmail." In the Philippines, the amount of third degree malnutrition was declared to be at a "disaster point." It was put to the decisionmakers that the country was, in effect, in a state of emergency because there were approximately 400,000 cases of third degree malnutrition. A "disaster" concept of severe malnutrition might be applied to the situation in any country, with the implication that this state of affairs could cause the leadership *political* trouble. Furthermore, the assignment of political responsibility can be made directly to individuals and to specific localities. For example, mayors in the Philippines were informed that if, within their jurisdiction, more than 5% of the children had third degree malnutrition and more than 50% among those third degree cases died, the locality would be considered to be in an "emergency" state.

Many Filipino nutritionists concede that the local problem had been known for a long time, but that attempts to solve it had been sporadic because there was no political decision. For concerted action to occur, national nutrition problems must first be recognized locally and then cast into a form usable by the political decisionmakers. Solon has done a masterful job of performing this function in the Philippines. "Don't give them journals," he says, and notes that he "translated" scientific articles into fact sheets for use by lay audiences. These were then distributed to cabinet members and to the president and the first lady who were thus able to understand the nutrition situation of their country. After the success of the first fact sheets, Solon's group made up sheets to enable economists to interpret the magnitude of malnutrition in terms of economic development. Only after all these sheets were presented was there a political decision and a political commitment.

Injecting nutrition into the four year plan of the country was accomplished by sitting down with the development planners in much the same fashion as had been done with the political leaders. By acknowledging the importance of long term economic development to the planners and at the same time convincing them that improved nutritional status is necessary for such development, nutrition advocates believed they were able to incorporate long term nutrition goals into long range national planning and could therefore hand over to the economists that portion of the planning. Politicians and planners, after all, are clearly already committed to economic development, whether or not such development is the solution to the nutrition problem. This approach is felt to complement the short term interventions, such as mass weighing, which, it is hoped, will grow into nationwide programs.

Nutritionists in the Philippines feel that politicians and planners should be responsive to the long term, medium term, and short term approaches, individualized as much as possible in the different communities. Having left the long term planning to the economists, however, nutrition planners can now concentrate on short term and medium term plans for a nutritional approach. In the next stage, planners will be trained, this time within the country, to design community participation projects.

The sequence of events in the Philippines demonstrates that, after the achievement of political support, the next immediate task is the development of local capacity to plan and implement programs. The issues involved in training the kind of personnel who can understand nutritional problems and plan for their solution in concert with politicians have been explored mostly through trial and error in different national contexts. The locus of training may, it seems, have profound implications for the relationship of nutrition advocates to the overall political system. In the Philippines, initially, high level nutrition workers were sent abroad to learn something about planning strategies, and expert advice came in from every corner of the world to provide trained manpower. Now, however, it is felt to be a mistake to recruit the top people for training in nutrition planning. A lot of money is spent to send such people abroad, yet on their return, they never serve full time, and give only scattered attention to nutrition. This pattern can then result in a situation where the country remains essentially without full-time planners. Frequently, it would appear, the most effective use of personnel is to have full-time planners paid by the nutrition council—or whatever body is responsible for nutrition in a given society. A relative lack of experience in these planners may not be detrimental, as long as their institutional and career loyalties are committed to nutrition.

Good planners must be complemented by good implementors, but they are not interchangeable. Workers caution against the attitude that "if we don't have enough planners in nutrition, we will use good implementors." Solon makes the analogy with construction of a building: the architect designs the plans and then the contractor must build. There must always, of course, be an association between the architect and the contractor so the job gets completed properly. The special skills of both are needed.

Maletnlema identifies another point of entry into the political system: the utilization of facets of the current powerful political ideology in developing a program. This strategy is applicable mainly where the leadership of the country articulates a particular social ideology to justify its legitimacy. Of course, the content of the message will differ considerably from one country to another, just as policies differ from country to country. The danger of this approach, in the end, is that nutritionists themselves will become, or at least be seen as, politicians and will run the risk of being thrown out if the government changes.

In some countries, choosing the facet of political ideology on which to hang nutrition may be easy. In Tanzania, for example, politicians have chosen to preach against what they call the "three enemies": poverty, disease, and ignorance. Advocacy of nutrition programs adapts to this emphasis quite easily. In a nearby country, with a different socioeconomic orientation, the nutrition program has a very different approach. It is based on outreach to the poorer people through a separate antihunger committee. This committee has grown so large and is handling so much money that it has become an independent power in the country. In this process, because of an advantageous financial situation, the nutritionists, with some attention to the political situation, should be able to get nutrition into the national plan quite effectively.

It is interesting that, even with very different ideologies, as in the two African countries just mentioned, the same kinds of programs may evolve. Examined from the point of view of the child, the specific projects underway in the two countries may not be that different. Considerations of local politics, finance, and administrative authority, may determine the shape of programs even where political ideology is the enabling tool in their initiation.

Economic Development and Nutrition

Ideology plays a prominent role in the literature on the relationship between general economic development and equity issues, including the welfare of the poor. In elaborating this theme, Wray cites the work of Irma Adelman and Cynthia Taft Morris, which looks at the economic outcome of the so-called First Development Decade,[5] and comes to the following conclusion: "The primary impact of economic development on income distribution is, on the average, to decrease both the absolute and the relative incomes of the poor. Not only is there no automatic trickle down of the benefits of development; on the contrary, the development process leads typically to a 'trickle up' process in favor of the middle classes and the rich."

Furthermore, Richard J. Barnet and Ronald E. Miller,[6] writing on multinational corporations, note that: "Particularly in those countries which experienced 'economic miracles,' the pattern was increasing affluence for a slowly expanding but small minority and increasing misery for a rapidly swelling majority. Concentration of income in Mexico, for example, has increased significantly during the 'Mexican miracle.' In the early 1950s, the richest 20% of the population had ten times the income of the poorest 20%. By the mid-1960s the rich had increased their share to seventeen times what the bottom 20% received. A 1969 UN study reports that in the Mexico City area the richest 20% of the population lived on 62.5% of the area's income while the poorest 20% attempted survival on 1.3% of the income. During the Decade of Development [1960s], according to US government estimates, the share in the 'Brazilian miracle' for the 40 million people at the bottom dropped from 10.6% to 8.1%." By 1970, a UN report indicated that the richest 5% in Brazil had increased their share of the national income from 44% to 50%. Adelman and Morris cite additional data showing that the richest 5% in many of these countries are garnering anywhere from 35% to 55% of the total income.

These statistics demonstrate well the previous assertions that even remarkable growth, when it is uninformed by a system of values favoring equitable distribution, does not seem to bestow benefit to the most needy in proportion to their numbers, their needs, or even their previous share of the "pie." According to Wray, the issue of values in the context of development is one of the things that the current Chinese government has addressed. The process of "moral reeducation" to which the Chinese submitted their elites has been described by Robert J. Lifton.[7] The new government did not line up technocrats and educated people to shoot them down, concludes Wray. Instead, the political leadership realized it had to have technical help, but demanded that help on new terms: namely, the elites were not going to have any special privileges or affluence. Wray comments that this is in sharp contrast to the Westernized technologic elites which do enjoy special privileges and affluence in both developed and developing nations.

Privileged socioeconomic status may create incentives for the elites to favor the status quo and, in the end, may prove a major stumbling block to reform. Wray describes a tendency for technocrats to dodge the moral issues of undernutrition: "We're afraid to confront economists on nutrition issues because they come down to moral questions, and these are nonscientific and hard to grapple with. So we slide away from them." At the root of the ideologic problem, then, he postulates a moral problem. Is it morally right to let vast numbers of people starve while others are enjoying an affluent and consumption-oriented pattern of life?

This was a crucial question in China, in 1949, because they were short of everything, Wray recounts. Their resources were extremely limited, so that the Chinese did not come to their present system in isolation from the moral question of equity. In the United States, for example, because there is more or less enough to go around, the system can get away with less discipline. Projecting 25 to 30 years in the future, however, as the whole world becomes increasingly short of resources, Wray predicts that these questions will have to be dealt with on a moral basis, even in relatively rich countries. He concludes that there will have to be "moral changes" on the part of those who are enjoying the luxuries. Exactly who will have to make the sacrifices—and to what degree—is left unspecified.

Mellor cautions, however, that, in examining the relationship between growth and income distribution, one must be very careful not simply to plot countries against growth rates and then look at distribution. There are a number of countries, in fact, which have experienced rapid economic development with an *improvement* in the distribution of income. Furthermore, he notes, such favorable development patterns can provide substantial quantities of food for essentially all the people in a society without having what is now-adays called a "Marxist ideology."

Taiwan is an interesting case in point, Mellor feels, which should not be dismissed on the basis that it has been the recipient of considerable foreign aid: First, he notes, it would be difficult to take the position that aid which was largely in support of a military establishment would normally be the explanation of broad-based economic growth. Second, in fact, the foreign aid was rather modest as a percentage of national economic activity even during the five year period when it seemed to be fairly large in absolute terms. The proportion of national investment which came from foreign aid is not that impressive in Taiwan as compared to a large number of other countries.

In addition, Mellor reminds us to be cautious of a hypothesis that suggests that the pattern of economic development is basically determined by foreign aid and that the stance of the recipient country itself is a minor point. Therefore, he argues, Taiwan itself had a strategy which was basically conducive to spreading the benefits of development. Throughout the last twenty years, disparity in income distribution has been declining, especially in the rural areas. There is also no evidence of rising income disparity in Hong Kong, Singapore, South Korea, or Japan. According to Mellor, these countries *have* had broadened participation in the growth process and *have* dealt with basic nutritional problems fairly effectively in association with economic growth. Such facts, too, must be kept in mind when making broad generalizations.

Moreover, Mellor finds an unsettling aspect of the Taiwan story the fact that growth and the distribution of that growth are *not* a post-World War II foreign aid success story. The basic strategy of growth was set far earlier by the Japanese and a good deal of development occurred before World War II. The lesson thus might be that one must build on a substantial base of literacy, over a sustained period of time, to produce broad-based growth. On the other side of the ledger, Mellor adds, development workers have learned much in the last years, with the result that many processes can be contracted in time and may no longer require generations to culminate in significant economic growth.

The Nutrition Advocate, the Economist, and the Politician

Many advocates are distressed by economists who try to force nutrition workers to make an *economic* case for nutrition and nutrition-related activities. Some workers have therefore adopted a strategy aimed at "pushing the economists to the wall," asking them whether the success of development activities can be evaluated properly *without* considering nutritional status. The whole of development, after all, is aimed at achieving certain goals, and adequate nutritional status is one of them. Instead of looking for sophisticated and sometimes weak arguments for nutrition as a factor in economic development, Sai challenges economists to make the negative case: that you can have development without any nutrition activities. He suggests further that certain nutrition indicators can be used as overall development measurements within a community. Then, nutrition programs would have leverage beyond their purely nutritional implications.

Mellor notes that, as an economist, he would be satisfied with a definition of economic development solely in terms of improvement of the nutritional status of the lower 50% of the population. On the other hand, he points out such a goal for development would necessitate major changes in the economy in order to provide, for example, 20% more calories for 50% of the population—and a diversified diet in addition. Such changes could not come about by spending half of one percent of the national income on specific nutrition programs, he stresses.

In addition, although many economists might accept nutritional status as an important goal and important measure of development, many of those same economists might be prepared to put off improvement in nutritional status for many years in favor of other goals. In other words, according to Latham, they would say one first wants economic growth, and that, in turn, will lead to improvement in nutritional status. The economists might thus comfortably talk themselves out of the need to see any immediate improvements in nutritional status. Historical perspective on the Chontalpa Plan (see chapter 1) showed improvement in agricultural production and improvement in incomes but no improvement in nutritional status in one circumscribed population. The potential for programs to produce this type of result cannot be ignored. It cannot be lightly assumed that, if economic indices improve, nutritional well-being will be automatically assured, even in a small target population.

Furthermore, the fashion of the times dictates that, even in countries that are *not* fully committed to general social development, nutrition and nutrition programs have become a glamorous, popular subject. Thus, one can see a political commitment to the idea of "nutrition" without commitment to deal with other social problems. Governments may find, however, that those very nutrition programs will fail unless there are other investments in social improvement. Latham points to experiences in the United States that illustrate this point: at the first White House Conference on Food, Nutrition, and Health, the Nixon Administration apparently felt that it would be very easy to solve the nutritional problems in the United States, that these would be unrelated to other problems, and that the administration would not have to do anything about poverty. It was very unsettling to officials when, at the conference, a group of nutritionists and representatives of the public focused on increasing income for the poor and the use of nutrition as a vehicle to stimulate other social change.

Similar dynamics occur in many countries that have made a hastily conceived commitment to nutrition: first, there is the impression that this will

require only palliatives or minor readjustments; then it becomes clear that
nutrition is tied to many other aspects of national life. Though nutritional
problems are unlikely to result in political revolutions, emphasis on nutrition
programs may act to shift governments into more humanitarian, socially
oriented activity. Even in countries without total commitment to eliminate
social and economic deprivations, pushing the nutrition effort can thus result
in benefits apart from improved nutritional status.

Thomson, in examining these interrelationships, counters criticism that
nutritionists have not tackled the "basic issues" by asserting that it is not the
nutritionists' job to do what the economic development planner should be
doing. Sandoval and others agree with this assessment but emphasize that in a
special sense, the nutrition planner must be aware of the whole picture. All
those who have attempted nutrition planning advocate pushing ahead, as far
as circumstances allow, with the measures and means at hand, aiming to improve the whole picture, whether in fact there is a real possibility to produce
change or not. Proper understanding of the probability of improvement is
important in order to avoid personal and technical frustration as well as creation of unrealistic expectations.

Obviously, it is crucial for the planner to have an operative definition of the
area of "nutrition." If it is defined so that nutrition tackles only a small part
of the problem, the task is easier, although potentially unproductive. On the
other hand, if one pursues the previous argument that nutrition and food
elements have to be inserted into the national development and socioeconomic policies, some individual must assume the responsibility for creating
awareness of nutrition problems on the part of those who act in other areas
of national policy. Nutritionists, historically, have been forced to do the
special pleading. When dealing with economists on their own ground, of
course, this is a formidable task, for it is extremely difficult—and may, in
fact, be impossible—to show cost-benefit ratios for a nutrition program.

It is Thomson's opinion that nutritionists have overstated their case in trying to impress development planners with the need to incorporate nutrition
into development planning. These advocates have not been very successful,
therefore, both because of the overstatement and because of a lack of evidence. Given more time, evidence may be developed to substantiate what is
being asserted, according to Thomson. He feels that understanding of the
relationships among nutrition, working efficiency, and productivity, and of
the relationship between nutrition and mental development, certainly will be
expanded beyond the present stage of being strongly indicative.

Antrobus maintains that while overstatement of the nutrition case has occurred, it has also been necessary. Nutrition, like public health in general, is a
minority discipline, perhaps somewhat unglamorous and with low visibility in
political eyes. Overstatement serves to raise visibility; this has been especially
important in recent times, when so many of the developing countries have

emerged to full independence. The infancy of statehood burdens governments with many preoccupations which are normally considered vastly more important than the question of nutrition. A little hyperbole may function to put health and nutrition questions back on par.

Having dealt with the problems of formulating the "nutrition case" to policymakers, Schlossberg proposes that three basic approaches can be taken by nutrition advocates to make a connection between nutrition and development. Those who must try to make that connection should have clearly in mind the possible paths: the political, the economic, and the moral. Arguments can be made on each of these grounds, and the arguments can be presented to different decisionmakers depending on which argument will be most effective, adds Schlossberg.

The politician, for example, might respond to the notion that, from a political point of view, food and nutrition programs are easy to implement and are often very popular. It would be a political error for an officeholder to have large numbers of people essentially unserved by government when there is a way to assist them easily.

Second, an economic argument can be structured to be advantageous to the nutrition advocate and not easily assailed by the traditional economist. Schlossberg recalls an expert witness who testified before the Senate Select Committee on Nutrition and Human Needs that, while there is no evidence that feeding children will make them smart, the evidence that keeping them hungry makes them dull is indisputable. This is the tactic of basic common sense: if feeding people makes them healthier and more alert, there is bound to be some economic benefit. On those grounds, the economist must at least go part of the way along the route. Furthermore, if a government functions by spending money on health, education, and other services for the malnourished, perhaps those other investments would not be as burdensome if people were not in poor nutritional condition in general.

Finally, one can make a moral argument, as Joe Wray also noted, above, on the simple ideological grounds that there is something fundamentally wrong with letting people go hungry. Some who would not be persuaded by a political or economic argument might be moved if the situation were presented in these terms.

Mellor points out what he terms "a fairly serious problem" with the "simple" economic argument outlined as a potential political tactic. He points out that if, in a particular society, the lowest 20 to 30% of income groups have no opportunity for employment, and there is also no real will to employ them, then improving their health and mental status does not contribute to economic development; it has no economic value whatever. In fact, those in the lowest 40% of the income distribution in many developing countries have poor prospects of employment, very few go to school, very few are receiving any public expenditure on health. They are essentially *no problem.* So, while

the public expenditure argument might be persuasive in certain special circumstances, for the poorest of the poor in most developing countries, it is
largely irrelevant. Only where the basic development goal is to have everybody employed productively will there be an economic argument on the
grounds of productivity.

On the other hand, the political aim of this "economic argument" is not to
make unassailable economic sense, but to force the economist to argue publicly that feeding people is not economically productive, a difficult position
to take. The economist might take the position that one cannot create new
employment for 30% of the population and still have economic growth. Further, he/she might assert that economic growth will not, for a long time,
provide enough employment to employ that lower 30%. This same economist
might view such a line of argument as a higher, more sophisticated interpretation of the overall public good than simply distributing food.

Schlossberg proceeds with the scenario, however, and envisions the nutrition planner returning to the political leader to report that, "The economist
has just told me that he has no intention whatsoever of making 30% of the
population productive. That is his economic policy. Is that what you want?"
Even if the politician is inclined to answer "yes," it may be politically impossible to say so publicly. At a certain point in time, the argument with the
economist hinges on whether it is morally justifiable to argue against nutrition on economic grounds instead of devoting attention to plans for improved
health and increased productivity of citizens. Of course, notes Mellor, if only
that type of "moral" economist is hired, the argument will not be necessary:
nutrition goals will be accepted immediately.

We are reminded again by those who have worked within governments that,
in the real world, there is no firm distinction between "the economist," "the
planner," "the nutritionist," and "the politician." Everybody concerned is a
little bit of everything, and it is difficult to tailor one argument for the economist and another for the politician. It seems to many nutrition workers a
fundamentally simple proposition: "plain common sense" would solve the
whole problem! A logical function of nutrition planners, therefore, is to list
possible ingredients, not to make recipes.

As each country defines its own recipe through complex political and socioeconomic processes, demonstrations of solutions may be located and examined for their applicability in other environments. Indonesia might borrow
organizational techniques from the Philippines; or Tanzania from China. It is
not necessary that the whole political situation be the same in order to use
features of others' plans. Dogma is not the answer, and learning *can* be translated across systems, although solutions must be developed within the context of the problem. Planning, of course, is a methodology and not a solution.
Defining answers requires knowing what it is one wants to do: goals and the
objectives must be clear. Evaluation of the achievement of those goals must
be made with newer indicators than "economic growth" alone.

Nutrition and improved health can be viewed as the centerpieces of economic development in contrast with the approach of many traditional professional nutritionists who argue only for a very small piece of the social welfare pie. The emphases on moral commitment and on distributing the gains of development both imply that health and nutrition need very major attention. Specific programs may be a very important part of that attention, but they are only a part of the whole.

20 PROGRAM AND POLICY: SOME SPECIFIC QUESTIONS   Beverly Winikoff

The following areas were not singled out for discussion prior to the Bellagio conference. They are addressed specifically here because, over and over, they seemed to be the areas that aroused the most interest, concern, and comment from participants. This attention was taken as a signal of the importance of these topics in current attempts to develop national approaches to nutrition problems. As a result, five specific areas are explored in more detail in this chapter:

- the targeting of nutrition programs to specific population groups
- the role of the professional medical and nutrition communities
- the functions of nutrition councils and coordinating bodies
- the role of universities, nutrition institutes, and training
- the uses and abuses of international aid and advice

TARGETING

Theoretical discussions of government "commitment" as well as the more nuts and bolts approaches to program development and implementation both bring up the question of whether "targeting" programs is of value. It comes to the attention of nutrition workers because of the apparent lack of target approaches often noted in the same countries which have been cited as nutrition success stories: China, Taiwan, South Korea, Cuba, etc. Is it possible that targeting, which would seem to be a rational approach—define the problem, the sufferers, and the remedy—is in reality a prescription for avoiding the solution?

Mellor notes that often the less committed a government is to improving nutrition in the masses of the vulnerable group, the more detailed and the more specifically targeted will be its plan for nutrition delivery programs. The reason for this is that all governments do, indeed, need to have programs to help the poor, but some structure them only in such a way that the underlying order is not disturbed. Two other forces may well contribute to this outcome. First is the realistic appraisal that limited resources—a problem for all governments, even those with sincere political commitments—virtually dictate the use of targeted strategies to increase the effectiveness of the programs in reaching those who need it the most. Second, on the political level, many of the dividends of a nutrition or food program can be reaped by government simply by announcing and beginning some activity. The ultimate effectiveness of that activity as a solution to the problem is often politically irrelevant.

In fact, of course, if it is accepted that essentially *all* countries do target their specific programs while *most* countries are unsuccessful in eradicating malnutrition, it is clear that there will be a high mathematical correlation between the two—probably without importance in terms of a causal relationship. Levinson argues that a formula stating that commitment and targeting are *always* mutually exclusive is naive and unfair. In some cases, obviously, targeting *is* done where there is no commitment to reduce the size of the problem. This makes sense because the more one targets, the smaller the population there is to deal with, and the less is expended in the way of resources.

On the whole, however, it is probably a conceptual error to use the term "targeting" as the opposite of commitment, because effective programs with any deliberate, conscious, rational interventions, do require "targeting." Without a target strategy, one never knows what one is doing, or whether goals are being reached. Although they may not be spelled out in detail, intermediate targets, in the sense of goals, are also necessary if one wants to evaluate a program.

In fact, of course, if a country *is* trying seriously to tackle the problem and *does* have a sense of commitment, it still makes infinite good sense to "target" in order to invest widely the limited resources available. As Levinson notes, those countries that have been called the "success stories" have done a great deal of targeting. Countries that *are* effective in their attention to overall nutritional concerns seem to have a different—perhaps one could say less targeted—targeting! In Cuba, in particular, much of the emphasis of the overall health effort has been directed to the young children. The food policy is also targeted. Milk is for children, and the food rationing system appears to target as well. Britain, at the time when it was doing best nutritionally, also had targeted rationing. Chinese targeting has been described as an attempt to reach all the women and all the children—"rather blunderbuss targeting" according to Mellor. But even though interventions relate to *all* children, one must remember that it is decided at the community level, who is going to *have* the next children. A lot of programs thus may be extremely targeted without looking targeted because they do not appear as such in a national plan.

Two types of targeting can be distinguished. One specifies the recipient *groups* to be reached. As noted above, the presence or absence of narrow program focus on the neediest groups clearly is not perfectly correlated with levels of government commitment. Specificity of program *goal* or program *aim* can, itself, be viewed as another type of "target." In this sense, targeting refers to the breadth of conception of the program itself, rather than to the groups it addresses.

A more comprehensive program, for example "social development," or a health-nutrition-agricultural development project, could be viewed as less "targeted." On the other hand, "a nutrition program," or a "vitamin A program"—especially one which is defined solely in medical terms—could be viewed as very targeted or specific and might signify less government commitment to social goals, as they are not intrinsic to such an approach. Labeling a program or problem "medical" may serve to remove it from the realm of the political and social. It may also dilute the government's sense of responsibility. Such a narrow definition might also be the symbol for an initial lack of commitment. The presence or absence of that kind of targeting, therefore, might more accurately predict a distinction between levels of commitment.

If pressured by the national economic or political situation, it may be necessary to short-cut or limit programs, because "general approach" solutions may not be acceptable. Yet, these very limited programs then might be used by nutrition advocates to demonstrate that the short-cut approach (a) is too marginal in its success, or (b) is, in fact, a criminal waste of resources because of its lack of success.

Sai feels that program and project mixes can be identified which will not only influence the nutrition situation but also, most probably, influence overall development. If, for example, there is only a small group of the population vulnerable or suffering from lack of vitamin A, then it might appear economically most reasonable to dose that group with vitamin A preparations. If, on the other hand, vitamin A deficiency is a generalized problem within a community, one can start with mass dosing but cannot hope to eradicate the problem by continuing that approach over the long run. It is possible to *alleviate* the vitamin A problem with medicine but, to maintain the benefits, the vegetable and fruit situation must be improved or fortification begun, for example. This may require a reorientation of agriculture, processing, and/or transportation within the country, and, according to Sai, these sectors must be mobilized to solve the problem. Thus, nutrition indicators and their improvement can be used to marshal support for other activities.

THE ROLE OF THE PROFESSIONAL MEDICAL AND NUTRITION COMMUNITIES

How do nutrition drives get started? What is behind the initial push to tackle nutrition problems in a country? What are the roles of the medical and nutrition communities in the dynamics of a successful push in this direction? Do all programs start with medical or professional surveys, concerns, proposals, that then get politicized? What is the relationship between technocrats and political will? And, what can be done through professional approaches in the absence of political will? All of these questions seemed important after consideration of the various country experiences. A better understanding of the role of the technical nutrition person in attracting national attention and facilitating national action might lead to new strategies, devised to use professional expertise more efficiently and effectively.

Montgomery proposes that, in general, it is necessary to have professional identification of the problem, and, then, as the recognition of the professionals themselves enlarges, they, in turn, bring more actors onto the stage. Thus, nutrition activity becomes deprofessionalized, politicized, bureaucratized, and, eventually, turned over to local community leaders. Finally, according to Montgomery, when concern reaches out into the peripheries of government intervention, the original core can either disappear, absorbed in a larger context, or it can move on to another phase, a deeper penetration into the problem. Before anybody, politicians, sector planners, or administrators, will take up the nutrition dimension, however, they have to become aware of the side effects and nutritional consequences of their actions through technical-medical evaluation.

An interesting illustration is provided by the history of government attention to endemic goiter in Indonesia. During the Dutch colonial period, there was recognition of the problem, and iodization of salt was carried out. After independence, because of the decentralization of salt production, national iodization became more difficult and was not continued. The goiter problem increased; yet there was no study, no medical alertness to the problem. All those in the medical field seemed to have forgotten goiter. Only in the '60s, after medical interest was rekindled and medically initiated surveys gathered data on goiter, were policymakers alerted to the resurgence of iodine deficiency. Now, action has been taken once again. This vignette lends support to the contention that only the medical technocrats can demonstrate nutrition problems effectively and in ways so that politicians may take action. Certainly, the case studies in this volume indicate that this has been the general pattern.

The history of Indonesian interest in overall nutrition problems also seems to fit the Montgomery model fairly well. Starting from goiter, recently reemphasized by doctors, the entire nutrition issue is being politicized now. This process may still be in a fairly early stage because nutrition in Indonesia remains relatively professionalized. There are some experiments going on, including trials of vitamin A delivery programs, some of which are very professionally oriented; but others are very dispersed and community-oriented.

Also, it should be noted, that there is a very interesting prior history in this particular case: there *was* iodized salt and only *later* there was *no* iodized salt, an unusual sequence. In other words, through mechanisms of the socioeconomic system, iodine had been added to the salt of the whole country. Then, because of political change, iodine was no longer added to the salt. The doctors were not monitoring this situation at all, however. They had been left out, in part, because the process was already entirely within the political and economic systems and no longer part of medical consciousness. In order to get iodine *back* into the salt, it took medical "reinterest" in the problem. This suggests further that professional and technical groups, even though they recognize that hunger is a social problem, must maintain continuing interest. It argues against the assertion that the "core" can disappear once the dynamic process has taken hold. Things may go astray if these medical and nutritional problems are not monitored by the professionals and are instead left wholly to social, economic, and political forces.

Program maintenance is generally seen as a function which involves identifying and dealing with the potential enemies of a particular activity. Historically, in the case of iodized salt in Latin America, producer "enemies" have occasionally been able to overwhelm and defeat the attempt at a fortification program. Proposals to iodize bread have also aroused the active antipathy of interested producer groups. The Indonesian situation was slightly different, however, and reversion to uniodized salt was based on an administrative change. Failure did not occur because the program had to go through single or monopoly producers, but because, after independence, production switched to small operations. Not organized opposition but social and political change—and a changed production system—finally reversed the program by altering the conditions in which it operated.

There is an equally interesting sequence of events in Zambia in which the role of the medical community might be studied. There, the initial highlighting of the nutrition problem was done by an anthropologist. It was then taken up by the copper industry, which introduced feeding programs for its labor force because that was found to pay in productivity figures. After World War II, the Ministry of Health, with no enthusiasm, appointed a *non-medical* nutritionist who was unable to do very much until the Commission of Community Development took up the question and sought *international* support. Only in the very late stages, in the second half of the 1960s, had the Ministry of Health anything directly to do with nutrition planning. In fact, after the first meeting of the Executive Committee of the National Nutrition Council, the representative from the Ministry of Health wished to resign on the grounds that health had no part in nutrition programs!

This anecdote would appear to illustrate that program development is not necessarily based on a medical approach, but the story speaks also to the extreme importance of the interest and concern of the medical professional community. Zambia, in fact, may illustrate a situation in which there is sustained interest from other professional sectors, but no wholehearted commitment of the medical community and, *as a result*, no success in resolving nutritional problems on a national scale. According to Thomson, the response from government, when it came, was due basically to the personal interest of the president. The Ministry of Health never took a strong leadership or advocacy position and nutrition concerns still have little leverage when they conflict with other government objectives. Nutrition problems seem to remain widespread and serious.

Again, at first glance, it would appear that the history of the United States in this area is an exception to the hypothesized crucial role of the medical/nutrition community. In the United States, as elsewhere, physicians are badly trained in nutrition and have tended to deny that nutritional problems exist among the poor. Essentially, they abandon the nutrition issue. As a result, it took socially active politicians and concerned community organizers to delve into poverty questions and *then* find sympathetic nutritionists and medical people who would believe there was a nutrition problem. That activity then led to the medical/nutritional surveys as a follow-up to sociopolitical consciousness about poverty and malnutrition.

In fact, however, it was probably precisely that absence of an active health/ nutrition community in the United States that was the major obstacle to getting a political decision by the government to tackle malnutrition. In retrospect, according to Schlossberg, one of the most important things that could have been done in the United States, and is now occurring in a limited way, is ongoing nutritional assessment with the involvement of health professionals as part of the regular collection of health statistics. If such projects are well-planned, they will provide just the kind of basic data that policymakers need in order to make decisions.

In the evolution of interest in malnutrition in the United States, there was a period of three or four years during which considerable discussion of nutrition problems among low income people took place in public forums. Evidence of malnutrition was presented by small groups of doctors who had gone out and conducted small surveys. These, as well as the few earlier surveys, were not yet sufficiently persuasive to cause a breakthrough in government policy. The Congress, however, did commission the Public Health Service to conduct a nutrition survey similar to those which had been conducted overseas but had never before been attempted in the United States. Only after the preliminary results of that survey were presented to the Congress in a dramatic, public way—with X-rays of bones of malnourished children and technical talk about skin-fold thickness and pictures of malformed skulls—did the people who were opposed to acting on the nutrition problem begin to yield ground.

After that initial presentation, which was only based, in fact, on the *smallest* part of the whole survey, the case had been made sufficiently and so dramatically—perhaps overly dramatically—that nobody cared what the rest of the survey showed. In the end, it was never finished, according to Schlossberg. The entire nutrition issue thus received a stamp of legitimacy and was taken seriously only after the technological/medical backing was there. In this case, it did not require concerted outcries from the whole medical profession but rather the activism of a concerned subset of the physician community to highlight the problem.

Solon believes that if the Department of Health in the Philippines had acted ten years earlier, the Philippines program could, in fact, have been mounted ten years earlier. The necessity for a nutrition decision was brought to the president *not* by the Department of Health, which might have been an embarrassing implicit admission of failure, but by the Department of Social Welfare. This group awakened consciousness and pointed out poor conditions and then asked the first lady for ₱4 million, after which the Philippines Nutrition Program was created.

When Operation Timbang, the national weighing program, began, there was immediate sentiment that the Health Department should take charge. Why? Because, the reasoning went, "This is a diagnostic procedure." At present, the Department of Health does run Timbang and coordinates all other agencies as "cooperators." The Department of Health has the responsibility for delivering the nutritional assessment of the whole country in terms of weight. This is still seen as a health function, not just because of prestige value, but also because the Health Department understands the nutritional status of individuals.

According to Solon, if the program were to start all over at this point in time, he would suggest that the Department of Health be designated to assess and diagnose the nutritional condition of the country. After this, that department would have to design approaches to deal with the problem: medical, social, and agricultural prescriptions. These ideas would be communicated to the economists, the agriculturists, and the social anthropologists.

Although malnutrition seems to need endorsement as a serious medical/ health problem before it receives political attention, and despite the fact that nutritional problems basically manifest themselves as health problems, too often, health professionals think they can solve the problem entirely alone. Yet it is clear that they cannot. Other actors do need to be involved, but the tendency to treat malnutrition as a disease limits the interest that these others have in the problem. For later recruitment of allies, it may be necessary to approach malnutrition as a socioeconomic condition—but one which health professionals can make a major contribution toward curing. Policymakers, economists, and planners may be more willing to participate in the solutions to the problem if it is viewed in such a light than if it is monopolized as a health issue.

Indeed, there are differences among who *finds* the problem, who *assesses* the problem, who *brings the problem to political attention*, and who *tries to ameliorate the situation.* These appear to be discrete functions. In part, of course, it is a matter of who is able to define the problem in such a way that a specific intervention is deemed possible. It seems, however, in terms of assessment—both initially and on a monitoring basis—that somehow governments take medical-technological evidence seriously in a way that cannot be replaced by social welfare pleadings.

NUTRITION COUNCILS AND COORDINATION

It seems, therefore, that a concerned community of medical and biochemical nutritionists can draw attention to nutrition problems, but over the long run, at the national level, responses have been largely ineffective in dealing with the great magnitude of the problem. Why? Perhaps some answers can be gleaned by a look at what happens after the issue of nutrition is identified publicly and placed within the realm of government concerns.

Identification of a "nutrition problem" involves professional attention. It appears to need heavy doses of professional influence because the exact dimensions of the situation have to be defined and made more focused. The real issue for effective action is what happens next, after identification. Once the solely technical interest is converted into a political decision, it becomes possible to have "nutrition" as a vested interest in the political system and the administrative system. Montgomery proposes four national strategies in nutrition interventions, each of which could be examined to learn (1) what kinds of projects are undertaken, (2) which targets are identified, (3) what sorts of organizations arise, as well as (4) what ultimate outcomes result from each approach. In the end, one hopes to learn if it makes any difference which one of these routes a country follows.

The four models outlined by Montgomery are exemplified by the different countries whose histories are related above. One is the specific target approach as used in the Philippines and Panama. Targets are identified professionally and governments zero in on them because those targets have serious problems. Second is the incremental approach. Early efforts envision a big, overarching program, but it soon becomes apparent that everything cannot be dealt with at once, so small parts are emphasized. This may be the process which is occurring in the United States: there is no plan, but advocates hope to peel the onion layer by layer, because that is the way the United States does everything, according to Schlossberg. Targeting eventually begins to take place, and thus, these two approaches run together and may even phase into one another.

The third approach is the broad-based planning approach. Nutrition is dealt with in terms of the government's overall development plans. In some of these cases, national councils attempt to orchestrate the different individual ministries, as in Zambia, Colombia, and Indonesia. According to Levinson, Pakistan is another example of a country which began to approach the problem in this fashion but recently has embarked on a new type of overall planning approach. Initially, in the mid-60s, Pakistan began by having biomedical nutritionists do a nutrition survey, form a nutrition coordinating committee, and then try to analyze the results of the nutrition survey. That process—between starting the survey and analyzing the results—took about seven years. As so often happens, at the end, no practical planning decisions were made on the basis of the original survey.

After the creation of Bangladesh, nutrition activity, which had largely emanated from the nutrition section of the Health Ministry, essentially disappeared in Pakistan because almost all the prime actors had been Bengalis. At the same time, however, the Planning Commission received a new mandate from President Bhutto. Probably influenced by the China model, Bhutto had become interested in peoples' health and work schemes. In part because of the lessons learned from the earlier nutrition experience, the president let it be known that he wanted things done differently: he wanted to have "consumption planning," a decentralized health system, and "health guards," a Pakistani approximation of barefoot doctors. In fact, according to Levinson, a number of these changes have come about.

Within the Planning Commission, and attesting to the relative lack of penetration that all the years of prior work had achieved, workers were generally oblivious to the fact that anything had happened previously in the nutrition field! Indeed, notes Levinson, the new group started very differently from the previous effort: not with surveys and coordinating committees but by figuring out what to do in the agricultural sector, in the employment area, and in food subsidies to assure that the poor get more to eat. Because of the lack of communication between the two efforts, it took some time before the knowledge that had been gathered previously by the rather isolated nutrition efforts of earlier years could be used in the decisionmaking of the Planning Commission. The Pakistani experience of successive but disconnected nutrition planning efforts might be exaggerated because of historical circumstances. In substance, however, it does not differ that greatly from the stories in other countries where, instead of building on each other, each new attempt to generate momentum for nutrition intervention starts from zero, in isolation, and too often in ignorance of what has gone before.

The fourth and last pattern Montgomery identifies, he proposes to call 'hidden policies." China and Cuba do not have any special policies or programs to call "nutrition" because they do the things that affect nutrition under different headings. These are examples of governments which prefer not to use the label "nutrition" at all. The activities which might be labeled as such under other systems are here subsumed under the general state activities in welfare and health.

Some of the four policy patterns may flow naturally into others. In fact, according to Montgomery, there might be some natural or necessary sequence of stages which countries go through as they begin to deal with nutrition problems. The relationship, if any, between strategies remain to be elucidated by further research. For the present, one can simply label observed patterns and create hypotheses.

The momentum of "What to do next?" after the problem has been identified must thus be translated into some institutional mechanisms. When the problem is addressed straightforwardly, and not through a strategy involving "hidden policies," a favorite structure of the nutrition community, with the official sanction of the government, has been the council or committee to coordinate nutrition activity. This type of organization has been described under at least four separate titles: nutrition council, nutrition coordinating body, nutrition center, nutrition committee, and so on. Historically, such groups have been dominated by nutritionists and other medical specialists. Historically, also, they labor to very little avail, but not for lack of trying: they make efforts to attract attention and power, but in most cases they are not successful.

In attempting to create institutions appropriate to the task at hand, it may be natural to fall back on such a committee structure for at least two reasons. First, as nutrition is never the exclusive mandate of any one bureaucracy, it does not naturally fall under one department's aegis. If the new nutrition interest were seen to be merely lip-service or diversionary, no bureaucrat would want to be saddled with the new responsibility, especially one doomed to obscurity and failure. If, on the other hand, nutrition activities were to be the beneficiaries of significant attention and funding, no official would want to see "nutrition" assigned to some *other* bureaucrat.

A second factor that might serve to increase the popularity of nutrition councils in less planned economies is the suggestion of democratic decision-making that the creation of such bodies represents. They appear, on the surface, to be a rational means of balancing competing claims in favor of the best interests of the community. For this reason alone nutrition councils have powerful appeal.

Thus, using nutrition committees and councils to coordinate nutrition activity has been advocated for a very long time. Over and over, great hopes have been raised, and then dashed, that some particular country had found in its council a model for success in nutrition. Colombia, for one example, has endured a series of attempts to coordinate nutrition, all initially appearing very hopeful and none successful in the long run. According to Latham, the fact that these promised successes never seem to arrive in any country is one reason for cautious assessment of current programs, even those that seem to offer the brightest hope for the future. No new approach can be automatically viewed as an improvement on previous strategies simply because of its newness.

In fact, of course, advocacy of nutrition councils as a rational institutional mechanism to deal with nutrition has been in vogue, internationally, for several decades. The result is that when political leadership is pressured by various groups, including international agencies, to solve nutrition problems but is unable to be committed to a serious effort, it often turns to superagency coordination as a way of putting a troublesome topic to rest. The upshot is, of course, that nothing happens, at least as much due to lack of commitment as to the innate difficulties of working through a council structure.

Sai raises the possibility that the absence of a tradition of successful coordination in many fields within developing countries may, in itself, militate against success in coordinating nutrition. In this framework, Sai stresses the importance of the local historical situation in which all institutional apparatus must function. He questions the common wisdom of a universal rule that nutrition coordinating committees will die, irrespective of how well intentioned, how well-organized, or how well supported by law. This may be the likely fate of councils only in those situations where no council for coordinating any sector has ever had a chance to succeed.

A further serious difficulty with coordinating councils is that, most often, they have a mandate to deal with *nutrition* but have no power to influence *food* policy. This amounts to an inherent contradiction in function: councils can advise and can point out the implications for nutrition of different food policies, but they cannot change the *food* policy, which may be much more important in determining nutritional status than *nutrition* policy per se. Solon, for one, has advocated that nutrition workers have some say in the price of oil and of milk and in the polishing of rice in order to be effective in their attention to nutrition in the Philippines.

Soekirman notes that both FAO and the Second Asian Nutrition Congress have dealt with problems of coordination and tried to analyze why nutrition councils have always failed. From past experience, Indonesian workers find that such bodies have failed and will continue to fail unless they more nearly approach Havelock's conditions for functioning as a system.[1] According to this analysis, nutrition committees most often lack crucial *methods* of functioning and occasionally never even develop a *reason* for functioning. Seven factors are held to be most important in adequate functional competence. First is linkage, the degree of collaboration among members and among institutions: with no relationships, there is also no hope that the system will work. The second is structure: the degree of systematic coordination, not simply detailed organizational charts. The third factor is openness: willingness and readiness to accept outside help, innovation, and new ideas. Isolation from other institutions will decrease effectiveness. The fourth factor is capacity: the capability, degree of authority, and intellectual training of the members. Then, fifth, is a reward system: planned and structured positive reinforcement for doing the job properly. Sixth, proximity: nearness in time and place among members and to counterparts outside of the institution. The seventh factor is synergy: willingness of each department or ministry to support the others.

The Freedom from Hunger Campaign Committee in East Africa is an example of a program which fails to meet several of Havelock's criteria: coordination with the overall government apparatus has been singularly lacking, according to some observers. Outside of government control, this coordinating group has acquired a large, autonomous financial base while within several ministries there are already established very strong nutrition divisions which have been largely ignored by the committee. Thus, coordinating powers are not used to best advantage: the program has grown colossally without sinking roots into functioning government agencies and has not become adequately integrated into the social fabric of the country. A critical difference, it is alleged, between "Freedom from Hunger" and the Tanzanian program, for example, is that if government input stopped in the first case, the program would die, and, in the second, the program would go on. In the first instance, activities are being *maintained* and not truly coordinated or integrated.

Although many guidelines can be written on the subject of structuring councils, one of the most important aspects is not the structure mapping out the nutrition council, or even the program in a country, but attention to human factors, especially as they relate to the functional requisites listed above. Few governments pay adequate attention to this. The analysis of the failures of four Indonesian nutrition commissions by Indonesian workers, for example, suggests that all failed because of human factors, not because of structural defects. Management specialists can organize structure but it takes the right individuals to develop the organization and make it work according to designated principles.

Wray emphasizes the crucial importance of having the key people in an organization be competent, committed, and cooperative. A coordinating body is needed because complex problems require activity on the parts of various segments of the government. With appropriate personnel, however, it may not matter exactly where the locus of power lies. Without such people, adds Wray, it also does not matter where the power lies because nothing will happen in any event.

Wray adds that the functional system, as described by Havelock, is in this instance a "team" of people scattered throughout government agencies. The preconditions for functioning would be those necessary for effective team-work. The first requisite, according to Wray, is that members of the team must understand and share the goals of the operation. Lack of this under-standing is very often a cause of failure because when officials function by merely mouthing the organization's goals no effective action results. A second requisite is well-defined responsibilities for each team member. For example, agricultural workers may be expected to collaborate and cooperate, but they may not really understand exactly what is expected in terms of human nutri-tion unless their tasks are spelled out. Similar problems exist with other per-sonnel from every agency. A third requisite is that responsible individuals know how to carry out their assigned tasks. Very often people are expected to do things that they really are not able to do. Either they do not know how to do their jobs or they do not have the support or equipment they need. Finally, both coordinating bodies and field personnel must have the flexi-bility to adapt to changing circumstances. Such principles are simpler than Havelock's but equally central to the functioning of a coordinating body, states Wray.

Solon's experience with the three recent councils in the Philippines has demonstrated to him the crucial importance of the origin of the coordinating body in determining its ultimate ability to operate effectively. One of the Philippine organizations, the National Coordinating Council for Food and Nutrition, originated from a Philippine nutrition association; another, the National Food and Agricultural Council, was created by executive order to replace the first. The latest, the National Nutrition Council, was established by presidential decree, and this last group is clearly the most powerful. Solon feels that a council can only have adequate strength if it is an enactment of a congress or parliament, or created by decree. Other mechanisms are too weak to allow the councils to carry out their difficult tasks.

Thomson adds that for councils to be useful, they should *not* be established simply for *coordinating*. They must, on the other hand, *administer* the political decisions of the cabinet or president. For this, particularly, such an institution must have the backing of law or decree to give it the power to operate. Without both the authority and the responsibility to implement policy the council will not go anywhere.

The power of the council is also reflected by the composition of the body. Functioning is often impeded if members are of lower rank than minister or cabinet member. A structure built on the highest level members of government ensures direct exposure of the government leaders to the functions of the council and the problems of nutrition. For example, in the Philippines, when the government members themselves saw pictures of marasmus, kwashiorkor, and keratomalacia, that was the turning point for the start of a program, according to many observers. Of course, there are potential problems with personalizing all issues and decisions: if cabinet members should change, advocacy would have to start all over again!

If the council should become both functional and powerful, Solon notes, problems of control may then arise. When health does not like agriculture to take the lead, and agriculture does not like health to take the lead, action becomes difficult. Experience in the Philippines teaches, moreover, that there *must* be action after a council is constituted. Many councils fail, in fact, because they have nothing to coordinate! Administrators become so engrossed in organizing the council that there are only pilot programs, and pilot projects do not often hold the attention of cabinet-level government officials. Subordinates are designated to attend meetings, attendance becomes irregular, and the highest levels of government leadership are no longer actively involved.

In addition, money and manpower are necessary for adequate functioning. Whatever agency has these resources, whether it be health, agriculture, or a national nutrition committee, is able to assume the leadership in nutrition. In the Philippines, teachers are recruited to fill the manpower needs of nutrition activities. Since teachers are already spread throughout the country, they need not be recruited through either health *or* agriculture. The teachers work at the grass roots level, and, with this system, even when there is little coordination with other departments at the start of operations. activities can still take place out in the communities.

Finally, notes Solon, a council must have an executive director. Any official who acts only as part-time chairman will be unable to keep abreast of all that is happening. From his own experiences in this area, Solon is an enthusiastic advocate of a full-time director who, working through deputies, can be truly in touch with all aspects of the program. Equally important, this chief executive for nutrition must be of sufficient status to carry weight within the hierarchy of government so that the council can be effective.

Even with these ingredients, one has to depend to a certain extent on the good will of the individual ministries. Accepting a program is one thing but implementing it is different, and good working relationships must be maintained. Solon has devised an organizational stratagem in which a signed memo of agreement makes official the contributions of all ministries at all levels to the nutrition program. He further advocates that performance audits based on such agreements be carried out quarterly—not yearly—to see if all is proceeding as planned. If it becomes necessary, one can then demonstrate that certain ministries or individuals are not doing their assigned part. This approach seems to work fairly smoothly in the Philippine context.

On the other hand, the Zambian council, in addition to the normal coordinating power, has recourse to the highest governmental authorities if it is blocked in implementing its program. Zambian law states that, if a program is approved by government but a particular minister does not implement the decision, such foot-dragging or obstruction can be reported to the whole cabinet. This system operates at a slightly higher level of political risk because, by lodging a public complaint with a superior authority, nutrition advocates might conceivably so antagonize the offending ministry that it would refuse to cooperate in any further aspects of the nutrition program.

Of course, as Antrobus points out and the previous points illustrate, the success of nutrition councils is very largely dependent on authority, funding, and manpower, and these attributes are assigned by the political leadership. In fact, the degree of authority of these councils can probably be related to the real commitment of the politicians when they speak about nutrition. In most countries, for various reasons and as part of normal political activity, leadership must at least make a show of taking an interest in issues such as nutrition. It then becomes relatively easy to set up bodies simply for "display" purposes. This, in turn, completes the full circle back to the importance of political will as the main determinant of whether councils in fact have the teeth to do the job.

Montgomery points out moreover that, as politics change, even duly created commissions may tend to fail after a few years. The way to circumvent such disintegration is to transfer the commission's aims into the goals of workers with career commitments to nutrition. This may mean making nutrition activities part of the local leadership or turning them into a bureaucratic process, either by creating one's own bureaucracy or "colonizing" a preexisting one with nutrition workers. This follows the received wisdom that the way to ensure long term operations in government is to bureaucratize those functions: we are told, for example, that the horse cavalry of the US Army existed for at least fifteen years after the army no longer had any horses! Instead of bureaucracies, however, "nutrition councils" often establish essentially a "federal" structure among ministries, a situation that requires cautious treading in order to work.

In spite of any other country's experience, of course, each nation seems likely to attempt to untie the Gordian knot of appropriate organization in its own way and to reserve the right to make all mistakes anew. In this context, advocates can be most useful by trying to relate experiences in generalizable form, pointing out the few lessons that can be derived so that each country, in attempting its national solution, can avoid at least the most obvious problems of the past.

One must acknowledge that coordination of any policy is a demanding and difficult task. In other areas, such as family planning, and at other levels, such as international organizations, cooperation and integration have been preached for years to little avail as far as national programs are concerned. As nutrition can gain from the experiences of other programs, perhaps further study of the problems of coordinating nutrition activities will find wider application in all areas of social program development.

UNIVERSITIES, NUTRITION INSTITUTES, AND TRAINING

Given political commitment and reasonable institutions to administer policy, leaders must still develop goals for nutrition activities. What, then, is the role of universities and teaching institutions in the establishment of national nutrition goals? What happens to national nutrition efforts when universities are included in planning and when they are not included? How do training and education contribute to the establishment of national goals?

In situations where there is a strong relevant university department or institute, such as in the Caribbean, training centers can have a catalytic role. They can help to sensitize governments to issues related to nutrition and to the nutritional needs of the people. At the very least, such academic centers can frame issues in ways that give governments a new slant on the subject, complementary to the more natural political point of view. These institutions can also educate Planning and related ministries about the ideas, goals, and methods of nutrition planning.

Specialized departments of institutes can also act as resource bases and in a technical advisory capacity if they have sufficient trained manpower. In addition, they can identify areas of training which are needed to fulfill the specific manpower needs of the countries. They may also give direction to relevant research which can assist, ultimately, in the development of nutrition strategies.

Truly appropriate training is a central requirement in making programs succeed, according to those who have had experience in directing such efforts. Both the skills taught and the utilization of nutrition personnel, however, sometimes reflect the fact that nutrition falls between ministries and either generates attitudes of neglect or competition. These reactions, often noted in regard to distribution of new funds or new powers, are often equally apparent in the training of new types of appropriate personnel for nutrition interventions. In Zambia, for example, educational programs train both home economists and nutritionists. While the home economists are readily accepted as extension workers in both education and in agriculture, trained nutritionists are often seen as misfits. Agriculturists note that they are not trained in agriculture. Educators feel that nutritionists have no role in the normal educational bureaucracy. Health workers do not know how to use them. In such a situation, it appears that there must be a combined training course whose product would be nutritionist-economists or some other type of multipurpose worker for many aspects of nutrition improvement.

In other circumstances, utilization of personnel may be inadequate. Schools of nutrition or field projects may train workers appropriately but these may be eagerly siphoned off into the regular ministries where there is no bureaucratic or career commitment to nutritional goals. Valuable trained workers thus get lost in a business-as-usual government hierarchy. On the other hand, numbers of economists, nurses, and so forth, whose work is closely related to the field of nutrition, are rarely taught any nutrition in the context of their formal training.

In planning for nutrition training and education, one must be aware of the related programs in universities and institutions of higher learning into which nutrition training ought to have been added but was not. Ghana, for example, decided a food and nutrition training institution was needed, and therefore set up a Department of Food Science and Nutrition in the Faculty of Science and Home Sciences together with Agricultural Extension within the Faculty of Agriculture. To back up this network, the Food Research Institute was created as a technology wing. Appropriate arrangement of personnel within and among these institutions depends on the particular mix of programs to be developed, according to Sai.

Whether to train nutrition workers in great numbers depends partly on the ideological and economic fabric within which one tries to solve nutrition problems, in Sai's view. Naturally, if the country chooses to bypass specialized activities or programs in favor of letting the nutrition issue solve itself in the context of broad economic development, needs for specific nutrition personnel will not be that great. In addition, at certain levels of economic development, Sai feels that large numbers of trained nutritionists might be too difficult for the employment system to absorb and many might be added to the ranks of the unemployed. In other words, one must have identified, a priori, a target use of specifically trained nutritionists in order to make training programs worthwhile. In much of Africa, according to Sai, what is really lacking are food scientists, food technologists, and food and nutrition planning personnel, rather than nutritionists who act as individual education and information providers. It would, in fact, be unwise, in many of Africa's countries, to train a large number of traditional nutritionists for whom there would be little productive use.

The question of personnel training undoubtedly requires dialogue between the nutrition agency, those agencies or implementing ministries that have need for the workers, and the training institutions. Manpower planning for the future, Thomson asserts, should give a clear idea both of the numbers to be trained and of the type of training to be given. This planning, he suggests, should extend to job descriptions for those to be hired and include the development of: (1) curricula to provide all the skills and training required to carry out those job descriptions, (2) a place for the trainees once they are trained, and (3) a career structure for these workers after they start. People trained to have a career commitment to nutrition must also have a realistic career ladder on which to function.

There is virtually unanimous agreement among experienced managers that *some* specifically trained nutrition workers are necessary, but that nutrition must also be integrated into the education of the regular personnel within ministries responsible for *any* activities that affect nutrition. It is generally advocated that the best place to start is with the students at the universities who will, in the future, have the responsibility for running programs. Such well-trained personnel will be much more likely to design the type of multidisciplinary approach which is viewed as most appropriate to nutrition programs. In order to achieve this goal, those who run the educational systems of the country must understand the significance of food and nutrition problems themselves: the educators must be educated.

Wray emphasizes also the process of developing appropriate personnel characteristics: "We talk about *training*, but we are really interested in *learning.*" One can break down the components of learning into: knowledge, or facts; psychomotor skills, or being able to do things; problem-solving, or being able to deal with day-to-day things as they come along; and finally, attitudes: commitments, sense of responsibility, and so on. In the acquisition of facts, the teaching method does not matter a great deal, according to Wray: lectures work, programed learning works, and films work. With psychomotor skills or problem-solving, none of these helps at all. The only way to learn is by doing. Attitudes cannot be changed by either lectures or films, Wray adds. Research reveals that attitudes change only in face-to-face, experiential, emotion-laden situations. This is true even in the "learning" of high government officials. In the advocacy processes for nutrition programs, testimony before the US Senate Committee moved people emotionally; in the Philippines, a fact sheet for cabinet members had a like emotional impact.

Unfortunately, according to Wray, much of what is done in the name of nutrition education and training is focused exclusively at the level of didactic lectures where people sit passively and words flow in, out, and around. There is very little opportunity in such "training" to learn how to function at the village level or to have the face-to-face experiences that will change attitudes. So, in addition to classrooms, on-the-job experience must be provided or much education and training will prove a wasted effort.

INTERNATIONAL AID AND ADVICE

The next subject covered was the role of international aid and international organizations in national nutrition programs. Participants hoped to discover the role of international advice in promulgating, setting up, and implementing programs. Is this aid useful in creating political support for the domestic nutritionists or in mobilizing other interest within the host country? Is there a potentially destructive influence in the current organization of international services? A recurrent theme in all the previous discussion was the need for coordination among government agencies. Is there an equally profound need for coordination among aid agencies? What, if anything, can be done about such a need?

Effects Within Local Political Contexts

International agencies can be seen to have a very important role as pressure and advocacy groups for the local government. This is parallel to the previously noted role of respected educational institutions, such as CFNI in the Caribbean. Sai argues that the international agency community *may* or *may not* be a relevant advocate depending on a country's particular level of awareness and education about its own problem. In Indonesia, for example, international agencies appear to have heightened policymakers' awareness of nutrition problems within the country. While efforts of the international nutrition community may have helped to heighten the sensitivity of national governments to the problem, the utility of the solutions prescribed remains for separate evaluation.

In fact, it seems impossible to discuss specifics of policy and program for national nutrition that are fixed for every country. Obviously, there is no recipe or prescription that fits every situation because nutrition is in fact based on the national environment. Comparing the failures and successes of several countries is useful only in order to develop new ideas—not to try to incorporate, en bloc, the successes of Cuba and China, for instance, in Indonesia. The problem of advocates is how to promote nutrition activities enough for them to be implemented by each government within the context of its own political and economic framework. Workers repeatedly express frustration at the plethora of books and memos by international agencies aimed at "educating" governments on how to solve nutritional problems. It is often difficult to fit this advice into national frameworks in part *because* the formulations are aimed at all countries. For instance, one UNICEF publication emphasized the "national commission" idea with complete and detailed structure of an ideal organization. If this type of advice is applied as a "bible" by laymen appointed to deal with nutrition problems, it will prove too rigid and be essentially useless.

Once again, this highlights the importance of ideology: those who work in the international field, attempting to assist in preparing a national nutrition program, have to work within the ideology of that country at that time. There is no other effective way of going about it, according to Thomson. In fact, if one recommends to a government that the first thing they should do is change the government, no amount of assistance will be very effective! Third World nationals see this point as very relevant to the structure of the international community. They stress the importance of definition of national policy by the nationals themselves: each country has to decide what it wants, and the international community should serve that desire.

On the other hand, few appear ready to argue the proposition that countries which desire to tackle nutritional problems would do better with no help at all. Many do assert, however, that international aid should be largely confined to coordinating roles. Involvement in implementation should definitely be downplayed. This refocusing would increase the utility of the contributions of international organizations. In the present structure, a worker in Zambia, for example, who is part of an FAO group, is supposed to produce work which is identifiable as FAO-supported. Career structures provide incentives for agency-oriented end products, whereas more "Zambian-ness" and less "FAO-ness" would be more useful in practice in Zambia. Changing the incentives so that more reward was received the more *locally* oriented the product, would both improve the product itself and increase the coordination of all international agencies, multinational and bilateral.

Coordinating International Efforts

One major shortcoming of the international agencies, in fact, has been that they lack coordination with each other. For instance, over a short period of two years, 16 agencies came to Indonesia with different proposals and different recommendations. Such uncoordinated influx may frighten and act as a disincentive to policymakers. Recommendations, proposals, and reports need coordination to assure consistency, but such coordination is often sorely lacking. In terms of relevant programing, the coordination of international groups *within* each country is held to be much more important than the coordination of the global funding contributions of the many donor institutions.

Local cooperation and coordination is a serious problem which occasionally takes on comic proportions. When the many international experts (including, among others, those from FAO, WHO, UNICEF, UNIDO, MIT, World Bank) visited Indonesia during 1974-75, a suggestion was made that the agencies should, among them, appoint one nutrition officer to work with the government and coordinate all the proposals of the different international groups. This proposal circulated around the various agencies, and the replies were quite typical. WHO replied, "Certainly, provided the coordinator is a doctor." FAO said, "Yes, provided that person takes professional and technical direction from FAO!" The final resolution in Indonesia was that the local coordinator would be on the Planning Board of the national government. Any agencies which want to deal with nutrition must talk with him, and he coordinates everything.

Some workers have felt the problem of lack of coordination so acutely that they have toyed with the proposal that all UN agencies dealing with nutrition should come under one umbrella organization. Salient points have been raised against such an arrangement. At the national level, it appears that whether or not one has a good national coordinating body, with authority, with money, and so forth, one still needs roots within the ministries. This need for solid relationships with executive agencies is also apparent on the international level. With the creation of an international umbrella agency, the imagination conjures up a scenario in which WHO's nutrition component is closed and FAO's nutrition division is removed, both placed under an "International Food and Nutrition Council." Then, WHO might refuse to deal with nutrition in its extension work. This clearly would be a step backwards. While there is certainly a need within the United Nations for coordination of nutrition assistance, Sai warns of a prescription which would effectively withdraw nutrition units and personnel from all of the agencies in order to put them into a new one with its own bureaucratic rigidities.

Montgomery cites two other ways that *have* been used successfully to coordinate multinational donor operations. One is the consortium system, by which the donors coordinate their activities offshore. This has worked reasonably well if donors, after coordination, restrain themselves, and let local workers alone inside the country. Second, there are a number of cases where effective coordination has been achieved by the host country itself. Attempts to coordinate the in-country work of donors when the coordination is done by UN or agency representatives themselves often results in a process whereby donors "gang up" on the host countries, agree on the conditions that each agency will impose unilaterally, and divide the projects up among the donors like illicit booty, according to Montgomery. This is clearly not the same procedure as coordination.

The International Planned Parenthood Federation's (IPPF) experience in a specific, multidisciplinary subject—population and family planning—similar in many ways to nutrition, is relevant here, according to Sai. IPPF operates through national family planning associations, analogous to the "nations" in the nutrition context. Coordination and requests for assistance have to originate *from* the national program. The aid—both assistance directly from IPPF or channeled through the IPPF but originally from another agency—is then coordinated within the executive office of each national program.

IPPF also has an assembly, analogous to an international coordinating body, where the countries themselves set up the priorities. There, the international community meets with the national representatives to decide what should be done next. Problems arise here, as they do in UN agency discussions, in voting and decisionmaking. Members of the "recipient community" sometimes appear to vie with each other for larger slices of the pie by being deferential to the developed donor countries. International economic pressures have changed the incentives somewhat in the past five years, but political considerations are still extremely important and the aid potential of richer countries has been known to force the hands of the recipients.

Managing Relationships with International Helpers

Some program planners view international agencies as "a necessary evil." Yet, they recognize that an additional problem often results from the fact that the country does not have its own program first. For this reason, Solon advocates that national coordinating bodies have the power to approve which international agencies are to be allowed into the country. Only in this way can Montgomery's second model, coordination from within, be used effectively. In the Philippines, for example, international agencies have to state their plans and receive approval from the National Nutrition Center. If international workers ask for something directly from a municipality, the municipality will refer the request back to the central body for permission. The coordinating body thus has the leverage to make the agencies distribute funding appropriately.

Once a country has an official program, it must still avoid letting any international agency *dictate* what should be *in* the program in exchange for aid, according to Solon. He believes that the local team should be very firm in its program, plans, and objectives. The national program should then call on agencies to make their individual contributions and not simply accept any aid or advice which is offered. For example, it is noted that if US AID is asked to send an officer, advice will be heavily oriented toward commodities. FAO's work, on the other hand, often produces an agriculturally based plan, and WHO is oriented to health. A total national plan is thus necessary to make best use of the planners who come to advise and teach.

Flexibility is a key ingredient both for the program administrator and for the agencies involved. When the donors rushed to participate in the Filipino program, Solon suggested that, as a method of cooperation, each agency assist with different parts of the single national plan. This approach seems to pay dividends in increased donor flexibility. For example, AID commodities were costing ₱10 million from the tight budget, but now AID is considering a modification in policy so that the requirement that the recipient country purchase commodities will not drain resources from the educational aspect of the program. UNICEF made the large sacrifice of stopping its Applied Nutrition Project and placing it within the Philippine Nutrition Program.

Even with basically amiable relationships, Solon notes that "Once in a while, you must be a little tough or you may fall into their hands. Working with international agencies is not really bad as long as they don't control *you*." He seems to describe here a creative adversary relationship—somewhat on the order of a free-press/government interaction under good working conditions. Solon feels that the best administrative stance is that, without being dogmatic, it is perfectly reasonable to reject some aid if it cannot be made to conform to the national program. Countries should not be forced into, nor should they accept, compliance with a rigid "international policy" set up by donors. International agencies, in sum, must have flexibility based on the countries' individual needs rather than having one set policy for the whole world.

From the administrative as well as the ideological side, then, it is perceived that a strong national decision and national program are necessary. This is borne out by the sequence of experiences in Indonesia. When many outside agencies wrote proposals, local scholars, who had no strong a priori perspectives, became inundated with conflicting advice. The result was much confusion. Since the national program has begun, however, donors are told that they must contribute to the stated national goals, as in the Philippines. Planners now find they can use this procedure as leverage with their own national policymakers by pointing out that without a good program the country cannot expect useful international assistance.

In making best use of international aid, Sai stresses the need not only for strong, coordinated ministries but for strong personalities with integrity. A strong commission with strong ideas may be in place, he notes, but some individual politician, perhaps close to the chief of state, might desire to have aid pour in irrespective of its utility, simply because it will all flow through his shop. "Such a powerful politician has the potential to subvert all the most well-intentioned plans, while the program planner or administrator may find his/her figurative head chopped off," says Sai. In South Vietnam, for example, a lot of "nutrition" aid arrived, but a large percentage was funneled off for other uses, without commitment to nutritional goals. Such problems have to be avoided or corrected if international aid is to fit properly within a national setting.

In addition, to be truly helpful, international agencies should be prepared to finance the important implementation and evaluation parts of programs as well as the survey and planning aspects. The commitment of the local government is essential here as well because, after the international agency has helped, the government itself must have the will to carry the program through. Those with experience in international program development note that programs are often planned on long term bases, and international agencies arrive bringing personnel and a simultaneous warning that the plan will phase out in three to five years. Part of the initial agreement, then, is that the local government will take over funding of the project and provide staff to take over from the international staff. All too often, however, there is only lip service commitment of both the government and the agencies concerned. In actual fact, after three to five years, when the agency withdraws its personnel, there often have been no funds and the whole scheme collapses.

International agencies, it must be recognized, have their own severe problems secondary to international economic difficulties. Program planners have noted two that are especially important. First, some agencies are running out of funds although they still have expertise to lend. As a result, two programs are often squeezed under one advisor. Second, the quality of advisors is not always high. Sometimes medium-to-low level technical advisors, old career hands within an organization, can prove a hindrance instead of a help. Local program executives must understand, moreover, that the employees of aid organizations frequently have their own personal survival problems. Many individuals want to do their work as well as possible but are caught in the middle between local and home office demands.

The political role of aid agencies can be, in fact, quite delicate, even when the overall ideology of the host country is clearly accepted as the basis for program development. Although these international organizations are generally well-intentioned, care must be taken because they can be used politically by different factions, or even different ministries, bureaucracies, and agencies within a country. Frequently, there is rivalry between the different groups looking at the same nutrition problem. One or more of these groups may look for and find ways to use international advisors for their own purposes, to co-opt the aid donors for the purposes of internecine political haggling.

Finally, the meaning of international aid must *not* be seen, in fact, as limited to monetary and technical assistance. A very important type of aid, likely to have a multiplier effect, is the interchange of information and the sharing of experiences that help prepare directions for research and training in the future. This brings to the surface an important element in international responsibility, according to Montgomery. It is archaic to conceptualize the international community as reaching up into a great storehouse of knowledge and technology and delivering it. That is no longer relevant, he states. On the other hand, the international community, while it is no longer primarily a community of donors, *is* a community of experience. Ideas may be drawn from one place and then interpreted, translated, applied to, and worked out with the experience of another place. There may well be a leveling of capacity between donors and receivers of aid: the aid-donor agencies are in decline and the quality of their staffs may be obviously deteriorating, whereas the local planning officers and government ministries that deal with the international agencies are visibly improving.

National planners and local workers within the countries can often see donor agencies pursuing patterns of aid which are not really meeting nutrition goals. For this reason, evaluation at the international level is a necessary adjunct to the overall understanding of nutrition problems. Students of nutrition planning therefore advocate that international agencies adopt a mechanism by which they can review seriously the nature, purpose, and effects of aid with the countries involved. One of the key responsibilities of the international community is, thus, to find ways of creating reservoirs of experience and continuing analyses of comparative successes, failures, and experiments.

In this context, the Bellagio gathering can be seen as a venture in creating forums where nutrition planners, administrators, advocates, and scientists can meet and exchange ideas. The scenario for the future of the nutrition community, as it can be derived from the preceding discussions, will consist of increasing efforts to see that specific attention is paid to nutrition problems as part of general development planning. Despite assertions that it has not been adequately demonstrated, the argument that nutritional improvement is a prerequisite for socioeconomic development seems to be accepted at many levels of political life and across many regions of the globe. This international consciousness constitutes a significant resource in the armamentarium of nutrition advocates.

Ideas and trends clearly cross political barriers and are adopted and adapted across ideological chasms through both formal and informal international networks of communication. Within the last year, for example, the Cuban government has established a National Nutrition and Food Commission whose principal function is the "definition and evaluation of a national policy" for nutrition. This flies in the face of a recurrent theme in the Bellagio discussions: that societies organized in the Cuban manner do not need to give specific attention to nutrition, as such, in the structure of government. The exact meaning of the creation of such a commission in Cuba and the role of nutrition policy in that particular socioeconomic context can only be a matter for speculation at present. The nutrition community will surely be alert as the story unfolds.

International interchange of experience and ideas creates the basis for increased ability to manage the challenges of the future. Those who deal with nutrition issues will face several sets of complex tasks over the coming years. Among these are the difficult ones involved in refining, guiding, and further elaborating the move toward inclusion of nutrition within general development concerns. Also important are more specific but equally perplexing and politically explosive issues such as the role and management of food reserves, the development of ways to deal with food shortage emergencies, the uses and control of international aid, and the whole range of questions raised by existing international trade relations and the transfer of advanced technologies. Essential to the continuing process of dealing with such globally important problems are accumulated experience, together with arenas for open discussion among knowledgeable, thoughtful, and concerned professionals, as exemplified by the meeting at Bellagio.

REFERENCES

CHAPTER 1 (INTRODUCTION)

1 *Final Report of the Mixed Committee of the League of Nations on the Relation of Nutrition to Health, Agriculture and Economic Policy.* Geneva, League of Nations, August 14, 1937, Official Document No. A.13.1937.II.A, p. 37

2 Elizabeth W. Etheridge, *The Butterfly Caste: A Social History of Pellagra in the South.* Westport, Conn.: Greenwood Press, 1972

3 M. Hernandez et al. 'Effect of Economic Growth on Nutrition in a Tropical Community.' *Ecology of Food and Nutrition*, vol. 3 (1974), pp. 283-91

4 Excerpt from an interview with Ambassador Edwin M. Martin on the World Food Conference; reported in "War on Hunger," October 1974

CHAPTER 2 (CHILE)

1 For further discussion of this point, see Peter Hakim and Giorgio Solimano, "Nutrition and National Development; Establishing the Connection." MIT International Nutrition Planning Program, Discussion Paper No. 5, July 1975

2 Marcos Cuminsky and Raquel Fleishman. Analisis de los trabajos realizados sobre el crecimiento de niños en Santiago Chile, Años 1940-1966. *Revista Chilena de Pediatria*, vol. 39 (1968), p. 891

3 Interdepartmental Committee on Nutrition for National Defense. *Chile: Nutrition Survey, March-June 1960.* Washington, D.C.: US Government Printing Office, 1971

4 The preliminary results of a more recent national survey, which was initially organized in 1972 and conducted in 1974 and 1975, have now been published. The findings are remarkably similar to those of the ICNND Survey (n.3). See *Encuesta Sobre el Estado Nutritional de la Poblacion Chilena, Julio de 1974, Primer Informe: Perfil Encuestal*, Ministerio de Salud Publica, March 1976

5 Monckeberg et al. Estudio del Estado Nutritivo y las Condiciones de Vida de la Poblacion Infantil de la Provincia de Curico. *Revista Chilena de Pediatria*, vol. 38 (1967), p. 491

6 Sergio Molina et al. *Mapa de Extrema Pobreza.* Instituto de Economia, Universidad Catolica, 1974

7 Guillermo Stegen and Manuel Barros. Consideraciones Sobre Medidas Antropometricas en el Niño Sano y Desnutrido. *Revista Chilena pediatria* vol. 31 (1960), pp. 132-39

8 Reported in Salvador Allende, *La Realidad Medico-Social de Chile.* Santiago: Imprenta, Lathrop, 1939, pp. 26-7

9 Alfredo Riquelme. Nutritional Problems of Chile and Their Implications with Public Health. Unpublished DPH dissertation, Harvard School of Public Health, 1955

10 Francisco Mardones. *Control de la Diarreas Infantiles: Recursos y Programas para su control en Chile.* Publicacion del Servicio Nacional de Salud, 1954

11 M.S. Arraño et al. Estudio Nutricional de 500 Escolares del Area Central (Escuela no. 45) a traves de Examen Clinico Antropometrico y Encuesta Dietaria, 1968. *Revista Chilena de Pediatria* vol. 41 (1970), p. 913

12 Alfredo Avendaño et al. Estado Nutricional de Poblacion Escolar Fiscal, Grupo Etario 8 a 10 años, Area Norte de Salud, Santiago, 1969. *Revista Chilena de Pediatria*, vol. 41 (1970), p. 1085. S. Valiente et al. *Estado Nutritivo y Desarrollo Psicomotor en Escolares Chilenos.* Departamento de Nutricion, Facultad de Medicina, Universidad de Chile, 1970

F. Baeza et al. El Adolescente Urbano Popular: Caracteristicas Biologicas. *Revista Chilena de Pediatria*, June 1968, p. 453

J. Rosselot et al. Desnutricion en el medio escolar. *Pediatria* (Santiago) 8:60-70, January/March 1965, p. 60

13   Carlos Montoya and Manuel Ipinza. Peso y Estatura de Preescolares Santiaguinos Pertenecientes a Dos Estratos Sociales Differentes. *Revista Chilena de Pediatria*, vol. 35 (1964), pp. 269-77

14   Ita Barja et al. Peso y Talla de Pre-Escolares Chilenos Urbanos de Tres Niveles de Vida. *Revista Chilena de Pediatria*, vol. 36 (1965), p. 526

15   Alberto Duarte et al. El Estado Nutritivo del Lactante y Las Condiciones de Vida de su Grupo Familiar. *Revista Chilena de Pediatria*, vol. 22 (1951), p. 119

16   Alfredo Avendaño. *Incidencias de Algunos Factores Psico-Sociales en la Desnutricion Infantil, Area Norte de la V Zona de Salud, 1968-1969.* Tesis Para Docente, Facultad de Medicina, Universidad de Chile, 1969

17   Ita Barja et al. *Disponsibilidad de Alimentos en Chile, Quinquenio 1965-69.* Departamento de Nutricion, Facultad de Medicina, Universidad de Chile, Publicacion 25/71, 1971

18   Population figures for this study were obtained from a projection of census data from 1960 in accord with estimated rates of growth. The 1970 census showed that actual growth rates had been lower than these estimates

19   S. Soto and A. Arteaga. *Estudio de Disponsibilidad de Alimentos en Chile 1963-67.* Departamento de Nutricion, Facultad de Medicina, Universidad de Chile, Publicacion 16/70, 1970

20   M. Autret et al. Protein Value of Different Types of Diet in the World: Their Approximate Supplementation. FAO *Nutrition Newsletter*, vol. 6 (1968), p. 1

21   *The State of Food and Agriculture: 1968.* FAO, Rome, 1968

22   Direccion de Estadistica y Censos, *Encuesta Nacional de Presupuestos Familiares, Distribucion del Gasto Familiar en el Gran Santiago, Septiembre 1968-Agosto 1969.* Santiago, 1970

23   Flavio Machicado. *The Redistribution of Income in Chile and its Impact on the Pattern of Consumption of Essential Foods (1970-1971).* Land Tenure Center, University of Wisconsin, Research Paper No. 69, 1974

24   I. Barja, M.A. Tagle, and G. Donoso. "Consumo de Alimentos por Nivel Socioeconomico: Analisis Alimentario-Nutricional de una Encuesta de Presupuestos Familiares (unpublished, 1973)

25   ICNND (see n. 3), p. 8

26   Recall that clinical surveys indicated higher rates of malnutrition among rural residents in Chile

27   Emmanuel De Kadt. Aspectos Distributivos de la Salud en Chile, in Centro de Estudios de Planificacion, *Bienestar y Pobreza.* Santiago: Ediciones Nueva Universidad, 1974

28   Molina et al. (see n. 6)

29   Cited in Atilio A. Boron, Economic Development and its Effects upon the Distribution of Goods: The Case of Chile, 1930-1970 (unpublished, 1975)

30   C. Dragoni and E. Burnet. L'Alimentation Populaire au Chili, Report to the League of Nations. *Revista Chilena de Higiene y Medicina Preventiva,* vol. 1 (1938)

31   ICNND (see n. 3)

32   Barja (see nn. 17, 24)

33   Machicado (see n. 23)

34   The results of the national survey done in 1974 and 1975 (see n. 3) reported some 37% of all Chilean families consuming less than 75% of their caloric requirements—a percentage similar to the findings of the two earlier surveys cited

35   It is only in the past few years that reliable information has been gathered on the influence of malnutrition on infant mortality. A Pan American Health Organization

Study (Ruth Puffer and Carlos Serrano, *Patterns of Mortality in Childhood*, 19 /5) from 1968 to 1970 reported that, for children under age five, moderate and severe malnutrition was a present and contributing cause in one out of 4 deaths in urban Santiago, and in one out of 3 deaths in adjacent rural areas. Low birth weight or malnutrition was present in 50% of all childhood deaths

36 G.J. Stolnitz. A Century of International Mortality Trends. *Population Studies*, vol. 9, no. 1 (July 1955), pp. 24-55; vol. 10, no. 1 (July 1956), pp. 17-43. Recent Mortality Trends in Latin America, Asia, and Africa. *Population Studies*, vol. 19, no. 2 (November 1965), pp. 117-38

37 DeKadt (see n. 27)

38 Emmanuel de Kadt, Mario Livingston, and Dagmar Raczynski. Politicas y Programas de Salud: 1964-1973, in Centro de Estudios de Planificacion Nacional, *Salud Publica y Bienestar Social*. Santiago: Imprenta Editorial de la Universidad Catolica, March 1976, pp. 132, 133, and 137

39 Jorge Mardones and Ricardo Cox. *La Alimentacion en Chile: Estudios de Consejo Nacional de Alimentacion*. Santiago: Imprenta Universitaria, 1942

40 Servicio Nacional de Salud. 15 Años Trabaja Intensamente el SNS para el Beneficio de la Comunidad, 1952-1967. Santiago: Instituto Geografico, n.d.

41 Hugo Behm et al. Tendencias Recientes en la Mortalidad en Chile. *Cuadernos Medico Sociales*, March-June, 1963, p. 21

42 Luis Marchant. *Cambios Recientes en la Mortalidad Infantil Chilena*. Santiago: Subdepartamento de Estadistica, Servicio Nacional de Salud, July, 1970

43 Jose M. Ugarte. Evolucion de la Mortalidad Infantil Chilena por Zonas Geograficas, 1920-47. *Revista Chilena de Pediatria*, vol. 22 (1951), p. 265

44 As cited in de Kadt, (see n. 27), p. 147

45 De Kadt, (see n. 27)

46 Boron (see n. 29)

47 Oscar Muñoz. Crecimiento Industrial de Chile 1914-1955. Instituto de Economica y Planificacion, Universidad de Chile, Publicacion No. 105, p. 32

48 Osval Sunkel. Change & Frustration in Chile, in Claudio Veliz (ed.), *Obstacles to Change in Latin America*. London: Oxford University Press, 1965

49 Boron (see n. 29), p. 32

50 Isabel Heskia. La distribucion del ingreso en Chile. Centro de Estudios de Planificacion Nacional, Documento No. 31, 1974

51 Ricardo French Davis. *Politicas Economicas en Chile: 1952-1970*. Centro de Estudios de Planificacion Nacional, 1972, p. 345

52 James Petras. *Politics and Social Forces in Chilean Development*. University of California Press, 1969, p. 30

53 Alejandro Foxley and Oscar Muñoz. Redistribucion del ingreso, crecimiento economico y estructura social: el caso Chileno, in Centro de Estudios do Planificacion Nacional, *Bienestar y Pobreza*. Santiago: Ediciones Nueva Universidad 1974, p. 147

54 These data are from Solon Barraclough and Juan Carlos Collarte, *El Hombre y la Tierra en America Latina* (Santiago: ICIRA-Editorial Universitaria, 1971), pp. 254-256 and from Barraclough, "The Structure and Problems of the Chilean Agrarian Sector" in J. Ann Zammit, ed., *The Chilean Road to Socialism* (Sussex: Institute of Development Studies, 1973

55 Zammit (see n. 59), p. 29

56 Thomas L. Edwards. Economic Development and Reform in Chile: Progress under Frei, 1964-1970. Latin American Studies Center, Michigan State University, Monograph Series, n. 8, March 1972, p. 25

57 Kalman Silvert. *Chile: Yesterday and Today*. New York: Holt, p. 123

58   Markos Marmalakis and Clark Reynolds. *Essays on the Chilean Economy.* Homewood, Illinois: Richard D. Irwin, Inc., 1965, p. 146

59   Sunkel (see n. 48), p. 124

60   Charles J. Parrish and Jorge I. Tapia-Videla. "Welfare Policy and Administration in Chile. *Journal of Comparative Administration*, vol. 1 (February 1970), p. 456

61   Ibid.

62   Ibid.

63   De Kadt (see n. 27), p. 8

64   Jose Pablo Arellano. El Gasto Publico en Salud y la Distribucion del Ingreso, in Centro de Estudios de Planificacion Nacional, *Salud Publica y Bienestar Social*. Santiago: Imprenta Editorial de la Universidad Catolica, March, 1976

65   Thomas Frejka. *Analisis de la Situacion Educacional en America Latina.* Centro Latino Americana de Demografia, series A, no. 122, April 1974

66   Peter Hakim. Education in Chile (unpublished, 1971)

67   Sunkel (see n. 48), p. 138

68   See for example, Jose Cademartori, *La Economia Chilena* (Santiago: Editorial Universitaria, 1971); David Felix, "Chile," in Adamantio Pepelasis et al., *Economic Development: Analysis and Case Studies* (New York: Harper, 1961), pp. 288-326, Parrish and Tapia-Videla (see n. 60); and Sunkel (see n. 48)

69   Maria Angelica Tagle et al. "Disponibilidad Alimentaria: Chile 1970, 1971, 1972. Departamento de Nutricion Facultad de Medicina, Universidad de Chile, Sede Santiago Norte. Publicacion 54/73. In their computations, the authors neglected certain food items which were included in the earlier survey by Barja et al. (see nn. 17, 24). The percentage increase reflects only those items included in both surveys. Tagle and Barja, incidently, participated in both surveys

70   Barja, et al. (see nn. 17, 24)

71   Solon Barraclough and Almino Affonso. Diagnostico de la Reforma Agraria Chilena. *Cuadernos de la Realidad Nacional*, April 1973, pp. 74-5

72   Machicado (see n. 23)

73   The Department of Economics of the University of Chile, which carries out regular surveys on development, estimated 19.8% of the work force was jobless in March 1976. The 30% figure is the private estimate of several researchers working on employment studies

74   Reported in private communications. The reader will understand that the current political situation in Chile requires discretion in the identification of sources

75   The 1974 survey cited earlier does report incidences of first-, second-, and third-degree malnutrition, but no comparative data exist for prior years

76   Jose Franco Mesa. Agriculture: El Dificil Año 75. *Mensaje*, March-April 1976

77   M. Chossudovsky. La Medicion del Ingreso Minomo de Subsistencia, y la Politica de Ingresos para 1974. Documento de Trabajo No. 18, Instituto de Economica, Universidad Catolica de Chile, November 1973

78   Patricio Meller and J. Ruiz Tagle. El Poder Adquisitivo de Los Sectores Populares y Medios. *Mensaje*, January-February 1975, p. 46

CHAPTER 3 (COLOMBIA)

1   ICBF (Instituto Columbiano de Bienstar Familiar). El Problema Nutricional y Alimentario de Colombia. Mimeo., Bogotá, 1974, p. 1

2   ICBF Hoja de Balance de Alimentos Colombianos, 1972. Mimeo., Bogotá, 1974. Such food balance sheets are prepared every two years and follow the methodology recommended by FAO

3   IIT (Instituto de Investigaciones Technologicas). Programa para Fomentar la Industri-

alización de Alimentos de Alto Valor Nutricional y Bajo Costo. Mimeo, vol. II, Bogotá, 1975, pp. 24-61

4 ICBF, El Problema, p. 6

5 DNP (Departamento Nacional de Planeación). Plan Nacional de Desarrollo, Sector Salud. Unpublished preliminary document, Bogotá, 1975, p. 4

6 Ministry of Health

7 Bank of the Republic: National Accounts

8 Ibid.; DNP, Evolución General de la Producción Agricola. Unpublished preliminary document, Bogotá, 1974, p. 12

9 DNP, Evolución General, p. 22

10 Gutiérrez, Néstor, and Hertford. Una Evaluación de la Intervención del Gobierno en el Mercado de Arroz en Colombia. Quoted in Fedesarrollo (Fundación para la Educación Superior y Desarrollo), La Politica Agraria en Colombia, 1950-1974, mimeo, Bogotá, 1975, p. 72

11 Fedesarrollo, p. 94

12 Eugene Havens. Income, Employment, and Occupational Structure in the Small Farm Sector in Colombia. Mimeo., University of Wisconsin, Madison, 1972, p. 3

13 Ibid., p. 3

14 Miquel Urritia and Albert Berry. La Distribución del Ingreso en Colombia. Medellín: La Carreta, 1975, p. 76

15 Ibid., p. 15

16 Alfonso López Michelsen. Informe Presidencial sobre el Estado de Emergencia Económica. Talleres Gráficos del Banco de la República, Bogotá, November 1974, p. 65

17 Gillis and McClure. The Colombian Tax Reform. IBRD (International Bank for Reconstruction and Development), mimeo. confidential paper, Washington 1975, p. 1. Quoted with the permission of IBRD

18 Ministry of Finance: Tax revenues collected during the first six months of 1975 were 50% higher than those collected over the same period in 1974. Also, IBRD, p. 4: The ratio of taxes to GDP for the period 1970-1974 are as follows. For 1970, T/GDP was 9.87%; for 1971, 9.73%; for 1972, 9.38%; for 1973, 8.94%; and for 1974, 9.06%. These ratios include the first effects of the tax reform

19 ICBF. Informe sobre Siete Años de Labores (1963-1970). Mimeo. Bogotá, 1970

20 ICBF, Nutrition Division

21 Reinaldo Grueso. El Programa Integrado de Nutrición Aplicada (PINA) en Colombia. ICBF, n.d.

22 This description of the plan follows that in DNP, Plan Nacional de Alimentación y Nutrición, and also descriptions evolved in working groups and meetings, coordinated by DNP concerning the plan

References not cited in text:

DANE (Departamento Administrativo Nacional de Estadistica), Banco de Datos

ICBF. Planificación del Sector Salud, Area Nutrición. Mimeo, Bogotá, 1975

CHAPTER 4 (GHANA)

1 Fiawoo. Growth Studies of Children—Rural, Urban and Peri-Urban. Mimeo, unpublished

2 F.T. Sai. The Impact of Urban Life on the Diets of Rural Immigrants and its Repercussions on the Nutritional Status of the Community. Ghana Med. J., December 1967

3 P. Davey. National Food and Nutrition Survey. Food and Nutrition Council, 1960-62

4 C. Williams. Kwashiorkor. Lancet, 1934 (?)

5   F.T. Sai. Health Service Prospects, an International Survey. The Lancet and the Nuffield Provincial Hospitals Trust, 1973, pp. 125-55

6   Survey of World Needs in Family Planning. IPPF Office of Evaluation and Statistics, 1974

7   S. Ofosu-Amaah. Health Manpower in Ghana. Paper read to Ghana Medical Association, March 1975

8   D.B. Jelliffe. Commerciogenic Malnutrition. *Nutrition Reviews,* vol. 30, no. 9 (September 1972), pp. 199-205

9   G. Bymers and F.T. Sai. Limitations of Price Controls in Ghana's Economy. To be published

10   *Ghana Today,* no. 10

References not cited in text:

D.Y. Dako and J.D. Watson. Baafi—A Case Study in the Assessment of Nutritional Status. Mimeo

S. Ofosu-Amaah and M. Katzarski. The Growth of School Children in Accra—1969/70. *Ghana Med. J.,* vol. 12, no. 1 and 3, March and September 1973

B.S. Platt and J. Mayer. Report of the Joint FAO/WHO Mission to Ghana, United Nations, October-December 1958

CHAPTER 6 (INDONESIA)

1   Ig. Tarwotjo. Personal communication, 1975

2   Ig. Tarwotjo, Gunawan, Sunardi, Wilardjo, J. ten Doesschate, S. Reedy, and S. Santoso. Prevention of Xerophthalmia by Massive Oral Doses of Vitamin A, A Preliminary Report. *Health Studies in Indonesia,* vol. 3, no. 1, p. 23

3   J.S. Saroso. Child Health Problems in Indonesia. *Paed. Indon.,* vol. 15, no. 1-2 (1975), p. 8

4   Soekirman. *Priorities in Dealing with Nutrition Problems in Indonesia.* Cornell International Monograph Series, no. 1, 1974

5   R.R.J.S. Djokomoeljono. The Effect of Severe Iodine Deficiency. Thesis, University of Diponegoro, Semarang, 1975

6   D. Karyadi, S. Martoatmodjo, and Husaini. Studies on Nutritional Anemia in Indonesia, WHO-SEA Consultation on Anemia (personal communication, 1974)

7   A. Birowo, W.L. Collier, A. Mintoro, S. Saropie, V. Manurung. Employment and Income in Coastal Villages on the North Coast of Java. *Agro. Econ. Survey,* Bogor, 1974

8   A. Birowo. BIMAS: A Package Program For Intensification of Food Crop Production in Indonesia. SEADAG Paper, Seminar on Food and Nutrition, Yogyakarta, 1975

9   Sajogyo. ANP-Evaluation Study, IPB, Bogor, 1974

10   Lauw Tjin Giok, I. Tarwotjo, Djokosaptono, and R. Rosidi. (1962). A Study of the Nutritional Status at Two Economic Levels in Tjiwalen and Amansari Villages of West Java, Academy of Nutrition, Bogor, 1962

11   Sutedjo, M. Sugiono, S. Muslichan, and Sudijanto, Mortality in Infants and Children of Indonesian Doctors. *Paed. Indon.,* vol. 9 (1969), p. 1

12   Rustamadji and R. Talogo. (1965), Public Opinion of Diarrhea in Breast-Fed and Artificially Fed Infants in Jakarta. *Paed. Indon.,* vol. 5 (1965), p. 55

13   J.E. Rohde. Human Milk in the Second Year. *Paed. Indon.,* vol. 14 (1974), pp. 198-207

14   M.G. Tan, D.A. Nain, Suharso, J. Rahardjo, Sunardjo, and S. Muljohardjo, "Social and Cultural Aspects of Food Patterns and Food Habits in Five Rural Areas in Indonesia, LEKNAS (National Institute of Economic and Social Research), 1970

15   Sudibyo, J. Husaini, Rachmat, and Djokosusanto. The Role of Tuberculosis in the

Nutritional State of Preschool Children at Mother Craft Center Cijengkol, West Java. Third National Paed. Congress, Surabaya, 1974

16 W.A.F.J. Tumbelaka. (1974), New Aspects of Malnutrition in Indonesia. *Paed. Indon.*, vol. 14 (1974), p. 189

17 G. Nugroho. A Community Development Approach to Raising Health Standard in Central Java, Indonesia, in *Health by the People*, WHO, Geneva., 1975, p. 91

18 WHO's figures for 91 developing countries, 1973, in: WHO Official Records, no. 205, Geneva, 1973, p. 96

19 Ibid., p. 79

20 Sajogyo. New Approaches in Community Nutrition Programs, SEADAG Paper, Seminar on Food and Nutrition, Yogyakarta, 1975

21 A. Berg, N.S. Scrimshaw, and D.L. Call. *Nutrition, National Development and Planning.* MIT Press, 1973

22 W.L. Collier, Soentono, G. Wiradi, and Makali. Tebasan System, High Yielding Varieties and Rural Change: An Example in Java. *J. Indon. Soc.Ec.Aff.*, vol. 1 (1975), p. 17

23 FAO. Report of the Technical Meeting on Nutrition in Food Policy and Planning in Asia and the Far East (Bangkok). FAO Nutrition Meeting Report Series, no. 28, 1961

24 R.G. Havelock. Planning for Innovation through Dissemination and Utilization of Knowledge. Crusk Inst. for Soc. Research, Univ. of Michigan, 1971

References not cited in text:

K.H. Reng. Optimism and Alertness in Bandung. *Xerophthalmia Club Bull.*, no. 8, 1975

S. Wahjudi and H. Tedjokusumo. Mengatasi Masalah Pangan. *Prospek Jangka Panjang,* vol. 2 (1975), p. 75

CHAPTER 7 (JAMAICA)

1 I.E. Johnson and H. Fox. The Nature and Magnitude of the Nutrition Problem in Jamaica. Mimeo., 1974

2 National Planning Agency. *Economic and Social Survey, Jamaica 1974.* Kingston: Government Printery

References not cited in text:

A. Ashworth and J.C. Waterlow. *Nutrition in Jamaica, 1969-70.* Kingston: University of the West Indies, 1973

A. Berg. *The Nutrition Factor.* Washington: Brookings Institution, 1973

J.M. Gurney. Available Data on the State of Food and Nutrition of the Peoples of the Commonwealth Caribbean. Mimeo., 1975

I. Johnson and M. Strachan. Agricultural Development in Jamaica. Mimeo., 1974

S.L. Lorde. Food Prices and Trade Policies. Mimeo., 1974

M. Manley. *The Politics of Change.* London: Andre Deutsch, 1974

Nutrition Advisory Council. A Food and Nutrition Policy for Jamaica: Mimeo., revised ed., 1975

West Indies and Caribbean Yearbook(1974). Thomas Skinner Directories

CHAPTER 8 (PANAMA)

1 Hoja de Balance de Alimentos. Año 1970 a 1972. Direccion de Estadística y Censo, Contraloría General de la Republica

2 Hoja de Balance de Alimentos. Año 1973. Dirección de Estadística y Censo, Contraloría General de la Republica

3 Evaluacíon Nutricional de la Población de Centro América y Panamá. Publicación

INCAP V-30, 1969

References not cited in text:

Plan Operativo del Gobierno Nacional para 1974. Ministerio de Planificación y Política Económica, Julio 1974

Informe sobre la Coyuntura Económica de Corto Plazo. Ministerio de Planificación y Política Económica, 1975

Panamá en Cifras. Años 1964 a 1974.

Direccion de Estadistica y Censo, Contraloria General de la Republica. Noviembre 1974

Nutritional Evaluations of the Population of Central America and Panama 1965-1967. Regional Summary—DHEW Publication No. (H.S.M.) 72-8120

Informe Preliminar de la Evaluación Nutricional de la Población Beneficiada con el Programa de Alimentación Complementaria en Cinco Distritos de Veraguas. Enero 1975

Dirección Nacional de Mercadeo. Ministerio de Desarrollo Agropecuario. Documento privado

Programa de Alimentación Complementaria para Grupos de Población con Alto Riesgo de Desnutrición. Abraham Saied, 1974

Boletín Informativo sobre, Salarios Mínimos Vigentes. Ministerio de Trabajo y Bienestar Social. 1974

Encuesta Especial sobre Ingresos a través de los Hogares: Año 1970 Dirección de Estadística y Censo, Contraloría General de la República, 1974

Segunda Edición del Atlas de Geografía Medica, Ministerio de Salud, 1975

Boletín de Estadísticas de Salud. Ministerio de Salud, 1973

Boletín de Estadísticas Vitales, Serie B

Dirección de Estadísticas y Censo, Contraloría General de la República, 1972

Recomendaciones Dietéticas Diarias para Centro América y Panamá, 1973. Publicación INCAP-E709

Situación y Perspectivas del Empleo en Panamá PRALC-OIT-1973

Algunos Aspectos sobre la Fecundidad en la República de Panamá. Araica: Hildebrando, 1974

CHAPTER 9 (THE PHILIPPINES)

1   Presidential Decree No. 491. Creating a National Nutrition Council. July 1974

2   National Nutrition Council. The Philippine Nutrition Program. National Media Production Center. 1975

3   Sec. 30, Exec. Order 94, 1947. Implemented by Administrative Order No. 81, 1949, of the President of the Philippines.

4   A. Tanco. Rice Enrichment. *Nutrition News*, vol. 12, no. 2 (April-June 1956), pp. 44-51

5   Republic Act No. 832. Rice Enrichment Law of 1955

6   Food and Nutrition Research Center. Reports on Regional Surveys. National Science Development Board, 1958-69

7   Food and Nutrition Research Center. Annual Report. National Science Development Board, 1972

8   Office of the President. Exec. Order No. 288, 1958

9   C.R. Pascual. A Coordinated Approach Toward More Effective Community Nutrition Program. *Phil. J. Nutr.*, vol. 16, no. 2 (1963), pp. 66-8

10   Florentino S. Solon. Organizing of the Community for Nutrition Programs. Delivered at the Nutrition Education Conference, Guadalajara, 1972

11   Executive Order No. 285. Office of the President, 1971

12   National Food and Agricultural Council. Four-Year Philippine Food and Nutrition Program, 1974-77

13   Philippine Business for Social Progress. Brochure

14   Department of Agriculture and Natural Resources and Bureau of Agricultural Economics. Crop Livestock and Natural Resources Statistics, 1973

15   National Economic Development Authority. The Philippine Food Balance Sheet 1973. Food Balance Series No. 1, 1975

16   Food and Nutrition Research Center. Nutrition Profile of the Philippines. Unpublished data, 1975

17   Rodolfo Florentino. *The Malnutrition Problem in the Philippines.* Food and Nutrition Research Center, National Science Development Board Publication, 1973

18   National Nutrition Council. Partial "Operation Timbang" (OPT) Results in 9 Regions Covering 31 Municipalities and 14 Cities. Unpublished data, July, 1975

19   Florentino S. Solon. Research to Determine the Cost and Effectiveness of Alternate Means of Controlling Vitamin A Deficiency (Xerophthalmia). 1970

20   V.O. Tantengco, A.M. Marzan, N. Rapanot, L.E. Villanueva, and C.R. de Castro. Nutritional Anemia in Filipino School Children. *Southeast Asian J. of Tropical Medicine and Public Health*, vol. 4 (1973), p. 524

21   Aida A. Padlan. The Endemic Goiter Control Project of the Department of Health. *Proceedings of the Conference-Symposium, Technology of Public Health Nutrition*, 1972, p. 42

22   Department of Commerce. Family Income and Expenditures, 1971. *BCS Survey of Household Bulletin.* Bureau of Census and Statistics, Manila, p. xviii

23   Edita A. Tan. Income Distribution in the Philippines. *Philippine Economic Problems in Perspective.* Institute of Economic Development and Research, School of Economics, University of the Philippines, Diliman, Quezon City, 1975, ch. 7

24   The Agrarian Reform Coordinating Council. Presidential Decree No. 2. Executive Order No. 347, 1971

25   P.O. Wolley, Jr., C.A. Perry, L.J. Gangloff, and P.L. Larson. *Syncrisis: The Dynamics of Health.* Analytic Series on the Interactions of Health and Socioeconomic Development. IV, Philippines. US Government Printing Office, Washington, DC, 1972, p. 20

26   Efren Yambot et al. *Philippine Almanac and Handbook of Facts.* Philippine Almanac Printers, Inc., 1975, p. 25

27   Helen A. Guthrie. Infant Nutrition in 4 Tagalog Communities. *Ateneo de Manila University,* Manila, 1969, p. 265

28   Department of Health and National Economic Development Authority. *National Health Plan*, vol. 1 (1975-78)

29   World Health Organization. *World Health Statistics Annual.*, vol. 1 (1972), p. 292

30   Mercedes B. Concepcion and Eliseo A. de Guzman. The Philippine Population: Trends and Prospects. *Philippine Economic Problems in Perspective*, 1975, ch. 3

31   Nutrition Foundation of the Philippines. Annual Report, 1973

32   C.L. Leones. The Case for the Fully Mechanized Large-Scale Farm. *Philippine Panorama*, June 1975

33   Mahar Mangahas and R. Rimando. The Philippine Food Problem. *Philippine Economic Problems in Perspective*, 1975, ch. 4

34   National Economic Development Authority. The Philippine Food Balance Sheet. Food Balance Series. No. 1, Manila, 1973

35   Development Academy of the Philippines. Measuring the Quality of Life: Philippine Social Indicators. 1975

36   National Economic Development Authority. Four-Year Development Plan, FY 1974-77. Office of the President. 1973

CHAPTER 10 (TANZANIA)

1   B. Egero and R.A. Henin. The Population of Tanzania. Published by BRALUP and the Bureau of Statistics

2   Maletnlema and Bavu. E.A. Med. J., vol. 51, no. 7 (1974), p. 515

3   W.K. Chagula and E. Tarimo. Meeting the Basic Health Needs in Tanzania, in *Health By the People*, Kenneth W. Newell, ed. Geneva: WHO, 1975

CHAPTER 12 (ZAMBIA)

References not cited in text:

D.A. Smith. *Report of a Nutrition and Health Survey in Kawambwa District.* Government Printer, 1950

A. Richards and E.N. Widdonson. A Dietary Study in Northern Rhodesia. *Africa*, vol. 10, no. 2 (1936)

D.M. Lubbock and J.A. Clague. Report to the Government of Zambia on Nutrition Improvement. FAO, TA 2368, 1967

J. Collins. Kwashiorkor: Some Reflections. *Med. J. of Zambia*, vol. 1, no. 4 (1967)

Unpublished Reports of Schools Medical Officers

B.P. Thomson. Report on Nutrition Survey of Fort Rosebery District. Unpublished

Hansard. Fourth Session of the First National Assembly

E.C. Thomson. The Primary Deterrent to Human Progress. Unpublished

_____ Outline of Nutrition Work in Northern Rhodesia. Unpublished

_____ Country Report: Nutrition in Zambia. Proceedings of the East African Conference on Nutrition and Child Feeding

M.J. Forman, D. Rosenfield, J. McKigney, and R. Shank. Possibilities for AID Programme to Combat Malnutrition in Zambia. Report of a Team Representing AID/WHO which visited Zambia, July 5-10, 1966

Ida David. Report to the Government of Zambia on Home Economics Extension/ Applied Nutrition Scheme. FAO CEP Report 36, 1966

J. McNaughton, L. Krikava, J. Perisse, F. Stoces, C. Paci, and M. Lorstad. National Food and Nutrition Programme, Zambia. FAO ESN:DP/ZAM/69/512. Technical Reports 1, 2, 3 and Terminal Report

Gerard Lof and Louise Los-Fresco. The Impact of Modern Changes on Food and Nutrition in the Rural Area of Zambia. Agricultural University, Wageningan

Michael C. Latham. Preliminary Report on Nutrition Status Survey in Zambia, July, 1972

F.P.C. Gonvea. Report to the Government of Zambia. FAO TA 2327, 1967

CHAPTER 13 (THE SYNOPSIS OF SCIENTIST, PLANNER, AND ADMINISTRATOR IN NUTRITION PROGRAM IMPLEMENTATION)

1   Assembly Debate, League of Nations, Sept. 1935

2   Statement of Development Policy, 1971-80. Government Press, Zomba, Malawi, 1971

3   Abraham Horwitz. *Opportunities for Inter-Agency and Inter-Ministerial Co-ordination in Nutrition Program Planning.* Ch. 33, Pre-School Child Malnutrition. NAS-NSC Publication 1282, 1966

4   Joe Wray. Private communication, 1974

5   Alan Berg. The Nutrition Factor. Brookings Institution

6   Hamish Davidson, Consultant Physician, Government of Zambia

7   David Henry. Food and Nutrition Planning, the Dilemma of 352,000,000 Pre-School Children. UNICEF

8   Joe Kreysler, Nutrition Research Officer, Tanzania Government. Private Communication

9   A. Kraay Kamp. A Study of the Use of Education on Dietary Change in the Chapananga Chiefdom. Unpublished thesis, 1973

10   Alfred G. Smith, ed. *Communication and Culture*. Holt, Rinehart, and Winston, 1966

11   John Bowers. *Educational Processes and Problems in Combatting Malnutrition in the Pre-School Child*. Ch. 27, Pre-School Child Malnutrition. NAS-NSC Publication 1282, 1966

12   Andreas Fuglesang et al. Communication as Nutrition Education. Commonwealth Conference on Education in Rural Areas, 1970

CHAPTER 14 (NUTRITION AND CULTURE)

1   B.M. Popkin and M.C. Latham. The Limitations and Dangers of Commerciogenic Nutritious Foods. *American Journal of Clinical Nutrition* vol. 26 (1973), pp. 1015-23

CHAPTER 15 (NUTRITION AND HEALTH POLICY)

1   Walsh McDermott. Environmental Factors Bearing on Medical Education in the Developing Countries. *Journal of Medical Education*, vol. 41, supplement 1, pp. 137-62, 1966

2   McKeown, Brown, and Record. An Interpretation of the Modern Rise of Population in Europe. *Population Studies*, November 1972, pp. 345-82

3   Richard M. Titmuss. *Birth, Poverty and Wealth: A Study in Infant Mortality*. London: Hamish Hamilton Ltd, 1943

4   Edward H. Kass. Infectious Diseases and Social Change. *Journal of Infectious Diseases*, vol. 123, no. 1 (January 1971), pp. 110-14

5   Ruth R. Puffer and Carlos V. Serrano. *Patterns of Mortality in Childhood. Report on the Inter-American Investigation of Mortality in Childhood*. Scientific Publication No. 262. Washington: Pan American Health Organization, 1973

CHAPTER 19 (POLITICAL COMMITMENT AND NUTRITION POLICY)

1   S. Reutlinger and M. Selowsky. *Malnutrition and Poverty: Magnitude and Policy Options*. Baltimore: The Johns Hopkins University Press, 1976

2   G. Solimano and P. Hakim. Nutrition and National Development: Establishing the Connection. Discussion Paper No. 5 in MIT International Nutrition Planning Program, Massachusetts Institute of Technology, July 1975

3   John O. Field. The Soft Underbelly of Applied Knowledge: Conceptual and Operational Problems in Nutrition Planning. *Food Policy*, vol. 2, no. 3 (August 1977), p. 228

4   Alan Berg. *The Nutrition Factor: Its Role in National Development*. Washington, DC: The Brookings Institution, 1973

5   I. Adelman and C.T. Morris. *Economic Growth and Social Equity in Developing Countries*. Stanford, California: Stanford University Press, 1973

6   R.J. Barnet and R.E. Mueller. *Global Reach: The Power of the Multi-National Corporation*. New York: Simon and Schuster, 1974, pp. 149-50

7   R.J. Lifton. *Thought Reform and the Psychology of Totalism: A Study of "Brainwashing" in China*. Norton, 1961

CHAPTER 20 (PROGRAM AND POLICY: SOME SPECIFIC QUESTIONS)

1   R.G. Havelock. *Planning for Innovation Through Dissemination and Utilization of Knowledge* (University of Michigan, Institute for Social Research, 1969); *Training for Change Agents* (University of Michigan, Institute for Social Research, 1973)

The outline reproduced on the following pages was prepared prior to the Bellagio Conference, and served as a guide for the preparation of the papers of the country case study authors.

OUTLINE FOR CASE STUDIES

(Note:

The outline below is intended to illuminate the interplay of government policy and the nutritionally vulnerable groups in society. In Section I, each item needs only a brief mention, not exhaustive description. We are more concerned with an analytic approach to the development, implementation, and results of national nutrition policies, outlined primarily in Part II.)

I.   THE ENVIRONMENT: Background for Case Study

A. Who are the nutritionally vulnerable? (Viewing clinical

     evidence of malnutrition as the end result of an interplay

     of various risk factors.)

  1. What are the risk factors in your country? (include

       demographic data, income figures, where appropriate.)

     age

     sex

     economic status

     occupational group

     geographical location

  2. To what extent does each factor contribute to the picture

       of malnutrition?

B. Relationship of Health System to the Nutritionally Vulnerable

  1. Extent of immunization services to children

  2. Numbers of prenatal vists and professional deliveries

  3. Population served by government services.

     a- in theory

     b- in fact

-2-

4. Utilization of health services by the nutritionally vulnerable
   groups

5. Health budget of country: total and

   a- to preventive medicine

   b- **to** curative medicine

   c- to hospital construction and maintenance

6. Types of health personnel active in country and their geographical distribution.

C. Food and Agriculture System

   1. Average family consumption figures for whole population and
      especially in reference to vulnerable groups.

   2. Diet patterns of vulnerable groups: Staple diet and diet
      as % of nutritional requirements.

   3. What is the "purchasing system" for vulnerable groups -
      how do they acquire food.

   4. Export and import of foods: national figures

   5. Problems of food transport and storage

   6. Pattern of land tenure

   7. Price controls and/or subsidies for production or purchase
      of food commodities.

   8. "Agrarian reform"

   9. Extent of use of new technology - who uses it, who benefits

D. Income Distribution

   1. What is relative distribution - in re vulnerable groups.

   2. What is the lowest level of income at which one can buy
      enough food to feed oneself? How many below this level?

   3. Any conscious policy toward change in income distribution?

   4. Any conscious price policy for foods?

-3-

5. <u>Trends</u> in relative purchasing power of nutritionally vulnerable
    groups.

6. How do general government policies of growth and development
    relate to purchasing power of nutritionally vulnerable?

II. <u>How does the environment mesh with government activity to affect the
     nutritionally vulnerable groups.</u>

A. Does the government recognize a nutrition problem?
    If yes, how was the problem identified and defined? Is it
    linked with health, welfare, agriculture, taxes, incomes,
    distribution of resources, etc.?

B. What have been the proposed solutions to the problem?
    What were accepted and what rejected as approaches to nutritional
    problems and why?

C. What are seen as the major roadblocks to effective action on
    the problem?
    Are there other roadblocks unrecognized by government agencies?

D. What groups in the society have the responsibility for dealing
    with the problem?
    How much power do groups responsible for nutrition have vis-a-vis
    competing claims for government or private resources?

E. Is there a separate national nutrition council or committee?
    How is it set up and how does it function? Problems with this
    structure?

-4-

F. Does the government recognize special problems groups, problem
    districts, or problems with particular nutrients?

G. Does the government have or has it had any programs to deal
    with nutrition problems? (focus on major nationwide effort.)
    Including experiences with:

                        Fortification

                        Food distribution

                        New foods

                        Agricultural Development Programs

                        Nutrition Rehabilitation or "Mothercraft"
                        Centers

                        Education Campaigns

                        Subsidies or Incentives

                        Health teams

For each program: (1) What is the history of the decision to
                        undertake the program?

                   (2) How was the form and content of the
                        program decided upon?

                   (3) To whom was it directed? What population
                        was actually covered?

                   (4) What is the legislative and institutional
                        history of the program?

                   (5) Evaluation of program: What were the
                        objectives and to what extent were they
                        achieved?

                        Reasons for successes and failures? What
                        defines success or failure for the
                        government?

                   (6) Who benefited from the program?

-5-

(7) Who suffered because of the program?

H. Legislative history of the government's involvement with nutrition?

Are there or have there been laws directed to nutrition?

History of the passage of those instruments

Provisions for enforcement

Problems with enforcement

I. Relationship of government policy to private sector in re nutrition:

Industry

Agriculture

Charities

Churches

Mass Media

International Agencies

J. Relationship of other government policy to nutrition

Were there any policies, designed for other sectors, which had

a notable impact on nutrition? (especially of large #'s of people)

Are there any significant recent changes in nutritional/diet patterns

in the country, as yet unexplained? Hypotheses to account for the

change?

What are the development strategies of government? Implications for

malnutrition.

nb: For countries which have had active nutrition programs over many years,

these questions may be too extensive in scope. If that is the case,

an in depth look at a few of the programs (decision-making, implemen-

tation and results) would be far preferable to sketchy answers to all

of the questions.

INDEX